Cardiac Emergencies in Children

AF713766

Ashok P. Sarnaik • Robert D. Ross
Steven E. Lipshultz • Henry L. Walters III
Editors

Cardiac Emergencies in Children

A Practical Approach to Diagnosis and Management

Springer

Editors
Ashok P. Sarnaik
Pediatrics, Division of Critical Care Medicine
Children's Hospital of Michigan & Wayne State University School of Medicine
Detroit, MI, USA

Steven E. Lipshultz
Pediatrics, Division of Cardiology
Children´s Hospital of Michigan & Wayne State University School of Medicine
Detroit, MI, USA

Robert D. Ross
Pediatrics, Division of Cardiology
Children's Hospital of Michigan & Wayne State University School of Medicine
Detroit, MI, USA

Henry L. Walters III
Pediatric Cardiovascular Surgery
Children's Hospital of Michigan & Wayne State University School of Medicine
Detroit, MI, USA

ISBN 978-3-030-08852-1 ISBN 978-3-319-73754-6 (eBook)
https://doi.org/10.1007/978-3-319-73754-6

© Springer International Publishing AG, part of Springer Nature 2018
Softcover re-print of the Hardcover 1st edition 2018
This work is subject to copyright. All rights are reserved by the Publisher, whether the whole or part of the material is concerned, specifically the rights of translation, reprinting, reuse of illustrations, recitation, broadcasting, reproduction on microfilms or in any other physical way, and transmission or information storage and retrieval, electronic adaptation, computer software, or by similar or dissimilar methodology now known or hereafter developed.
The use of general descriptive names, registered names, trademarks, service marks, etc. in this publication does not imply, even in the absence of a specific statement, that such names are exempt from the relevant protective laws and regulations and therefore free for general use.
The publisher, the authors and the editors are safe to assume that the advice and information in this book are believed to be true and accurate at the date of publication. Neither the publisher nor the authors or the editors give a warranty, express or implied, with respect to the material contained herein or for any errors or omissions that may have been made. The publisher remains neutral with regard to jurisdictional claims in published maps and institutional affiliations.

This Springer imprint is published by the registered company Springer International Publishing AG part of Springer Nature
The registered company address is: Gewerbestrasse 11, 6330 Cham, Switzerland

Foreword 1

You are a pediatrician, a family practice physician, an emergency department physician who sees children, a pediatric hospitalist, a trainee, or a nurse practitioner caring for children and you encounter a cardiac emergency—it's somewhat uncommon and scary. Other than the little experience you receive during training, there are limited resources to help you to navigate the approach to care for such a patient, including no textbooks that focus on this problem, until now.

In this textbook, *Cardiac Emergencies in Children: A Practical Approach to Diagnosis and Management*, the editors and authors cover the pathophysiology of, diagnostic approaches to, and therapeutic rationale for children presenting with life-threatening conditions from a diverse group of congenital and acquired heart lesions, as well as the failing heart. They discuss topics ranging from the emergency presentations and recognition of cardiovascular disease in childhood in countries with resources and those with limited resources, to issues occurring in the child recovering from a surgical repair of congenital heart disease, to the use of mechanical circulatory support and problems seen in children after heart transplantation. In addition, emergencies in children with pulmonary hypertension, inflammatory heart disease, cyanotic heart disease, shunts, and arrhythmias are all detailed, and the practical approaches to their care are described. In delivering the needed information, the editors have utilized the talents of renowned leaders in the field of congenital and acquired heart disease, heart failure, and transplantation, including highly respected pediatric cardiologists and cardiac surgeons, pediatric and cardiac intensivists, and pediatric radiologists. The textbook they have produced will educate a wide variety of clinicians and trainees for many years to come and will become a "go-to" book for the current and future generations of clinicians planning to take care of children at risk for cardiovascular emergencies. Pediatric medicine owes its gratitude to the editors, Drs. Sarnaik, Ross, Lipshultz, and Walters III, as well as the authors of the excellent topical chapters, for their visions, insights, and recommendations which will undoubtedly help to care for children exposed to cardiac emergencies.

Memphis, TN, USA — Jeffrey A. Towbin, M.D.

Foreword 2

Ashok Sarnaik, Robert Ross, Steven Lipshultz, and Henry Walters III have set out to edit a unique book tailored to physicians who might encounter cardiac emergencies in children, but to whom such encounters are not their daily preoccupation. Some note of who these editors are helps to clarify their purpose.

Ashok Sarnaik is a senior pediatric intensivist whose preoccupations include the care of children who suffer cardiac emergencies. In the course of a day's work, he commonly receives transfers from physicians who have provided initial management. He recognizes the challenges they face and the limits to their expertise in this highly specialized clinical area. Robert Ross is a senior pediatric cardiologist with a grand overview and broad expertise in the pathophysiology of pediatric cardiac disease. Steven Lipshultz is a pediatric department chair who is also a senior pediatric cardiologist. As a pediatric department chair, Dr. Lipshultz has a broad overview of the skill sets of non-cardiologist pediatricians and others who see sporadic examples of pediatric cardiac emergencies. Henry Walters III is a pediatric heart surgeon with a broad understanding of the medical and surgical options for children who suffer or are prone to cardiac emergencies.

Together, the editors have undertaken to highlight the background needed to understand the nature of these emergencies, their basis in physiology, and their diagnostic elements and therapeutic options. The topics presented are tailored to the needs of the practitioners who face these challenging crises sporadically: adult and pediatric emergency physicians, hospitalists, primary care physicians, midlevel providers, and nurses.

This text is unique in its targeted readership, scope of content, and level of detail. It is both archival and educational. It can be used both to launch further literature inquiry and to quickly inform in a crisis. It is both problem oriented and diagnostically categorized.

It teaches both what to do and what not to do.

El Paso, TX, USA — Bradley Fuhrman

Preface

> **"There is no disease more conducive to clinical humility than aneurysm of the aorta."**
>
> **Sir William Osler**

Facing a critically ill child with a life-threatening cardiac emergency is extremely challenging for first responders. Children with either known or suspected heart disease most often present to an emergency department, including departments that predominantly serve adults, and some may present in a primary care provider's office. Many of these children have undiagnosed heart disease with congenital or acquired origins. The emergency manifestations of heart disease in a critically ill child can often mimic other common pediatric illnesses such as bronchiolitis, asthma, pneumonia, dehydration, shock, and sepsis, resulting in misdiagnosis and delays in beginning appropriate therapies, delays that can have catastrophic consequences. Also, commonly used therapies such as bronchodilators, fluid expansion, and supplemental oxygen can adversely affect the outcome in some situations.

With advances in surgery techniques, many children with complex congenital heart diseases are surviving with improved life expectancy and quality of life. Some of these children present with emergencies between several stages of cardiac surgical palliation. These patients have unique pathophysiological considerations and require individualized management approaches. Certain therapies that are life-saving in one situation can be paradoxically life-threatening in another. One such example is the potential danger of using supplemental oxygen in an infant who has recently undergone a first-stage Norwood procedure versus its potential benefit when used in that same infant, later in life, after undergoing a completion Fontan procedure. First responders without familiarity in managing such emergencies need a practical guide on how to quickly evaluate, stabilize, and initiate treatment on these patients and to know when to get immediate cardiology consultation.

Historically, pediatric cardiovascular surgery has often been limited in the developing world where children with heart disease received only supportive care. This is no longer the case; patients with heart defects such as septal defects, valvar stenoses, and vascular anomalies are now routinely operated on in developing countries. Even cardiac transplantation is now available with great success in many parts of the developing world. Thus, a normal life expectancy is an attainable goal for many such children. At the same time, with increasing globalization and international travel, technologically advanced countries have much to learn from countries with limited resources about cardiac involvement in conditions that are uncommon to them, such as vitamin D deficiency cardiomyopathy and dengue myocarditis. The authors of the chapter "Cardiac Emergencies in Countries with Limited Resources" have addressed some of the special challenges they routinely face in their practice.

In this book on pediatric cardiac emergencies, we attempt to bridge the gap between cardiac critical care subspecialists and the emergency care providers in various settings. The goal is to provide the pathophysiological basis of cardiac dysfunction, improve clinical reasoning to facilitate the diagnosis, and explain the rationale for stabilizing and managing cardiac emergencies in children. We emphasize the importance of history and physical examination and interpreting ECG and chest radiographs and describe situations where there is a need to consult subspecialists. We do so by presenting real-life case scenarios and practical guidelines.

This book is aimed primarily at pediatric and adult emergency physicians who do a yeoman's work in diagnosing and stabilizing patients. Primary care physicians and pediatric hospitalists who encounter cardiac emergencies in their practice will also find the information valuable. The book will also be beneficial for nurses and physicians at all levels of training including students, residents, fellows, and other health-care professionals.

Finally, we must acknowledge that this book is a result of true team effort. Experts from various institutions and specialties have willingly and selflessly provided their knowledge and expertise with the sole purpose of improving outcomes of children with heart disease throughout the world. We thank them from the cockles of our hearts!

Detroit, MI, USA — Ashok P. Sarnaik
Detroit, MI, USA — Robert D. Ross
Detroit, MI, USA — Steven E. Lipshultz
Detroit, MI, USA — Henry L. Walters III

Contents

Contributors

Tageldin Ahmed, M.D. Division of Critical Care Medicine, Children's Hospital of Michigan, Wayne State University School of Medicine, Detroit, MI, USA

Shahnawaz M. Amdani, M.B.B.S., M.D. Division of Pediatric Cardiology, St. Louis Children's Hospital, Washington University School of Medicine, St. Louis, MO, USA

Division of Cardiology, Department of Pediatrics, Children's Hospital of Michigan, Wayne State University School of Medicine, Detroit, MI, USA

Harbir Arora, M.D. Division of Infectious Diseases, Department of Pediatrics, Children's Hospital of Michigan, Wayne State University School of Medicine, Detroit, MI, USA

Basim I. Asmar, M.D. Department of Pediatrics, Children's Hospital of Michigan, Wayne State University School of Medicine, Detroit, MI, USA

Neha Bansal, M.D. Division of Cardiology, Department of Pediatrics, Children's Hospital of Michigan, Wayne State University School of Medicine, Detroit, MI, USA

Christian Bauerfeld, M.D. Division of Critical Care Medicine, Children's Hospital of Michigan, Wayne State University School of Medicine, Detroit, MI, USA

Katherine Cashen, D.O. Department of Pediatrics, Division of Critical Care Medicine, Children's Hospital of Michigan, Wayne State University School of Medicine, Detroit, MI, USA

Monika Chauhan, M.D. Division of Critical Care Medicine, Children's Hospital of Michigan, Wayne State University School of Medicine, Detroit, MI, USA

Saurabh Chiwane, M.B.B.S., M.D. Division of Critical Care Medicine, Department of Pediatrics, Cardinal Glennon Children's Hospital, Saint Louis University, St. Louis, MO, USA

Manish Chokhandre, M.D. Department of Pediatrics, Fortis Child Heart Mission, Mumbai, India

Jeff Clark, M.D. Division of Critical Care Medicine, Department of Pediatrics, Children's Hospital of Michigan, Wayne State University School of Medicine, Detroit, MI, USA

Ralph E. Delius, M.D. Division of Pediatric Cardiovascular Surgery, Children's Hospital of Michigan, Wayne State University School of Medicine, Detroit, MI, USA

Thomas J. Forbes, M.D. Department of Pediatrics, Wayne State University School of Medicine, Detroit, MI, USA

Division of Cardiology, Children's Hospital of Michigan, Detroit, MI, USA

Chapel Hill, NC, USA

James M. Galas, M.D. Division of Cardiology, Department of Pediatrics, Children's Hospital of Michigan, Wayne State University School of Medicine, Detroit, MI, USA

Swati Garekar, M.D., B.C. Division of Pediatric Cardiology, Fortis Child Heart Mission, Mumbai, India

Marjorie Gayanilo, M.D. Division of Cardiology, Department of Pediatrics, Children's Hospital of Michigan, Wayne State University School of Medicine, Detroit, MI, USA

Sabrina M. Heidemann, M.D. Intensive Care Unit, Division of Critical Care Medicine, Department of Pediatrics, Children's Hospital of Michigan, Wayne State University School of Medicine, Detroit, MI, USA

Patrick Hines, M.D., Ph.D. Division of Critical Care Medicine, Children's Hospital of Michigan, Wayne State University School of Medicine, Detroit, MI, USA

Aparna Joshi, M.D. Pediatric Radiology, Children's Hospital of Michigan, Wayne State University School of Medicine, Detroit, MI, USA

Nirupama Kannikeswaran, M.D. Division of Emergency Medicine, Children's Hospital of Michigan, Wayne State University School of Medicine, Detroit, MI, USA

Peter P. Karpawich, M.Sc., M.D., F.A.A.P., F.A.C.C. Cardiac Electrophysiology Services, Division of Cardiology, Department of Pediatrics, Children's Hospital of Michigan, Wayne State University School of Medicine, Detroit, MI, USA

Daisuke Kobayashi, M.D., F.A.A.P., F.A.C.C. Department of Pediatrics, Wayne State University School of Medicine, Detroit, MI, USA

Division of Cardiology, Children's Hospital of Michigan, Detroit, MI, USA

Chapel Hill, NC, USA

Steven E. Lipshultz, M.D. Division of Cardiology, Department of Pediatrics, Children's Hospital of Michigan, Wayne State University School of Medicine, Detroit, MI, USA

Deemah R. Mahadin, M.D. Division of Cardiology, Department of Pediatrics, Children's Hospital of Michigan, Wayne State University School of Medicine, Detroit, MI, USA

Prashant Mahajan, M.D., M.P.H., M.B.A. Department of Emergency Medicine, CS Mott Children's Hospital of Michigan, University of Michigan School of Medicine, Ann Arbor, MI, USA

Christopher W. Mastropietro, M.D. Pediatric Cardiovascular Intensive Care Unit, Riley Hospital for Children at Indiana University Health, Indiana University School of Medicine, Indianapolis, IN, USA

Eric McGrath, M.D. Division of Infectious Diseases, Department of Pediatrics, Children's Hospital of Michigan, Wayne State University School of Medicine, Detroit, MI, USA

Kathleen L. Meert, M.D. Critical Care Medicine, Children's Hospital of Michigan, Wayne State University School of Medicine, Detroit, MI, USA

Matthew J. O'Connor, M.D. Cardiomyopathy, Heart Failure and Heart Transplantation Section Pediatric Cardiology, Department of Pediatrics, Children's Hospital of Philadelphia, University of Pennsylvania Perelman School of Medicine, Philadelphia, PA, USA

Kristen Richards, C.P.N.P.-A.C. Pediatric Nurse Practitioner, Department of Pediatric Cardiovascular Surgery, Children's Hospital of Michigan, Detroit, MI, USA

Robert D. Ross, M.D. Pediatrics, Division of Cardiology, Children's Hospital of Michigan and Wayne State University School of Medicine, Detroit, MI, USA

Raya Safa, M.D. Divisions of Cardiology and Critical Care Medicine, Department of Pediatrics, Children's Hospital of Michigan, Wayne State University School of Medicine, Detroit, MI, USA

Yamuna Sanil, M.D. Division of Cardiology, Department of Pediatrics, Children's Hospital of Michigan, Wayne State University School of Medicine, Detroit, MI, USA

Ajit A. Sarnaik, M.D. Division of Critical Care Medicine, Children's Hospital of Michigan, Wayne State University School of Medicine, Detroit, MI, USA

Ashok P. Sarnaik, M.D., F.A.A.P., F.C.C.M. Division of Critical Care Medicine, Department of Pediatrics, Children's Hospital of Michigan, Wayne State University School of Medicine, Detroit, MI, USA

Syana Sarnaik, M.D. Emergency Department, Children's Hospital of Michigan, Wayne State University School of Medicine, Detroit, MI, USA

Swati Sehgal, M.D. Department of Pediatrics, Division of Cardiology, Children's Hospital of Michigan, Wayne State University School of Medicine, Detroit, MI, USA

Usha Sethuraman, M.D. Division of Pediatric Emergency Medicine, Children's Hospital of Michigan, Wayne State University School of Medicine, Detroit, MI, USA

Robert E. Shaddy, M.D. Keck School of Medicine of the University of Southern California, Children's Hospital Los Angeles, Los Angeles, CA, USA

Rekha Solomon, M.D. Critical Care Medicine, BJ Wadia Hospital for Children, Mumbai, India

Chenni Sriram, M.D. Division of Cardiology, Department of Pediatrics, Children's Hospital of Michigan, Wayne State University School of Medicine, Detroit, MI, USA

Curt Stankovic, M.D. Division of Emergency Medicine, Children's Hospital of Michigan, Wayne State University School of Medicine, Detroit, MI, USA

Lloyd Y. Tani, M.D. Department of Pediatrics, Division of Pediatric Cardiology, University of Utah School of Medicine, Primary Children's Hospital, Salt Lake City, UT, USA

Bradley Tilford, M.D. Division of Critical Care Medicine, Children's Hospital of Michigan, Wayne State University School of Medicine, Detroit, MI, USA

Susan P. Tourner, M.D. Department of Pediatrics, ProMedica Toledo Children's Hospital, University of Toledo College of Medicine, Toledo, OH, USA

Dongngan T. Truong, M.D. Department of Pediatrics, Division of Pediatric Cardiology, University of Utah School of Medicine, Primary Children's Hospital, Salt Lake City, UT, USA

Daniel R. Turner, M.D. Department of Pediatrics, Wayne State University School of Medicine, Detroit, MI, USA

Division of Cardiology, Children's Hospital of Michigan, Detroit, MI, USA

Chapel Hill, NC, USA

Henry L. Walters III, M.D. Department of Cardiovascular Surgery, Children's Hospital of Michigan, FTA, Wayne State University School of Medicine, Detroit, MI, USA

Adam L. Ware, M.D. Department of Pediatrics, Division of Pediatric Cardiology, University of Utah School of Medicine, Primary Children's Hospital, Salt Lake City, UT, USA

Celeste T. Williams, M.D. Henry Ford Hospital, Wayne State University School of Medicine, Detroit, MI, USA

Emergency Presentation of Heart Disease

1

Syana Sarnaik, Katherine Cashen, and Ashok P. Sarnaik

Introduction

Congenital heart defects (CHD) are the most common congenital malformations with an estimated prevalence of 6–8 per 1000 live births [1]. Advances in fetal ultrasound and echocardiography have improved the prenatal detection of CHD. In addition, screening for critical congenital heart disease (CCHD) was added to the US Recommended Uniform Screening Panel in 2011. Since that time, CCHD screening with pulse oximetry has become nearly universal for newborns born in the United States [2]. Approximately 25% of neonates with CCHD will not be detected by pulse oximetry alone, and many children will not be diagnosed until after discharge from the hospital. Reasons for undiagnosed CHD at birth include the lack of prenatal diagnosis due to no or poor prenatal care, standard ultrasonography missing CHD, postnatal detection failure through pulse oximetry, or home birth. Most cardiac emergencies due to CHD in undiagnosed children most often present in neonates and infants less than 1 year of age. When previously undiagnosed children present with life-threatening cardiac emergencies, it is often the physicians in the ED (including those who predominantly care for adults) or the primary care providers in an office setting who will first see the patient. Also, with improved surgical outcomes of complex CHD, there are more adults than children with CHD in developed countries. Emergency presentations of CHD often masquerade as other common entities delaying diagnosis and prompt institution of lifesaving therapy.

S. Sarnaik, M.D. (✉)
Department of Pediatrics, Division of Emergency Medicine, Children's Hospital of Michigan, Wayne State University School of Medicine, Detroit, MI, USA
e-mail: ssarnaik2@dmc.org

K. Cashen, D.O. • A. P. Sarnaik, M.D., F.A.A.P., F.C.C.M.
Department of Pediatrics, Division of Critical Care Medicine, Children's Hospital of Michigan, Wayne State University School of Medicine, Detroit, MI, USA
e-mail: kcashen@med.wayne.edu; asarnaik@med.wayne.edu

© Springer International Publishing AG, part of Springer Nature 2018

A. P. Sarnaik et al. (eds.), *Cardiac Emergencies in Children*,
https://doi.org/10.1007/978-3-319-73754-6_1

Pediatric cardiac emergencies may result from anatomic abnormalities (congenital or acquired) or electrophysiological dysfunction. The latter is discussed in Chap. 8.

Symptomatology of Cardiac Emergencies in Children

There are three major symptom complexes that children with previously undiagnosed heart disease present with life-threatening emergencies. These are (1) respiratory distress, (2) shock, and (3) cyanosis. The clinical manifestations and pathogenesis of these symptom complexes and responsible underlying pathophysiologic states are outlined in Table 1.1. Of these symptom complexes, respiratory distress and shock are fraught with many diagnostic pitfalls and may be mistaken for other commonly encountered entities in children such as asthma, bronchiolitis, pneumonia (respiratory distress), dehydration, and sepsis (shock) (Table 1.2). The physician must look for diagnostic clues whenever presented with such scenarios.

Chronology of Presentation of Heart Disease in Children

Neonatal and infantile cardiopulmonary adaptation has a profound influence on the likelihood of a specific congenital heart lesion presenting at a given age. Before birth, the fetal circulation is in parallel circuits. The airless lungs have

Table 1.1 Emergency presentation of heart disease in children

Symptom	Clinical manifestations	Pathophysiology	Underlying state
Respiratory distress	• Tachypnea • Retractions • Wheezing • Grunting	• ↓ Lung compliance • Metabolic acidosis • Respiratory alkalosis	• Pulmonary edema • Airway obstruction • Anxiety • Baroreceptor stimulation
Shock	• Tachycardia • Poor perfusion • Hypotension	Decreased cardiac output	• Obstructive lesions • Decreased contractility • Increased afterload
Cyanosis	Central cyanosis	Hypoxemia	Right-to-left shunt

Table 1.2 Cardiogenic shock: diagnostic pitfalls

• Most present with respiratory distress (metabolic acidosis, stimulation of baroreceptors): misdiagnosed as asthma, bronchiolitis, pneumonia
• Early manifestations of pulmonary edema: wheezing, hyperinflation
• Treatment with bronchodilators worsens clinical state
• Apparent dehydration leads to inappropriate fluid expansion
• Lack of obvious findings such as jugular venous distension (JVD) or hepatomegaly
• Shock state is often blamed on sepsis especially in neonates
• Metabolic acidosis is blamed on hypovolemic state or sepsis
• Lack of cardiomegaly on chest X-ray in early stages of myocarditis

*Avoid low index of suspicion

suprasystemic vascular resistance accepting only 10% of cardiac output. A large portion of venous return to the right side of the heart is shunted across the foramen ovale (FO) and ductus arteriosus (DA) to the left side of the heart. The systemic circulation including the placenta accepts 90% of total cardiac output. The fetus tolerates complex congenital heart lesions as the FO and DA allow the right side of the heart to take over the function of the left side of the heart and vice versa.

Early Neonatal Period (1–7 Days)

Soon after birth, with initiation of air-breathing and oxygen-induced pulmonary vasodilation, the pulmonary vascular resistance (PVR) falls to 50% of systemic vascular resistance (SVR) which rises as placental circulation ceases to exist. Also, the FO and DA initially close functionally and then subsequently close anatomically. The circulation changes to being in series as the right ventricular stroke volume approaches that of the left ventricle with very little if any blood being shunted across the FO or DA. In this phase of early neonatal hemodynamic adaptation, several groups of congenital lesions are prone to manifest. These are:

Systemic arteriovenous fistula: The increasing systemic venous return flowing into the lung allows greater shunting across arteriovenous (AV) fistulae resulting in high-output congestive heart failure. The two places to look for AV fistula in a young infant with high-output failure are a) aneurysm of the vein of Galen and b) liver. It is important to auscultate for a bruit on the head and on the liver when dealing with such situations.

Left-sided obstructive lesions: Because of the functional closure of DA, the right ventricle cannot push blood into the descending aorta to maintain systemic perfusion. Lesions such as hypoplastic left heart syndrome, critical aortic stenosis, and interrupted aortic arch are likely to present in 1–7 days of life with systemic hypoperfusion, cardiogenic shock, and lactic acidosis. This hypoperfusion predominately manifests in the child as a gray and listless appearance rather than overt central cyanosis.

Right-sided obstructive heart lesions: Pulmonary blood flow can be maintained at a sufficient level for adequate oxygenation as long as the left ventricle can pump enough blood across the DA into the pulmonary artery. As the DA begins to close, an increasing amount of systemic venous return is shunted into the systemic arterial circulation. Lesions such as tricuspid atresia, hypoplastic right heart syndrome, and pulmonary atresia present in the early neonatal period with central cyanosis as the DA begins to close. Some cyanotic heart diseases such as tetralogy of Fallot may not manifest until a few weeks after birth as long as the right ventricular outflow tract (RVOT) is not too severely obstructed and allows reasonable amount of pulmonary blood flow. These patients are sometimes missed during the initial neonatal pulse oximetry screening. Cyanosis develops when RVOT obstruction worsens resulting in increased shunting across the ventricular septal defect.

Independent circuits: Transposition of the great vessels (TGV), where the aorta and pulmonary artery are transposed, presents soon after birth when functional closure of FO and DA prevent mixing of blood in the two circuits resulting in cyanosis.

Pulmonary venous obstruction: As pulmonary arterial flow increases after birth so does the pulmonary venous flow back to the left atrium. Lesions associated with obstruction to pulmonary venous flow such as total anomalous pulmonary venous return (TAPVR) and cor triatriatum will present in the early neonatal period with increasing pulmonary venous hydrostatic pressure and pulmonary edema resulting in respiratory distress and cyanosis. If the pulmonary venous return is less severely obstructed, such lesions may not manifest until later in life.

Early Infancy (6 Weeks–3 Months)

In the first 6 weeks to 3 months of life, the pulmonary vascular resistance continues to fall as the pulmonary arterial tunica media muscle continues to involute. By 3 months of age, the PVR declines to about 15% of SVR, a relationship that is maintained into adulthood. Since the tunica media muscle is mainly deposited in the last trimester of pregnancy, prematurely born infants have a more rapid fall in PVR compared to infants born after full term. The following lesions are more likely to become symptomatic at the age of 6 weeks to 3 months:

Left-to-right shunt: Ventricular septal defect (VSD), atrial septal defect (ASD), and patent ductus arteriosus (PDA) allow increasing pulmonary blood flow with decreasing pulmonary vascular resistance. The result is an increase in pulmonary blood flow (Qp) compared to systemic blood flow (Qs), hyperdynamic circulation, and congestive heart failure. Clinical manifestations include respiratory distress, tachycardia, bounding pulses, and eventually cardiac decompensation. If left untreated, left-to-right shunts result in hypertrophy of the medial musculature and intimal changes which lead to a rise in PVR and pulmonary hypertension limiting the amount of shunt. Without surgical intervention such children are at risk of developing suprasystemic PVR and Eisenmenger complex and right-to-left shunting.

Anomalous origin of left coronary artery from pulmonary artery (ALCAPA): While children are born with ALCAPA, the lesion does not manifest itself at birth. Even though the left coronary artery is carrying deoxygenated blood, myocardial oxygen consumption is not compromised as long as the pulmonary artery pressure (PAP) remains sufficiently elevated. The myocardial oxygen consumption is more dependent on coronary perfusion pressure compared to coronary oxygen content since the heart is one of the most efficient extractors of oxygen. It is when PVR, and therefore the PAP, falls below a critical level, the anomalous left coronary artery fails to perfuse the myocardium with sufficient blood flow to maintain its oxygen demands. The manifestations are those of episodic screaming (angina), feeding difficulty (effort intolerance), and overt cardiogenic shock (myocardial infarction).

Any Age

Certain conditions are not dependent on postnatal cardiovascular adaptation. They can present at any age. Infection (myocarditis, pericarditis, sepsis) and cardiomyopathies should be considered at any age when cardiac dysfunction is suspected (Table 1.3).

Table 1.3 Age-specific lesions and most common ED presentations

Age	Lesion	Presentation
Newborn (less than 1 month)	Ductal-dependent pulmonary blood flow lesions • Tricuspid atresia • Pulmonary atresia • Tetralogy of Fallot • Critical pulmonary stenosis • Ebstein's anomaly • D-transposition of the great arteries • Double outlet right ventricle with severe pulmonary stenosis	Cyanosis, gray appearance, eventually shock
Newborn (less than 1 month)	Ductal-dependent systemic blood flow lesions • Critical coarctation of the aorta • Critical aortic stenosis • Aortic atresia • Interrupted aortic arch • Double outlet right ventricle with aortic stenosis	Hypoperfusion, shock, and pulmonary edema
Young infant (2–6 months)	Lesions dependent on pulmonary vascular resistance • Ventricular septal defects • Atrioventricular canal defects • Large patent DA • Unobstructed TAPVR	Volume overload, congestive heart failure • Tachypnea • Tachycardia • Poor feeding • Hepatomegaly • Pulmonary edema • Facial edema • Increased work of breathing, diaphoresis
Young infant (2–6 months)	Lesion dependent on pulmonary arterial pressure • Anomalous left coronary artery from the pulmonary artery (ALCAPA)	Shock
Any age	Acquired heart disease • Myocarditis • Cardiomyopathy • Pericarditis • Cardiac tumor Arrhythmias • Supraventricular tachycardia • Heart block	May present with mild, vague symptoms, older children may present with dyspnea, exercise intolerance Younger children may present with poor feeding, irritability, or shock

Table 1.4 Risks of commonly employed treatment strategies

• Oxygen—pulmonary vasodilator: worsening pulmonary edema, pulmonary circulation steal from systemic circulation—peripheral vasoconstrictor, increased afterload
• Fluid bolus—worsening pulmonary edema—decreased coronary perfusion (CPP = MAP–CVP)
• Albuterol—increased myocardial oxygen consumption—worsening tachypnea and metabolic acidosis
• Furosemide—worsened relative hypovolemia
• Treatment with bronchodilators worsens clinical state
• Apparent dehydration leads to inappropriate fluid expansion

Practical Considerations for Initial Care Providers

Ductal-dependent lesions should be a consideration in all neonates presenting in shock and/or cyanosis in the neonatal period. Alprostadil (PGE1) infusion may be lifesaving if instituted even prior to an established diagnosis. FO-dependent lesions (TGV, obstructed TAPVR) may need balloon atrial septostomy. All patients with suspected CCHD should be promptly transferred to tertiary care centers.

Oxygen administration, which is a common intervention for life-threatening pediatric emergencies, may have deleterious consequences in certain cardiac lesions. Elevated PaO_2 results in constriction of DA and pulmonary vasodilation. In left-sided obstructive lesions of the heart, constriction of DA would result in worsening of systemic hypoperfusion, shock, and lactic acidosis. Pulmonary vasodilation in single ventricle physiology (e.g., Norwood surgery for hypoplastic left heart syndrome) may result in a greater proportion of cardiac output going to the lungs (Qp) at the expense of the rest of the body (Qs). Also, in left-to-right shunts, pulmonary overcirculation resulting from vasodilation may worsen pulmonary edema. Oxygen administration in such situations must be carefully monitored to maintain SaO_2 around 75–80% in single ventricle physiology and around 90% in left-to-right shunts.

Administration of albuterol in a child whose respiratory symptoms are secondary to myocardial dysfunction will lead to increased oxygen demands on an already compromised heart. Excessive fluid resuscitation for decreased cardiac output and apparent dehydration in a situation with a failing heart will have similar adverse consequences (Table 1.4). Early identification of cardiac etiology as the underlying mechanism of life-threatening manifestations is of utmost importance.

Important Historical Findings in Infants with Heart Disease

Unlike older children and adults, infants and young children are unable to articulate their symptoms. The clinician needs to seek from the caretaker certain historical findings that may act as surrogates for symptoms that older children may complain about (Table 1.5). Tachypnea, rapid or congested breathing, and wheezing are suggestive of pulmonary edema from congestive heart failure. Feeding difficulty and

Table 1.5 Important historical findings of heart disease in infants

Symptoms/signs	Cardiac relevance	Condition
Fast breathing	Decreased lung compliance Pulmonary edema	Congestive heart failure
Wheezing/coughing/congested breathing	Pulmonary edema Compression of airways Vascular compression	Congestive heart failure Chamber enlargement Vascular ring/sling
Turning blue spells	Right-to-left shunting	Pink tetralogy Cyanotic heart disease
Chest pounding	Hyperdynamic circulation	Left-to-right shunt Cardiomegaly
Excessive sweating	Increased sympathetic activity	Heart failure
Episodes of screaming	Angina	Coronary ischemia
Feeding difficulty Failure to thrive	Effort intolerance Increased work of breathing	Congestive heart failure

failure to thrive could be manifestations of effort intolerance and increased work of breathing. Excessive sweating may result from increased sympathetic activity and obvious chest "pounding" could be a result of hyperdynamic circulation. Episodes of screaming may signify angina from coronary ischemia.

Case Presentation 1

A 4-day-old, full-term neonate is brought to the ED by his parents for poor feeding and lethargy. His vital signs are as follows: temperature 36.2 °C, heart rate (HR) 192 beats per minute, respiratory rate (RR) 63 breaths per minute, and blood pressure (BP) 62/37 mmHg with oxygen saturation (SpO2) of 92% on room air. On examination, the baby appears lethargic with cool extremities and capillary refill time of 4 s. He has nasal flaring with intercostal retractions. Liver edge is palpable 3 cm below the right costal margin. The saturations improve to 97% on 100% oxygen. Repeat vital signs after initiation of oxygen administration show a HR of 212 beats per minute, RR of 75 breaths per minute, and a right upper extremity BP of 54/23 mmHg. A chest radiograph demonstrates pulmonary edema and cardiomegaly (Fig. 1.1). An initial arterial blood gas (ABG) demonstrates pH 7.15, PCO_2 28 mmHg, PaO_2 94 mmHg, bicarbonate 10 mEq/L, and lactate 12 mmol/L.

The neonate in this vignette has signs of shock, severe metabolic acidosis, and marked hyperlactatemia. The etiology of shock in an infant needs to be determined and lifesaving measures employed rapidly. Cardiogenic shock should be suspected in all such infants in addition to hypovolemia and sepsis. In this infant presenting with shock in the first week of life, there are no historical findings to account for hypovolemia, hypotension, and poor perfusion. Therefore treatment for an underlying ductal-dependent cardiac disease is imperative. Obstructive lesions of the left side of the heart such as HLHS, critical aortic stenosis, coarctation of the aorta, and interrupted aortic arch are at the top of the list of differential diagnosis. The infant may appear relatively normal at birth as long as the DA remains open, and the

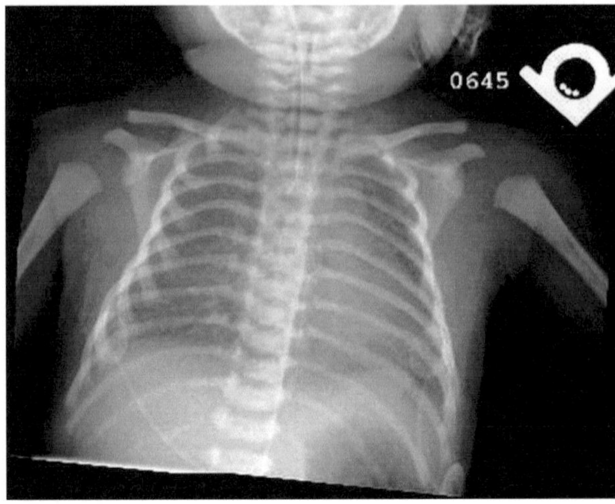

Fig. 1.1 Chest radiograph showing cardiomegaly and early pulmonary edema

postobstructive systemic circulation is maintained by the right ventricle through the pulmonary artery and DA. Symptoms appear when closure of the DA leads to systemic hypoperfusion. These children are not cyanotic but rather appear ashen gray because of hypoperfusion and increased peripheral oxygen extraction. In order to maintain ductal patency and establish systemic blood flow, alprostadil infusion must be started. Since alprostadil is a systemic vasodilator, judicious intravenous fluid expansion may be necessary to maintain normal blood pressure for age.

The use of oxygen in a child with shock due to a left-sided obstructive lesion can be of particular harm as oxygen itself is a potent DA constrictor which may further limit blood flow through a compromised DA. Ductal patency is a major factor that determines the difference between survival and death in a child dependent on the DA for systemic blood flow.

Unlike the infant in the vignette, a child with right-sided obstructive lesions (pulmonary atresia, tricuspid atresia,) or independent circuits (TGA) will present with central cyanosis and often has PaO_2 ~40 and oxygen saturations ~75%. In cyanotic infants, the hyperoxia test may be utilized as a clinical tool to differentiate between pulmonary and cardiac disease. The test is based on the principle that 100% oxygen will increase alveolar PO_2, leading to an increase in systemic arterial PO_2 in the absence of a fixed cardiac shunt. In cyanotic congenital heart disease, little or no rise in PaO_2 would be expected after breathing 100% O_2. An arterial blood gas analysis done both before and after the administration of 100% O_2 demonstrating an increase in PaO_2 to more than 100 mmHg would suggest a respiratory disease, while an increase of PaO_2 of less than 80 mmHg would require evaluation for cyanotic CHD. Thus, persistent hypoxia refractory to 100% oxygen supply would indicate cyanotic CHD rather than a primary pulmonary disease. It should be noted that the hyperoxia test should be utilized only in cyanotic infants to differentiate cyanosis from pulmonary vs. cardiac etiology. It should not be used in infants who are in shock and therefore appear gray but have SpO_2 above 90%. These patients should be suspected of ductal-dependent left-sided obstructive lesion in whom 100% oxygen administration could be detrimental.

The most important first step in managing a neonate presenting within the first week of life with either shock or cyanosis necessitates that the ED physician considers a ductal-dependent cardiac lesion and initiates the administration of an alprostadil drip to improve patency of the DA.

Case Presentation 2

A 3-month-old, full-term male presents to the ED due to tachypnea and poor feeding for the last 12 h. His vital signs are temperature 37 °C, HR 170 beats per minute, RR 50 breaths per minute, BP 78/50 mmHg, and oxygen saturation 94% on room air. On examination he is fussy and showing signs of respiratory distress. Extremities are cool with prolonged capillary refill time. He has grunting, retractions, and wheezing bilaterally. Liver edge is palpable at 4 cm below the costal margin. His cardiac examination is significant for a gallop. Capillary blood gas reveals pH 7.28, PCO_2 20 mmHg, sodium bicarbonate 11 mEq/L, and lactate 5.8 mmol/L. Chest radiograph shows cardiomegaly and left lung atelectasis (Fig. 1.2). The EKG is obtained (Fig. 1.3). What is the most likely diagnosis? What are the risks of albuterol, 100% oxygen, and fluid boluses?

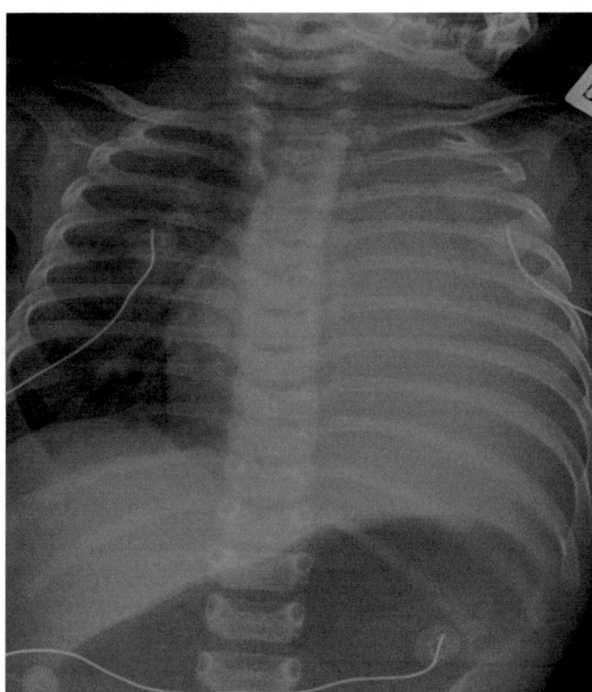

Fig. 1.2 Chest radiograph showing marked cardiomegaly and left lung atelectasis

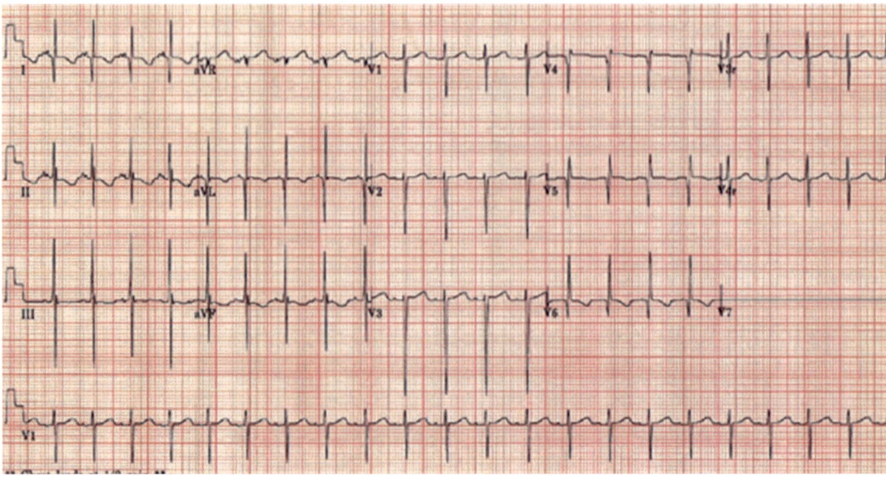

Fig. 1.3 Electrocardiogram showing deep Q waves in left-sided chest leads

The infant in this vignette is presenting with signs of uncompensated heart failure and systemic hypoperfusion. Infants 1 month to 6 months of age with undiagnosed congenital heart disease usually present to the ED with signs of heart failure due to decreasing pulmonary vascular resistance (PVR). In lesions with large intracardiac left-to-right shunts (large ventricular septal defects, atrioventricular canal defects, large patent DA), the continued decline in PVR results in increasing pulmonary blood flow. This increased pulmonary blood flow may cause the child to present with volume overload and signs and symptoms of congestive heart failure (poor feeding, tachypnea, grunting, retractions, cardiac wheezing, tachycardia, hepatomegaly, gallop, metabolic acidosis with respiratory alkalosis, and cardiomegaly on chest radiography). These infants often show evidence of hyperdynamic circulation with bounding pulses and increased pulse pressure.

The infant in this vignette exhibits cardiogenic shock with peripheral vasoconstriction and decreased pulse pressure. EKG shows myocardial infarction evidenced by deep Q waves in left-sided leads. This clinical picture is pathognomonic of ALCAPA which is typically unmasked during the early infancy period. As PVR and PAP decrease, the coronary perfusion pressure is compromised resulting in myocardial ischemia and infarction. Symptoms of a failing left ventricle and congestive heart failure progressing to shock develop around 2–4 months of age. The diagnostic clues include the signs of shock and the deep Q waves on left-sided leads on EKG.

An infant who presents with heart failure may be misdiagnosed as having viral bronchiolitis, bacterial pneumonia, or asthma. These infants may be treated with fluid boluses due to tachycardia or concern for sepsis. This may worsen the clinical status of a child in shock from congestive heart failure. Similar to Case Presentation 1, a careful history and examination to differentiate the etiology of shock must be undertaken with attention to tachypnea, gallop rhythm, jugular venous distension (JVD), hepatomegaly, and weak pulses. This assessment could prevent the inappropriate excessive administration of fluids to a child in CHF. The use of oxygen in an infant with CHF can be of particular harm as oxygen itself is a pulmonary vasodilator and may worsen left-to-right shunting and further increase pulmonary overcirculation and worsen pulmonary edema. Finally, administration of albuterol with resultant tachycardia in a child whose respiratory symptoms are secondary to myocardial dysfunction will lead to increased oxygen demands on an already compromised heart.

Acute management of infants with CHF includes optimizing hemodynamic status, decreasing oxygen consumption, maintaining optimal preload, decreasing afterload, and improving contractility. Decreasing oxygen consumption is achieved by taking away the work of breathing by sedation and mechanical ventilation, achieving atrioventricular synchrony, and avoiding β-agonists bronchodilators and other medications that may cause tachycardia. Maintaining optimal preload may require an isotonic intravenous fluid bolus. This requires frequent assessments of the clinical response to fluid. Excessive fluid administration will not be well tolerated and may worsen pulmonary edema. Improving contractility with the addition of inotropic support may be necessary.

Case Presentation 3

A 16-year-old female presents to the ED with difficulty breathing, emesis, and progressive listlessness. She has had a previous ED visit for progressive wheezing and shortness of breath 7 days ago. She was given an albuterol inhaler and dexamethasone. Despite the use of his inhaler every 6 h, her shortness of breath and wheezing worsened. Her temperature is 38.2 °C, HR 118 beats per minute, RR 23 breaths per minute, BP 102/70 mmHg, and SpO_2 92% on RA. On examination, she has mild respiratory distress and is taking shallow, quick breaths. Her lung fields are notable for diffuse crackles and wheezing. Her cardiac examination reveals tachycardia with a gallop rhythm and capillary refill of 3 s. Her rhythm strip suggests sinus tachycardia. She is given an albuterol treatment and fluid bolus of 20 mL/kg of normal saline. During the breathing treatment and fluid bolus, she suddenly develops hypotension and worsening respiratory distress. Repeat vital signs are as follows: HR 145 beats per minute, RR 45 breaths per minute, and BP 72/42 mmHg. She is somnolent, with rapid breathing and diffuse wheezing. Cardiac exam reveals tachycardia with poor peripheral pulses. She has hepatomegaly 4 cm below costal margin. CXR reveals pulmonary infiltrates and cardiomegaly (Fig. 1.4.) What are the diagnostic approach and management strategies in this patient?

This child is presenting with signs of acute decompensated heart failure. Similar to the infant in the earlier vignette, this child has signs and symptoms of heart failure including difficulty breathing, wheezing, tachycardia, gallop, hepatomegaly, and cardiomegaly. The differential diagnosis includes dilated cardiomyopathy (due to genetic causes, chronic hypertension, etc.), large pericardial effusion, and myocarditis. This child was previously healthy but had a preceding viral illness 7 days prior to the ED visit suggesting myocarditis. Myocarditis may occur at any age although studies indicate that infants and teenagers are more commonly affected. Common pitfalls include misdiagnosis as asthma or bacterial pneumonia and initiation of steroids or β-agonist bronchodilator therapy which will be harmful. Immediate management is centered around optimizing cardiac output (contractility, preload, and afterload) and transfer to a tertiary care pediatric cardiac center.

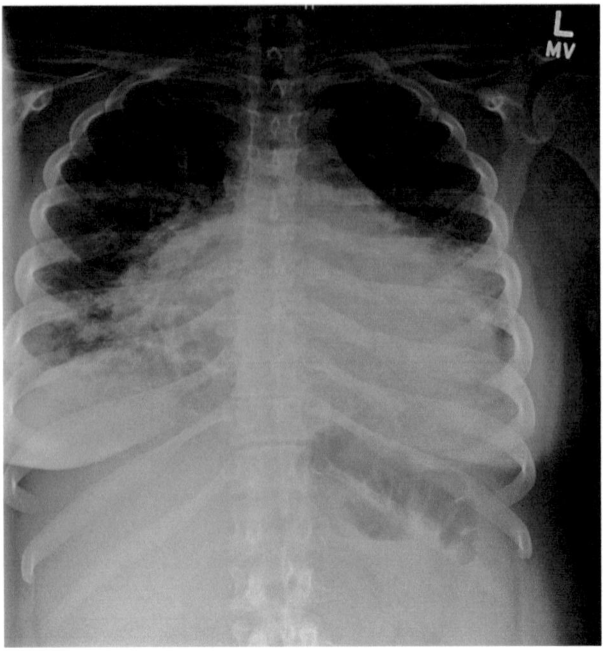

Fig. 1.4 Chest radiograph showing marked cardiomegaly and pulmonary edema

ED Management

The goals of ED management are to stabilize the airway, obtain vascular access, and support the circulation and in neonates and infants to establish and maintain patency of the ductus arteriosus. Age and physical examination findings will be the most helpful clues toward diagnosis in the initial assessment period (Table 1.3). Alprostadil infusion should be considered in infants <1 month who present in shock or cyanosis where ductal-dependent lesion is strongly suspected based on history and clinical findings. While echocardiography is necessary to make the diagnosis, awaiting echocardiography to initiate therapy may result in wasting valuable time to open the ductus and may contribute to mortality. Side effects of alprostadil include hypotension from systemic vasodilation, apnea, and fever. Blood pressure should be closely monitored, and hypotension should be treated with judicious intravascular fluid expansion. Most of these infants require prophylactic intubation and mechanical ventilation during transport.

Neonates and infants with shock, respiratory distress, or profound cyanosis may require positive pressure ventilation. Unlike older children and adults, noninvasive positive pressure (NIPPV) will rarely be an option. More likely the patient will need a definitive airway via endotracheal intubation. Prior to intubation ED physicians should prepare for further deterioration due to cardiopulmonary interactions after intubation, the effects of intubation medications, and supplemental oxygen on the pulmonary vascular bed. Pulmonary arterial reactivity and risk for pulmonary hypertensive episodes in response to medications and the unavoidable peri-intubation trauma are important considerations.

Positive pressure ventilation (PPV) has advantages and disadvantages due to cardiopulmonary interactions. Disadvantages include peri-intubation trauma, decrease in venous return leading to decreased RV preload, and increase in RV afterload. The advantages of PPV include decrease in LV afterload, limitation of left-to-right shunting, improvement in pulmonary edema, and reduction in work of breathing. The goal of PPV is to minimize the risks and maximize the benefits.

Careful selection of intubation medications is important. Many sedatives decrease systemic vascular resistance (SVR) and are myocardial depressants which contribute to hypotension, reduced aortic diastolic pressure, and poor cardiac output. Yet, sedation is needed to minimize the risk of pulmonary hypertensive crisis and for safe intubation. Intubation agents should be chosen thoughtfully and are discussed in detail in Chap. 7. In addition, supplemental oxygen should be considered similar to a drug that can have desirable effects (pulmonary vasodilation in infants at risk for pulmonary hypertension) and undesirable effects in other situations (constriction of the DA, pulmonary vasodilation, and worsening of left-to-right shunting).

Summary

ED presentations of pediatric heart disease are age and lesion specific. Children with cardiac emergencies present with respiratory distress, shock, or cyanosis. The likelihood of a given disease entity depends on the age at presentation. Tachycardia, sweating, poor feeding, cyanosis, hepatomegaly, wheezing, and cardiomegaly may be important diagnostic clues. Common pitfalls are misdiagnosis as other respiratory disorders commonly encountered in children such as asthma, bronchiolitis, and pneumonia and conditions such as sepsis and dehydration. Routinely employed ED therapeutic agents such as oxygen, bronchodilators, fluid administration, etc. may be potentially harmful in this patient population, and a high index of suspicion is necessary to manage these complex patients in the acute setting.

Clinical Pearls

- Neonates with ductal-dependent lesions typically present early within the first weeks to a month of life.
- Initiation of alprostadil (PGE1) should not be delayed in a neonate who presents in shock or with cyanosis.
- Infants with large left-to-right shunts and ALCAPA present to the ED with acute heart failure as pulmonary vascular resistance drops between 1 and 6 months of age.
- Myocarditis and arrhythmias may occur at any age.
- Goals of management include stabilizing the airway, initiating alprostadil therapy promptly when indicated, optimizing preload, decreasing afterload, and improving contractility.
- Acute management of heart failure is based on optimizing preload, reducing systemic vascular resistance, and reducing myocardial oxygen consumption.

Board Exam Questions

1. A 3-week-old male born at full term presents to the ED with tachypnea. He was well until yesterday when he stopped feeding. On physical examination he is irritable and tachypneic with a respiratory rate of 60 breaths per minute with a HR of 170 beats per minute. He is afebrile and right upper extremity blood pressure is 70/50 mmHg. Extremities are cool with delayed capillary refill and femoral pulses are difficult to palpate. Oxygen saturations are 94% on room air. What is the most important next step in managing this patient?
   (A) Intubation and mechanical ventilation
   (B) Systemic antibiotics
   (C) Albuterol treatment with administration of 100% oxygen
   (D) **Initiate alprostadil (PGE-1) infusion**
2. The neonate from question 1 has an echocardiogram performed in the ED showing severely depressed LV function and no evidence of a patent ductus arteriosus. The next most appropriate treatment for this child is to initiate:
   (A) Calcium chloride infusion
   (B) Vasopressin infusion
   (C) Continuous albuterol inhalation
   (D) **Epinephrine infusion and reassess end organ perfusion**
3. The neonate from question 1 most likely has which one of the following diagnoses?
   (A) Total anomalous venous return (TAPVR)
   (B) Anomalous coronary artery from the left pulmonary artery (ALCAPA)
   (C) Myocarditis
   (D) **Critical coarctation of the aorta**
4. A 4-month-old with known unrepaired atrioventricular septal defect presents to the ED with poor feeding and respiratory distress. On arrival to her bedside, you see a small infant with tachypnea, retractions, and nasal flaring. Vital signs show a T 37 °C, HR 160 beats per minute, RR 60 breaths per minute, BP 80/40 mmHg, and SpO_2 92% on high-flow nasal cannula at 8 L per minute with 70% FiO_2. On respiratory examination, the liver is 4 cm below the costal margin, and a systolic murmur over the precordium and bilateral wheezes are heard. The nurse asks you if FiO_2 should be raised because of the low SpO_2. Which of the following is the best response?
   (A) Increase the FiO_2 to 80%
   (B) Increase the FiO_2 to 100% and prepare for intubation
   (C) Increase in FiO_2 will not help because of right-to-left shunting
   (D) **Titrate the FiO_2 downwards as long as SpO_2 remains > 90%**

Conflicts of Interest *Disclosures*: The authors have not disclosed any potential conflicts of interest.

Selected Reading

1. Allan L, Benacerraf B, Copel JA, et al. Isolated major congenital heart disease. Ultrasound Obstet Gynecol. 2001;17(5):370–9.
2. Kemper AR, Mahle WT, Martin GR, et al. Strategies for implementing screening for critical congenital heart disease. Pediatrics. 2011;128:1259–67.
3. Mastropietro CW, Tourner SP, Sarnaik AP. Emergency presentation of congenital heart disease in children. Pediatr Emerg Med Pract. 2008;5(5):1–31.
4. Pickert CB, Moss MM, Fiser DH. Differentiation of systemic infection and congenital obstructive left heart disease in the very young infant. Pediatr Emerg Care. 1998;14(4):263–7.
5. Hoke TR, Donohue PK, Bawa PK, et al. Oxygen saturation as a screening test for critical congenital heart disease: a preliminary study. Pediatr Cardiol. 2002;23(4):403–9.
6. Ross RD, Bollinger RO, Pinsky WW. Grading the severity of congestive heart failure in infants. Pediatr Cardiol. 1992;13(2):72–5.
7. McCrindle BW, Shaffer KM, Kan JS, et al. Cardinal clinical signs in the differentiation of heart murmurs in children. Arch Pediatr Adolesc Med. 1996;150(2):169–74.
8. Freed MD, Heymann MA, Lewis AB, et al. Prostaglandin E1 infants with ductus arteriosus-dependent congenital heart disease. Circulation. 1981;64(5):899–905.
9. Freedman SB, Haladyn JK, Floh A, et al. Pediatric myocarditis: emergency department clinical findings and diagnostic evaluation. Pediatrics. 2007;120(6):1278–85.
10. Durani Y, Eagan M, Baffa J, et al. Pediatric myocarditis: presenting clinical characteristics. Am J Emerg Med. 2009;27:942–7.

Recognizing, Stabilizing, and Managing Children with Heart Failure in the Emergency Department and Other Acute Care Settings

2

Matthew J. O'Connor, Robert E. Shaddy, and Robert D. Ross

Clinical Vignette

A previously healthy 9-year-old boy was admitted from the emergency department to the general pediatric unit after a week of daily episodes of vomiting, diarrhea, decreased oral intake, and decreased energy and activity. In the emergency department, his blood pressure for age was normal, although tachycardia was present (heart rate 155/min). Cardiac auscultation revealed a gallop versus splitting of the second heart sound. He was given a 500 mL IV fluid bolus, admitted for rehydration, and discharged 24 h later with a diagnosis of gastroenteritis.

He was readmitted to the hospital 1 week later with ongoing vomiting, new epigastric abdominal pain exacerbated by activity, and dyspnea exacerbated by laying supine. Blood pressure was normal, but he continued to be tachycardic. A chest radiograph revealed cardiomegaly and pulmonary edema. He was given an IV fluid bolus and again admitted to the general pediatric unit. Examination after admission was notable for hepatomegaly. His B-type natriuretic peptide concentration was markedly elevated, at 8578 pg/mL. An echocardiogram subsequently revealed a dilated left ventricle and severely diminished left ventricular systolic function, with an ejection fraction (EF) of 15%. He was transferred to the intensive care unit and started on diuretics and inotropic drugs.

M. J. O'Connor, M.D. (✉) • R. E. Shaddy, M.D.
Division of Cardiology, The Children's Hospital of Philadelphia, University of Pennsylvania Perelman School of Medicine, Philadelphia, PA, USA
e-mail: oconnorm@email.chop.edu; rshaddy@chla.usc.edu

R. D. Ross, M.D.
Pediatrics, Division of Cardiology, Children's Hospital of Michigan and Wayne State University School of Medicine, Detroit, MI, USA
e-mail: RRoss@dmc.org

© Springer International Publishing AG, part of Springer Nature 2018

A. P. Sarnaik et al. (eds.), *Cardiac Emergencies in Children*,
https://doi.org/10.1007/978-3-319-73754-6_2

Clinical Vignette Comment

The clinical course of this patient highlights the fact that heart failure (with a subsequent diagnosis of dilated cardiomyopathy in the patient described above) in children may initially present with symptoms manifested primarily through other organ systems (e.g., gastrointestinal, respiratory). Given the high incidence of viral, self-limited gastrointestinal and respiratory illnesses in the community, particularly in children, such symptoms are likely to be attributed to common causes. Children with heart failure are often evaluated several times before the diagnosis is established.

Introduction

The clinical syndrome of heart failure (HF) is defined by the American Heart Association (AHA) as symptoms or signs attributable to inadequate ventricular filling or ejection of blood [1]. This definition encompasses HF with reduced ejection fraction (EF), or systolic dysfunction, as well as HF with preserved EF, frequently referred to as diastolic dysfunction. This latter entity is uncommon in children and is not discussed here. Although HF is generally uncommon in unselected populations of children, it often initially presents in acute care settings, such as the emergency department or urgent care clinic [2]. For this reason, clinicians working in such environments need to know the symptoms, signs, causes, and initial management of HF in children.

Definition of Pediatric Heart Failure

There is no formal definition of HF in children, although several professional societies have published diagnostic classifications for various HF syndromes in children [3, 4]. The definition of HF proposed by the AHA for adults can be applied to children. The different presentations of HF are often classified with various staging criteria, such as the AHA/American College of Cardiology HF staging classification, which includes elements of risk classification, symptomatology, and treatment, and the New York Heart Association (NYHA) HF criteria, which are symptom-based [1] (Table 2.1). Given the unique developmental characteristics of children, however, these classifications may not be as relevant. The original Ross criteria classified HF in children by their developmental status [5] (Table 2.2), and recently, other parameters have been added, such as serum natriuretic peptide concentrations and the results of exercise testing (for older children and adolescents).

Table 2.1 Heart failure classification systems in adults

ACCF/AHA stages of heart failure		NYHA functional classifications	
A	At high risk for HF but without structural heart disease or symptoms of HF	None	
B	Structural heart disease but without signs or symptoms of HF	I	No limitation of physical activity. Ordinary physical activity does not cause symptoms of HF
C	Structural heart disease with prior or current symptoms of HF	I	(as above)
		II	Slight limitation of physical activity. Comfortable at rest, but ordinary physical activity results in symptoms of HF
		III	Marked limitation of physical activity. Comfortable at rest, but less than ordinary activity causes symptoms of HF
		IV	Unable to carry on any physical activity without symptoms of HF or symptoms of HF at rest
D	Refractory HF requiring specialized interventions	IV	Unable to carry on any physical activity without symptoms of HF or symptoms of HF at rest

ACCF American College of Cardiology Foundation, *AHA* American Heart Association, *HF* Heart failure, *NYHA* New York Heart Association

Reprinted from reference [1], with permission from Wolters Kluwer

Table 2.2 Original and Revised Ross classifications for heart failure in children

Original Ross classification
Class I: Asymptomatic
Class II: Mild tachypnea or diaphoresis with feeding in infants; dyspnea on exertion in older children
Class III: Marked tachypnea or diaphoresis with feeding in infants; prolonged feeding times with growth failure resulting from HF; marked dyspnea on exertion in older children
Class IV: Symptoms such as tachypnea, retractions, grunting, or diaphoresis at rest
Revised Ross classification • Defined age groups (0–3 months, 4–12 months, 1–3 years, 4–8 years, 9–18 years) • Ten clinical variables, each scored 0, 1, or 2 – Score 0–5: **Class I** – Score 6–10: **Class II** – Score 11–15: **Class III** – Score 16–20: **Class IV** • Clinical variables – Feeding (infants—3 years), growth (1–8 years), nausea/vomiting (9–18 years) – Breathing – Respiratory rate – Heart rate – Perfusion – Hepatomegaly – NT-proBNP – Ejection fraction – AV valve insufficiency – Maximum percent oxygen consumption (9–18 years)

Reprinted and adapted from reference [6], with permission (Springer publication)

Causes of Heart Failure in Children

Heart failure in children has several causes, and an in-depth discussion of each is beyond the scope of this chapter. Broadly speaking, HF can be caused by primary heart muscle disease (i.e., cardiomyopathy), toxic or inflammatory conditions (i.e., myocarditis, sepsis), acquired heart disease (i.e., Kawasaki disease, rheumatic fever), and congenital conditions (i.e., congenital heart disease, metabolic disease, or inborn errors of metabolism; Table 2.3). The probability a particular diagnosis depends in

Table 2.3 Causes of heart failure in children

Neonates and infants
Congenital heart disease
Obstructive lesions
Aortic stenosis
Aortic arch obstruction
After closure of PDA in critical left-sided heart obstruction
Volume overload
Left-to-right shunts (VSD, AV canal, PDA, truncus arteriosus)
Valvular dysfunction
Atrioventricular valve regurgitation
Semilunar valve regurgitation
Complex defects
Single ventricle
Pulmonary hypertension (right ventricular failure)
Cardiomyopathy
Primary (dilated, noncompaction)
Secondary (arrhythmia, hypothyroidism, hypoglycemia, sepsis, hypoxemia)
Inflammatory
Myocarditis
Kawasaki disease
Metabolic disease (inborn errors of metabolism, mitochondrial disease)
Children and adolescents
Unoperated congenital heart disease (all defects)
Status post surgery for congenital heart disease
Residual defects
Residual atrioventricular or semilunar valve regurgitation
Ischemic injury
Failure of systemic ventricle in single-ventricle congenital heart defects
Pulmonary hypertension (right ventricular failure)
Cardiomyopathy
Primary (dilated, noncompaction; less commonly hypertrophic, restrictive)
Secondary (arrhythmia, sepsis, toxins/chemotherapy, muscular dystrophy, Friedreich ataxia)
Inflammatory
Myocarditis
Kawasaki disease
Metabolic

PDA Patent ductus arteriosus, *VSD* Ventricular septal defect, *AV* Atrioventricular

large part on age at presentation. For example, metabolic disease and congenital heart disease are relatively common causes in infants, whereas cardiomyopathies and myocarditis tend to predominate in adolescents. However, these are broad guidelines, and it is important to recognize that most causes of heart failure can present in any age group. A more in-depth discussion of HF causes and epidemiology in children can be found in several recent reviews, important original papers, and book chapters [6–9].

Pathophysiology

Failure of myocardial pump function decreases cardiac output, which leads to decreased tissue oxygen delivery and metabolic stress in end organs and tissues. However, the clinical syndrome of HF is not simply an imbalance between tissue oxygen supply and demand caused by myocardial dysfunction; rather it encompasses a broad array of compensatory and adaptive responses that involve a number of metabolic, hormonal, and neutrally mediated pathways. An in-depth discussion of these mechanisms is beyond the scope of this chapter, but a simplistic characterization follows. Decreased tissue oxygen delivery leads to the release of endogenous catecholamines, which when released in the circulation act to stimulate the myocardium and increase cardiac output through increasing cardiac contractility and heart rate. While initially effective, this response eventually proves maladaptive by way of increasing myocardial oxygen consumption and myocardial calcium concentration, both of which lead to cellular damage and fibrosis. In the setting of decreased cardiac output, there is a resultant increase in extracellular fluid volume. In the renal circulation, this leads to the activation of the renin-angiotensin-aldosterone pathway, which has a number of downstream effects including natriuresis and diuresis, but also activates metabolic pathways that lead to myocardial fibrosis and scarring, a process referred to as remodeling. While alteration of the abovementioned pathways is not critical in the acute management of decompensated HF, they are important in the therapy of chronic HF. For example, blockade of the renin-angiotensin-aldosterone system with angiotensin-converting enzyme inhibitors and the mineralocorticoid receptor antagonist aldosterone are mainstays of the management of chronic HF. Further discussion of the various mechanisms involved in HF can be found in several excellent reviews [10, 11].

Clinical Presentation

The clinical presentation of children with HF in the acute setting varies with its cause, the age of the child, and the timing of disease onset (acute versus chronic), in addition to several other factors. As highlighted in the opening clinical vignette, practitioners must recognize that HF in children often masquerades as common childhood maladies, particularly in the early stages of disease, which of course can have serious outcomes. For example, wheezing caused by left atrial and pulmonary venous hypertension and resultant transudation of fluid into the interstitial space between alveoli in left ventricular dilation and systolic dysfunction could readily be mistaken for reactive airway disease, asthma, or bronchiolitis. In addition, vague gastrointestinal complaints, such as vomiting, abdominal pain, and fussiness during feeding are common in infants and children with HF [2]. Despite the high index of suspicion needed to discriminate children with HF from more common, self-limited conditions, all children presenting with common signs and symptoms should not be suspected of having HF or undergo targeted evaluation for it. A detailed history and physical examination with appropriate imaging and laboratory studies, however, should be able to distinguish children with self-limited conditions from those with more serious underlying disease. In particular, HF should be considered in children with repeated presentations of the same signs and symptoms or those who have not responded to usual therapies.

Heart failure is often associated with systemic or pulmonary venous congestion and impaired cardiac output. However, the balance of these factors varies among patients, as do compensatory responses. Conceptually, children with HF can be placed into one of four categories, depending on the adequacy of systemic perfusion ("warm" or "cold"), as well as the presence or absence of venous congestion ("wet" or "dry") [12]. These four categories include "wet and warm" (the most common presentation), "dry and warm," "dry and cold," and "wet and cold." The appropriate category can be determined rapidly at the bedside by physical examination without the need for diagnostic testing. For example, a patient may conceptually be described as "wet" on the basis of peripheral edema, hepatomegaly, or the presence of tachypnea or rales on auscultation of the lungs. The distinction between "cold" and "warm" may be made by assessing the quality and amplitude of the peripheral pulses and duration of the capillary refill time. In addition, as discussed below, placing patients into one of these four categories can help guide initial therapy.

Diagnostic Evaluation

History

The first steps in diagnosis are the history and physical examination. Children with acute HF often have prodromal symptoms suggesting a viral infection, with lethargy, poor oral intake, and varying degrees of dyspnea. Fever may be present in the setting of viral myocarditis, rheumatic fever, or Kawasaki disease. Children with more chronic and indolent symptoms, such as those of the dilated cardiomyopathies, often have vague symptoms, such as slowly worsening fatigue, weight loss or gain, and dyspnea on exertion. Heart failure may occur in children and young adults with certain forms of congenital heart disease, particularly those with prior palliative surgery for single-ventricle physiology (Fontan operation) and survivors of other complex surgical reconstructions (e.g., atrial switch procedures [Mustard/Senning] for transposition of the great arteries). Children with a history of cancer who have received chemotherapy, particularly anthracycline agents, are at risk for the development of HF. In these patients, HF may become apparent many years after receiving chemotherapy. A pediatric cardiologist should be involved early when HF is suspected.

Physical Examination

In addition to the "warm and wet" categories described above, the vital signs and physical examination can indicate the degree of hemodynamic compensation. "Compensation" refers to the extent to which normal blood pressure and perfusion are maintained, where normotension is a surrogate for adequate tissue oxygen delivery. Children with "decompensated" heart failure will be hypotensive according to age-specific norms. Hypotension in children with HF is an ominous sign of impending cardiovascular collapse or cardiac arrest. In these children, tachycardia is a primary compensatory mechanism. Persistent tachycardia despite appropriate treatment for HF may indicate the presence of an associated arrhythmia.

Assessing vital signs in neonates warrants special discussion. In all neonates with symptoms or signs of HF, blood pressure and oxygen saturation should be measured in all four extremities, or, at a minimum, the right arm and either leg. A systolic blood pressure higher in the arms than in the legs, in conjunction with differential cyanosis (lower oxygen saturation in the legs), strongly suggests aortic arch or left-sided heart obstruction with a closing ductus arteriosus. If the ductus arteriosus has closed, the blood pressure differential may persist in the absence of differential cyanosis. All neonates with critical left heart obstruction will have right-to-left shunting at the ductus arteriosus, leading to differential cyanosis, which forms the basis for neonatal pulse oximetry screening for critical congenital heart disease [13, 14].

Other physical signs should raise concern for HF in children. Most (but not all) children with HF will have some degree of tachypnea and hepatomegaly. Thus, careful examination of the abdomen and accurately assessing liver size are critically important. Although a murmur may not be a common finding in pediatric HF, the presence of gallop rhythm should alert the clinician for the presence of ventricular dysfunction.

Chest Radiograph

After the initial diagnostic assessment and stabilization, appropriate initial studies include a chest radiograph and electrocardiogram. Classic findings in children with HF include cardiomegaly, pulmonary edema, and lung hyperinflation (Fig. 2.1). Cardiomegaly may be subtle, and its absence does not rule out HF with acceptable sensitivity or specificity. Also, the chest radiograph indicates the size of the cardiothymic silhouette and, if enlarged, could represent a pericardial effusion, rather than actual cardiomegaly.

Electrocardiogram

The electrocardiogram will frequently show sinus tachycardia, and clinicians should specifically look for arrhythmias, such as ectopic atrial tachycardia and other supraventricular arrhythmias that are often difficult to distinguish from sinus tachycardia.

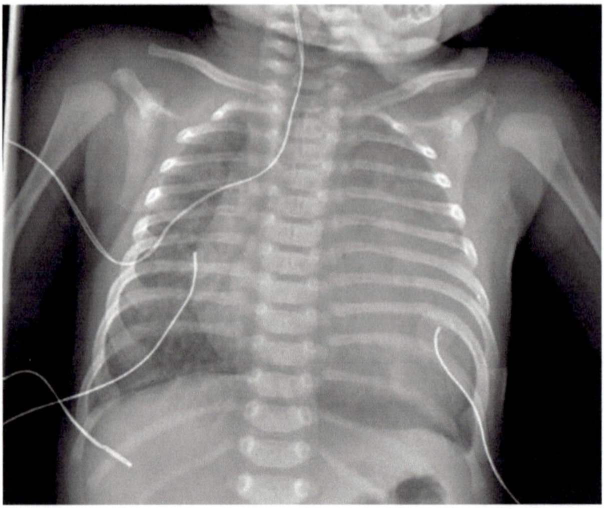

Fig. 2.1 Typical anteroposterior chest radiograph of a 2-month-old infant with acute heart failure, tachypnea, and poor feeding. There is marked cardiomegaly, lung hyperinflation, and pulmonary edema

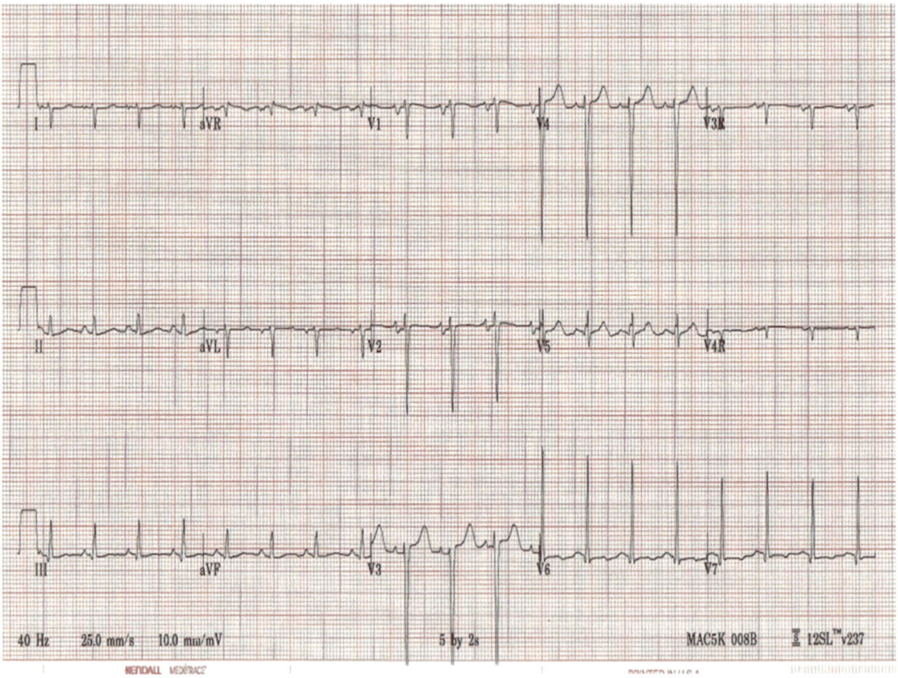

Fig. 2.2 A 15-lead electrocardiogram of a 3-month-old male with dilated cardiomyopathy showing LVH with nonspecific ST segment and T wave changes. The ST segments and T wave are flattened in precordial leads V1 and V6 and in inferior limb leads II, III, and avF

Frequently, ECG changes in HF will be nonspecific, such as diffuse T wave flattening and ST segment changes in children with dilated cardiomyopathy (Fig. 2.2). However, acute inflammatory conditions, such as myocarditis, may have strikingly

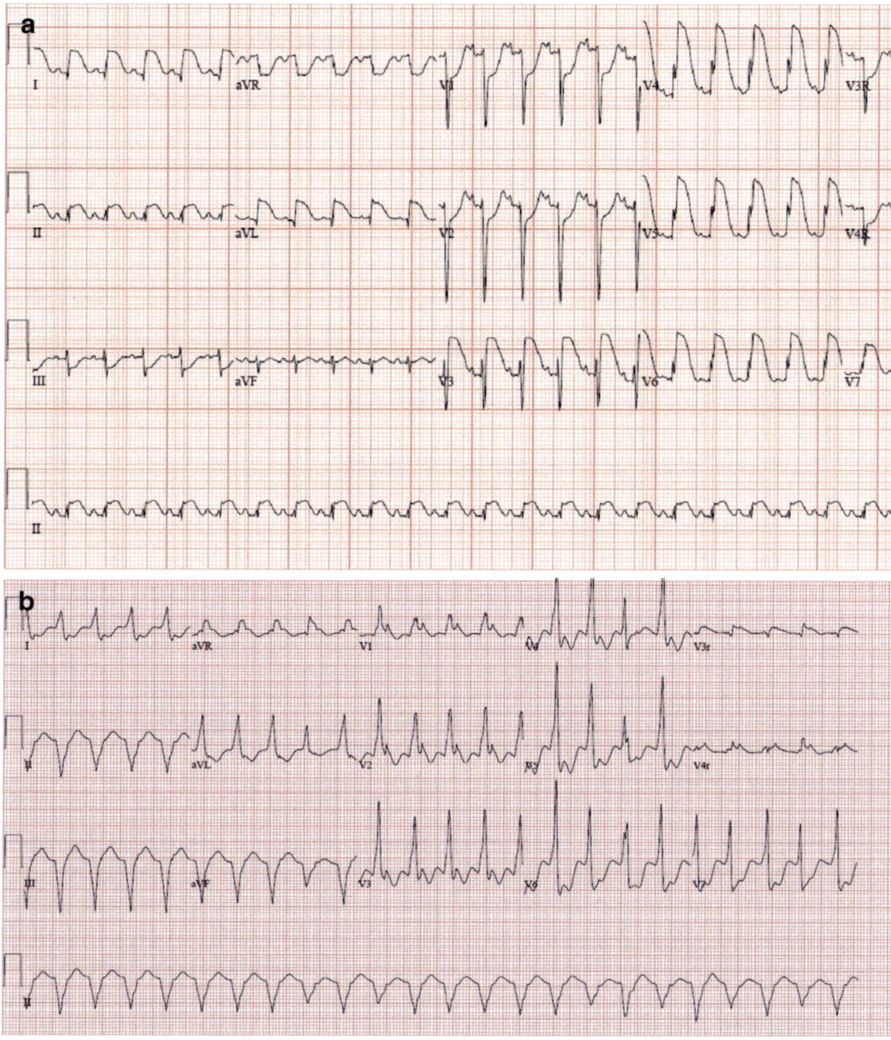

Fig. 2.3 Examples of marked ECG abnormalities in two patients with myocarditis. (**a**) Diffuse ST segment elevations and depressions in a 2-year-old boy with parvovirus myocarditis. (**b**) A wide complex tachycardia (ventricular tachycardia) in a teenage boy with giant cell myocarditis

diffuse ST segment changes, low voltages (R waves <5 mm tall each) in all of the limb leads, or arrhythmias, such as ventricular tachycardia (Fig. 2.3). Heart rate and rhythm should be monitored continuously in children with suspected HF.

Echocardiogram

Noninvasive imaging modalities are critical in assessing children with suspected HF. Echocardiography can provide information about cardiac function and insights into the cause of HF. Echocardiography can reliably measure left ventricular EF in most children, with a value of less than about 55% generally considered to be abnormal. Care should be taken to distinguish EF (percent volume change in the left ventricle over a single cardiac cycle) from shortening fraction (SF, percent diameter change in the left ventricle over a single cardiac cycle), as EF and SF have different values defining normal. Echocardiography can also assess cardiac chamber size, which is important in HF as left ventricular dilation commonly, but not always, accompanies new-onset HF. Given that children vary widely in size, absolute measurements of left ventricular cavity size can be normalized by using a "Z-score," which represents the standard deviation of the absolute measurement relative to age and body surface area [8]. In addition to assessing ventricular function and valve regurgitation, echocardiography can rapidly identify pericardial effusions, which are often encountered with inflammatory processes, such as myocarditis and Kawasaki disease (Fig. 2.4). The advent of focused, bedside echocardiography performed by non-cardiologists in acute care settings has been important in rapidly identifying ventricular dysfunction and pericardial effusions in both children and adults [15–17]. Echocardiography has important limitations, including an inability to readily quantitatively assess ventricular function in patients with the right ventricle serving as the systemic ventricle, as is encountered in patients with various forms of CHD (e.g., hypoplastic left heart syndrome or patients with Mustard or Senning operations for transposition of the great arteries). In addition, image quality may be limited in very large or postoperative patients, many of whom have poor acoustic windows.

Laboratory Evaluation

Laboratory tests should be obtained in all patients, including a complete metabolic (chemistry) panel; complete blood count with differential, type, and screen; and troponin and B-type natriuretic peptide concentrations. In selected patients, arterial or venous blood gas analysis may be warranted. Mixed venous oxygen saturation reliably indicates the adequacy of cardiac output if the sample is obtained from an upper-body central vein, such as the internal jugular or superior vena cava. Serum troponin and B-type natriuretic peptide concentrations are only two of an ever-growing list of cardiac biomarkers that can be rapidly obtained in most acute care settings and that provide additional diagnostic and prognostic information. Serum troponin concentrations are usually elevated, sometimes markedly so, in inflammatory (i.e., myocarditis) and ischemic conditions [18, 19], whereas B-type natriuretic peptide concentrations are elevated in response to increased ventricular wall stress (myocardial "stretch"), which accompanies ventricular dilation and systolic dysfunction. Either the B-type natriuretic peptide or an inert relative, N-terminal pro-B-type natriuretic peptide can be measured in the clinical setting; the preferred test often varies among hospitals and ordering clinicians. The normal values for these two assays differ and may be a source of confusion; the normal B-type natriuretic peptide concentration is <100 pg/mL, while the normal N-terminal pro-B-type natriuretic peptide concentration is <300 pg/mL; values below these cutoffs have

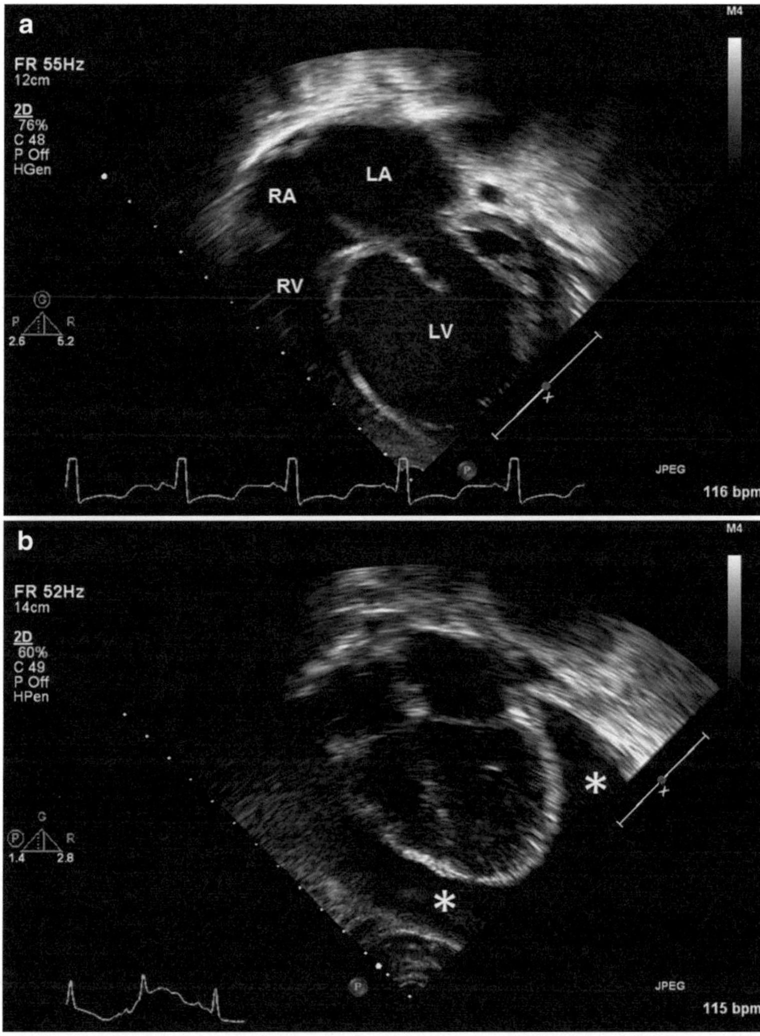

Fig. 2.4 Echocardiographic abnormalities in children with heart failure. (**a**) Marked dilation of the left atrium (LA) and left ventricle (LV) in a 9-year-old girl with newly diagnosed dilated cardiomyopathy. The right atrium (RA) and right ventricle (RV) are unaffected. (**b**) A large pericardial effusion (asterisks) in a 7-year-old girl with acute myocarditis

very high negative predictive value for a diagnosis of HF [20, 21]; the assays have also been validated in children in acute care settings [22, 23]. The use of natriuretic peptides in the diagnosis of HF is discussed in detail in this excellent review [24]. In children with a history of a prodromal viral upper respiratory illness, PCR analysis of nasal secretions and blood samples for the presence of common viruses causing myocarditis (e.g., adenovirus, parvovirus B19, human herpesvirus-6, and Coxsackievirus) is indicated.

Stabilization and Management

When HF is suspected or diagnosed, cardiac output should be maintained, and symptoms of congestion (if present) should be treated. Once again, the early involvement of a pediatric cardiologist is necessary, particularly if complicating factors are present, such as arrhythmias or congenital heart disease. Intravenous or intraosseous access should be established, and the child should be placed on continuous cardiorespiratory monitoring. Providing 100% oxygen through a nasal cannula or face mask may help increase systemic oxygen delivery in children with impaired cardiac output. However, in infants with ductal-dependent, single-ventricle physiology, 100% oxygen can sometimes further reduce systemic blood flow.

For children in more advanced respiratory distress, tracheal intubation and mechanical ventilation should be considered, but only after consulting a critical care specialist or anesthesiologist. Although positive pressure mechanical ventilation can be beneficial to children with severe left ventricular dysfunction and impaired cardiac output, the antecedent events necessary for intubation (sedation, analgesia, paralysis) and the physical act of intubation may profoundly destabilize a hemodynamically unstable patient and provoke cardiac arrest. In the acute care setting, intubation and mechanical ventilation should be avoided when possible, until hemodynamic stability is achieved and advance care providers can evaluate the child.

Diuretics may relieve symptoms in children with "wet" presentations of HF (see above). Intravenous furosemide is useful for children with systemic or pulmonary venous congestion and may improve symptoms of respiratory distress that often accompany acute presentations of HF. Diuretics should be avoided in children without symptoms or signs of congestion or if preload to the right or left ventricle is inadequate, as in hypertrophic cardiomyopathy. However, in general, early administration of diuretics in a child with symptomatic congestive HF is recommended and often quite effective in improving symptoms and stabilizing cardiovascular function. In children with chronic HF, consideration should be given to long-term alterations in renal and hepatic function that may accompany chronic HF. The "cardiorenal syndrome" is a state of impaired renal function provoked by decreased renal blood flow in the setting of chronically depressed cardiac output [25]. In such patients, administration of diuretics to relieve symptoms of congestion may be ineffective or even harmful to renal function. In a somewhat analogous fashion, chronic HF may lead to hepatic congestion and impaired hepatic blood flow, which can compromise hepatic synthetic and metabolic functions and alter the response to medications administered for relief of HF signs and symptoms [26].

Children with decompensated HF require treatment to increase blood pressure. A common question in acute care settings is whether intravenous fluid administration is advisable in children with HF. In general, small fluid boluses (i.e., 5 mL/kg) can be administered safely to children without symptoms or signs of pulmonary venous congestion. However, large, rapidly administered fluid boluses, particularly when given repeatedly, can clearly be detrimental. Determining the appropriate approach to fluid management in children with HF can be challenging, particularly in the setting of myocarditis or sepsis in conjunction with myocardial dysfunction. In these situations, prompt transfer to a pediatric intensive care unit is crucial for hemodynamic monitoring and further therapy.

Typical inotropic agents used in acute care for decompensated HF include epinephrine, dopamine, dobutamine, and milrinone. Epinephrine, dopamine, and dobutamine are all catecholaminergic agents that provide varying degrees of systemic vasoconstriction and rapid increases in blood pressure. Tachycardia or arrhythmias are major concerns with all of these agents because they increase myocardial oxygen consumption which is likely harmful to an injured myocardium.

Milrinone is a phosphodiesterase inhibitor that augments cytosolic cAMP to increase calcium influx in the sarcoplasmic reticulum of cardiac myocytes, thereby increasing cardiac contractility. In the peripheral vasculature, however, milrinone has a vasodilatory effect. Vasodilation may be beneficial in children whose condition is consistent with vasoconstriction ("cold" presentation), but in other children, the resultant hypotension may limit the use of this drug. Milrinone also has a long half-life (from 4 to 6 h), so it cannot be rapidly titrated in children with unstable conditions and marginal hemodynamics.

Children unresponsive to the above measures or who experience cardiac arrest in the acute care setting may benefit from mechanical circulatory support (MCS). Although MCS for children is clearly not available (or feasible) in many hospitals, it can be a lifesaving for children with severe decompensated HF. The primary modality for MCS in the acute care setting is venoarterial extracorporeal membrane oxygenation (ECMO), which has been used in the emergency department as well as in the ICU to rescue children from cardiogenic shock and cardiac arrest as presentations of HF [27, 28]. An advantage of ECMO is that it can be rapidly implemented and can be used in children of all age groups, down to a weight of about 3 kg. In older adolescents and young adults, percutaneous short-term MCS has been used in selected centers, using devices such as the TandemHeart as a bridge-to-recovery or cardiac transplantation.

A management algorithm for management of HF in children in the emergency department or other acute care settings is presented in Fig. 2.5.

Conclusion

Heart failure in children has a range of causes; however, the "syndrome" of HF can usually be readily recognized by a careful, thorough history and physical examination and by the appropriate diagnostic tests. Quickly identifying children with HF can be challenging in acute care settings because of its similarity to other, more benign conditions. However, early recognition and administration of appropriate therapy may be lifesaving and prevent missed diagnoses, readmissions, and excess morbidity and mortality in these children.

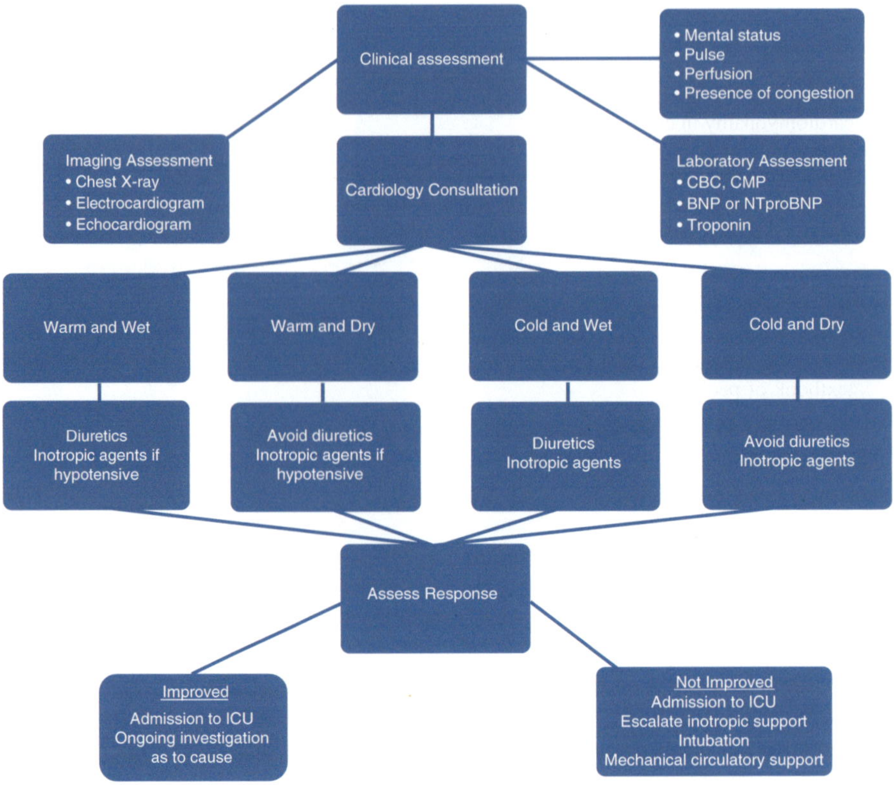

Fig. 2.5 Management algorithm—heart failure in the emergency department

References

1. Yancy CW, Jessup M, Bozkurt B, Butler J, Casey DE Jr, Drazner MH, Fonarow GC, Geraci SA, Horwich T, Januzzi JL, Johnson MR, Kasper EK, Levy WC, Masoudi FA, McBride PE, McMurray JJ, Mitchell JE, Peterson PN, Riegel B, Sam F, Stevenson LW, Tang WH, Tsai EJ, Wilkoff BL, American College of Cardiology Foundation/American Heart Association Task Force on Practice Guidelines. 2013 ACCF/AHA guideline for the management of heart failure: a report of the American College of Cardiology Foundation/American Heart Association Task Force on Practice Guidelines. Circulation. 2013;128:e240–327.
2. Macicek SM, Macias CG, Jefferies JL, Kim JJ, Price JF. Acute heart failure syndromes in the pediatric emergency department. Pediatrics. 2009;124:e898–904.
3. Kantor PF, Lougheed J, Dancea A, McGillion M, Barbosa N, Chan C, Dillenburg R, Atallah J, Buchholz H, Chant-Gambacort C, Conway J, Gardin L, George K, Greenway S, Human DG, Jeewa A, Price JF, Ross RD, Roche SL, Ryerson L, Soni R, Wilson J, Wong K, Children's Heart Failure Study Group. Presentation, diagnosis, and medical management of heart failure in children: Canadian Cardiovascular Society guidelines. Can J Cardiol. 2013;29:1535–52.
4. Kirk R, Dipchand AI, Rosenthal DN, Addonizio L, Burch M, Chrisant M, Dubin A, Everitt M, Gajarski R, Mertens L, Miyamoto S, Morales D, Pahl E, Shaddy R, Towbin J, Weintraub R. The International Society of Heart and Lung Transplantation Guidelines for the management of pediatric heart failure: executive summary. J Heart Lung Transplant. 2014;33:888–909.

5. Ross RD. The Ross classification for heart failure in children after 25 years: a review and an age-stratified revision. Pediatr Cardiol. 2012;33:1295–300.
6. Towbin JA, Lowe AM, Colan SD, Sleeper LA, Orav EJ, Clunie S, Messere J, Cox GF, Lurie PR, Hsu D, Canter C, Wilkinson JD, Lipshultz SE. Incidence, causes, and outcomes of dilated cardiomyopathy in children. JAMA. 2006;296:1867–76.
7. Wilkinson JD, Landy DC, Colan SD, Towbin JA, Sleeper LA, Orav EJ, Cox GF, Canter CE, Hsu DT, Webber SA, Lipshultz SE. The Pediatric Cardiomyopathy Registry and heart failure: key results from the first 15 years. Heart Fail Clin. 2010;6:401–13.
8. Lipshultz SE, Cochran TR, Briston DA, Brown SR, Sambatakos PJ, Miller TL, Carrillo AA, Corcia L, Sanchez JE, Diamond MB, Freundlich M, Harake D, Gayle T, Harmon WG, Rusconi PG, Sandhu SK, Wilkinson JD. Pediatric cardiomyopathies: causes, epidemiology, clinical course, preventive strategies and therapies. Futur Cardiol. 2013;9:817–48.
9. Rusconi PG, Harmon W, Wilkinson JD, Lipshultz SE. Heart failure. In: McInerny TK, Adam HM, Campbell DE, DeWitt TG, Foy JM, Kamat DM, editors. American academy of pediatrics textbook of pediatric care. 2nd ed. Elk Grove Village, IL: American Academy of Pediatrics; 2017. p. 2868–77.
10. Leopold JA. Aldosterone, mineralocorticoid receptor activation, and cardiovascular remodeling. Circulation. 2011;124:e466–8.
11. Eapen Z, Rogers JG. Strategies to attenuate pathological remodeling in heart failure. Curr Opin Cardiol. 2009;24:223–9.
12. Nohria A, Tsang SW, Fang JC, Lewis EF, Jarcho JA, Mudge GH, Stevenson LW. Clinical assessment identifies hemodynamic profiles that predict outcomes in patients admitted with heart failure. J Am Coll Cardiol. 2003;41:1797–804.
13. Ewer AK, Middleton LJ, Furmston AT, Bhoyar A, Daniels JP, Thangaratinam S, Deeks JJ, Khan KS, PulseOx Study Group. Pulse oximetry screening for congenital heart defects in newborn infants (PulseOx): a test accuracy study. Lancet. 2011;378:785–94.
14. Thangaratinam S, Daniels J, Ewer AK, Zamora J, Khan KS. Accuracy of pulse oximetry in screening for congenital heart disease in asymptomatic newborns: a systematic review. Arch Dis Child Fetal Neonatal Ed. 2007;92:F176–80.
15. Marin JR, Abo AM, Arroyo AC, Doniger SJ, Fischer JW, Rempell R, Gary B, Holmes JF, Kessler DO, Lam SH, Levine MC, Levy JA, Murray A, Ng L, Noble VE, Ramirez-Schrempp D, Riley DC, Saul T, Shah V, Sivitz AB, Tay ET, Teng D, Chaudoin L, Tsung JW, Vieira RL, Vitberg YM, Lewiss RE. Pediatric emergency medicine point-of-care ultrasound: summary of the evidence. Crit Ultrasound J. 2016;8:16.
16. Gaspar HA, Morhy SS, Lianza AC, de Carvalho WB, Andrade JL, do Prado RR, Schvartsman C, Delgado AF. Focused cardiac ultrasound: a training course for pediatric intensivists and emergency physicians. BMC Med Educ. 2014;14:25.
17. Labovitz AJ, Noble VE, Bierig M, Goldstein SA, Jones R, Kort S. Focused cardiac ultrasound in the emergent setting: a consensus statement of the American Society of Echocardiography and American College of Emergency Physicians. J Am Soc Echocardiogr. 2010;23:1225–30.
18. Harris TH, Gossett JG. Diagnosis and diagnostic modalities in pediatric patients with elevated troponin. Pediatr Cardiol. 2016;37:1469–74.
19. Eisenberg MA, Green-Hopkins I, Alexander ME, Chiang VW. Cardiac troponin T as a screening test for myocarditis in children. Pediatr Emerg Care. 2012;28:1173–8.
20. Maisel AS, Krishnaswamy P, Nowak RM, McCord J, Hollander JE, Duc P, Omland T, Storrow AB, Abraham WT, Wu AH, Clopton P, Steg PG, Westheim A, Knudsen CW, Perez A, Kazanegra R, Herrmann HC, McCullough PA. Breathing not properly multinational study investigators. Rapid measurement of B-type natriuretic peptide in the emergency diagnosis of heart failure. N Engl J Med. 2002;347:161–7.
21. Januzzi JL Jr, Camargo CA, Anwaruddin S, Baggish AL, Chen AA, Krauser DG, Tung R, Cameron R, Nagurney JT, Chae CU, Lloyd-Jones DM, Brown DF, Foran-Melanson S, Sluss PM, Lee-Lewandrowski E, Lewandrowski KB. The N-terminal pro-BNP investigation of dyspnea in the emergency department (PRIDE) study. Am J Cardiol. 2005;95:948–54.

22. Cantinotti M, Storti S, Crocetti M, Assanta N, Murzi B, Clerico A. Decision levels for plasma B-type natriuretic peptide assay to diagnose significant cardiovascular disease in children. J Am Coll Cardiol. 2010;55:1166–7.
23. Maher KO, Reed H, Cuadrado A, Simsic J, Mahle WT, Deguzman M, Leong T, Bandyopadhyay S. B-type natriuretic peptide in the emergency diagnosis of critical heart disease in children. Pediatrics. 2008;121:e1484–8.
24. Weber M, Hamm C. Role of B-type natriuretic peptide (BNP) and NT-proBNP in clinical routine. Heart. 2006;92:843–9.
25. Sarraf M, Masoumi A, Schrier RW. Cardiorenal syndrome in acute decompensated heart failure. Clin J Am Soc Nephrol. 2009;4:2013–26.
26. Samsky MD, Patel CB, DeWald TA, Smith AD, Felker GM, Rogers JG, Hernandez AF. Cardiohepatic interactions in heart failure. J Am Coll Cardiol. 2013;61:2397–405.
27. Yamamoto LG, Young LL. Acute-onset dysrhythmia heralding fulminant myocarditis and refractory cardiac arrest treated with ED cardiopulmonary bypass and extracorporeal membrane oxygenation. Am J Emerg Med. 2007;25:348–52.
28. Posner JC, Osterhoudt KC, Mollen CJ, Jacobstein CR, Nicolson SC, Gaynor JW. Extracorporeal membrane oxygenation as a resuscitative measure in the pediatric emergency department. Pediatr Emerg Care. 2000;16:413–5.

3 Hypoplastic Left Heart Syndrome

Monika Chauhan, Susan Tourner, and Christopher W. Mastropietro

Introduction

The incidence of hypoplastic left heart syndrome (HLHS) is 0.2–0.4 per 1000 live births. In early reports, untreated HLHS accounted for 25% of deaths related to congenital heart disease that occurred in the first few weeks of life [1, 2]. Despite advances in antenatal detection of congenital heart disease, some children with HLHS are born undiagnosed and continue to present to pediatric providers in extremis. For those who survive the immediate postnatal period and undergo surgical intervention, they remain fragile throughout infancy and early childhood. This chapter focuses on the emergency presentation and management of infants with HLHS.

Genetics and Embryology

The etiology of HLHS remains unclear, although evidence for a genetic influence is mounting. The recurrence risk in families with one affected child is 0.5–2%, which is more than 25 times the incidence in the general population. There is a strong

M. Chauhan, M.B.B.S. (✉)
Division of Critical Care, Department of Pediatrics, Children's Hospital of Michigan, Wayne State University School of Medicine, Detroit, MI, USA
e-mail: mchauhan@med.wayne.edu

S. Tourner, M.D.
Department of Pediatrics, University of Toledo College of Medicine, Toledo, OH, USA

ProMedica Toledo Children's Hospital, Toledo, OH, USA

C. W. Mastropietro, M.D.
Indiana University School of Medicine, Riley Hospital for Children at Indiana University Health, Indianapolis, IN, USA
e-mail: cmastrop@iu.edu

© Springer International Publishing AG, part of Springer Nature 2018

A. P. Sarnaik et al. (eds.), *Cardiac Emergencies in Children*,
https://doi.org/10.1007/978-3-319-73754-6_3

familial correlation between HLHS and aortic valve abnormalities [3–5]. Many genetic syndromes are associated with HLHS. The genetic factors and embryological origins of HLHS remain an important focus of research in contemporary pediatric cardiology [5, 6].

During embryonic development, blood flow is crucial for growth of cardiac structures. For example, left ventricle (LV) hypoplasia could arise secondary to flow obstruction across the aortic or mitral valves due to stenosis or atresia. The severity of LV hypoplasia correlates with the severity of the obstruction. Consequently, the ascending aorta is hypoplastic due to the paucity of blood ejected from the left ventricle.

Likewise, LV underdevelopment can ensue from premature closure of the foramen ovale. Fetal blood predominantly flows from the right atrium across the foramen ovale to the left atrium and subsequently to the LV. In the setting of a restrictive or absent foramen ovale, blood flow to the left ventricle is minimal, and the LV is hypoplastic.

Anatomical Subtypes

HLHS is a spectrum of congenital cardiovascular malformations characterized by underdevelopment of the left heart with significant hypoplasia of the left ventricle including atresia, stenosis, or hypoplasia of the aortic and/or mitral valve and hypoplasia of the ascending aorta and aortic arch. The hypoplastic left side structures, such as the mitral valve, aortic valve, and ascending aorta, cannot support systemic blood flow and require either single ventricle palliation or cardiac transplantation. A list of the different anatomical subtypes of HLHS is provided in Table 3.1.

Pathophysiology

Normally, the pulmonary and systemic circulations are connected in series. The right ventricle pumps deoxygenated blood into the pulmonary circulation, and the left ventricle pumps oxygenated blood into the systemic circulation. A hypoplastic LV is inadequate to support the systemic circulation, so the right ventricle (RV) must pump blood to both circulations in a parallel configuration (Fig. 3.1). Oxygenated blood from the pulmonary veins flows into a small left atrium, traverses an obligate atrial septal defect, and mixes with deoxygenated blood in the right

Table 3.1 Anatomical variants of hypoplastic left heart syndrome (HLHS)

HLHS with mitral atresia/aortic atresia (MA/AA)
HLHS with mitral stenosis/aortic stenosis (MS/AS)
HLHS with mitral stenosis/aortic atresia (MS/AA)
HLHS with mitral atresia/aortic stenosis (MA/AS)
Right ventricle (RV) dominant complete atrioventricular canal defect (CAVCD)
Some variations of double outlet right ventricle (DORV)

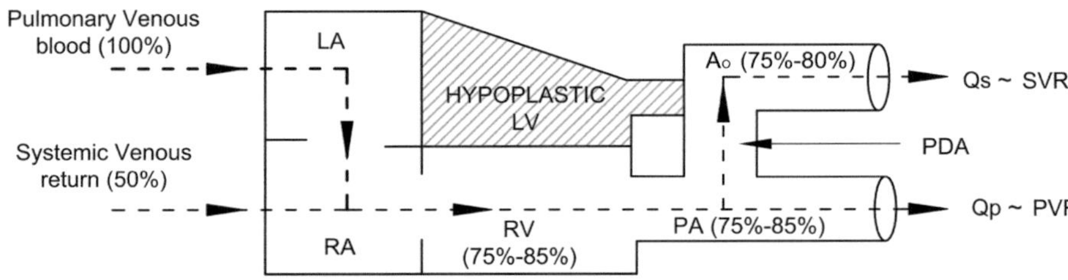

Fig. 3.1 A line diagram illustrating the parallel circulation in a patient with unoperated HLHS where blood exiting the right ventricle divides between the pulmonary (Qp) and systemic (Qs) circulations based upon the respective resistances of these two vascular beds. *LA* left atrium, *RA* right atrium, *RV* right ventricle, *LV* left ventricle, *Ao* aorta, *PA* pulmonary artery, *PDA* patent ductus arteriosus, *Qp* pulmonary blood flow, *Qs* systemic blood flow, *SVR* systemic vascular resistance, *PVR* pulmonary vascular resistance

atrium. This partially oxygenated right atrial blood passes into the right ventricle and is pumped into the main pulmonary artery. A portion goes directly to the lungs, through the right and left pulmonary arteries, and a portion enters the systemic circulation through the patent ductus arteriosus (PDA). The ratio of pulmonary-to-systemic blood flow, referred to as the Qp:Qs, is determined by the resistances of the two circulations. The resistances in pulmonary and systemic vascular beds must be balanced to provide adequate blood flow to both the pulmonary and systemic circulations. Ideally, similar proportions of mixed blood are ejected into the systemic and pulmonary circulations, resulting in arterial oxygen saturation 75%–85%.

- In patients with HLHS, the pulmonary and systemic circulations are connected in parallel, such that blood ejected from the right ventricle is distributed to both circulations concurrently. Under ideal circumstances, this physiology results in adequate blood flow to each circulation resulting in arterial oxygen saturation of 75–85%.

Case Example 1

A previously healthy full-term 6-day-old infant is brought to the emergency department (ED) at a community hospital with a 12-h history of poor feeding and listlessness. Of note, the infant received little antenatal care and was delivered at home by a community midwife. Vital signs upon arrival included an axillary temperature of 35.6 °C, a heart rate of 174 beats per minute, a blood pressure of 62/41 mmHg, and a respiratory rate of 72 breaths per minute. The oxygen saturation as determined by pulse oximetry (SpO_2) was 80% in room air. The physical examination was remarkable for tachypnea with marked subcostal retractions; a palpable liver edge 3 cm below the right costal margin; full anterior fontanelle; weak, thready pulses in all extremities; and cool, mottled extremities with capillary refill time of approximately 5 s.

The infant was placed on oxygen therapy via nasal cannula while ED staff was preparing for endotracheal intubation and intraosseous line placement. Shortly after the initiation of oxygen therapy, the infant became bradycardic and pulseless.

Clinical Presentation

Most neonates with HLHS are diagnosed by antenatal ultrasound allowing for optimal parental counseling, controlled delivery, and timely resuscitation. After birth, intravenous access is immediately achieved, and an infusion of prostaglandin E1 (PGE1) is initiated to maintain patency of the ductus arteriosus. An echocardiogram confirms the diagnosis and delineates the specific anatomy.

In a subset of neonates, as in this vignette, an antenatal diagnosis is not made. At birth, a patent ductus arteriosus ensures adequate blood flow to the systemic circulation and the neonate appears well. Cyanosis may not be visible when the arterial oxygen saturation is 80% or greater. In some cases, these infants are discharged home undiagnosed. Clinical presentation of these infants depends on following factors: restriction of blood flow at the atrial level, patency of the ductus arteriosus, and pulmonary vascular resistance (PVR).

A patient with an absent or small (restrictive) atrial septal defect develops severe left atrial hypertension and consequent pulmonary venous congestion. Symptoms of respiratory distress appear immediately or soon after birth, regardless of ductal patency. Urgent atrial septostomy (to allow unimpeded blood flow from the left atrium to the right atrium) or extracorporeal life support may be needed for survival.

For infants with an adequate atrial septal defect, presentation is not as abrupt. In infants with a normal heart, functional closure of the ductus arteriosus occurs within the first few hours after birth [7]. Patients with HLHS however require patency of the ductus arteriosus to provide systemic blood flow. High-volume blood flow through the ductus arteriosus temporarily delays ductal closure, so the infant is often initially asymptomatic. The clinical presentation depends upon the timing of ductus arteriosus closure, typically in the first 1–2 weeks of life. As the ductus arteriosus begins to close, a patient with HLHS may initially have increased arterial oxygen saturations, even greater than 90%. This relatively high arterial oxygen saturation is due to an imbalance between the systemic and pulmonary circulations, with an increase in pulmonary blood flow. Pulmonary overcirculation eventually leads to pulmonary edema, decreased oxygen saturation, tachypnea, and respiratory failure. Concomitantly, ductus arteriosus closure also leads to decreased systemic perfusion. Initial symptoms include poor feeding and lethargy and quickly progress to life-threatening shock. The neonate will appear ashen with cool extremities, feeble pulses, delayed capillary refill time, hepatomegaly, facial edema, and full fontanelle. Metabolic acidosis due to poor systemic perfusion further exacerbates tachypnea and respiratory failure.

- An adequately sized interatrial communication and a patent ductus arteriosus are required for neonate with HLHS to survive until surgical intervention.

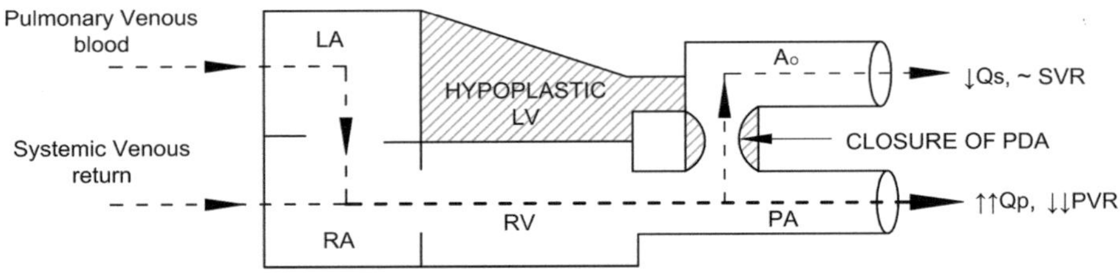

Fig. 3.2 A line diagram illustrating the anatomy in a patient with unoperated HLHS with preferential blood flow to the pulmonary circulation (pulmonary overcirculation), as the ductus arteriosus is closing and the pulmonary vascular resistance is decreasing, thus causing systemic hypoperfusion. *LA* left atrium, *RA* right atrium, *RV* right ventricle, *LV* left ventricle, *Ao* aorta, *PA* pulmonary artery, *PDA* patent ductus arteriosus, *Qp* pulmonary blood flow, *Qs* systemic blood flow, *SVR* systemic vascular resistance, *PVR* pulmonary vascular resistance

PVR decreases at birth and continues to decrease to its nadir between 2 and 8 weeks of age [8]. As the PVR decreases in patients with HLHS, a greater proportion of the cardiac output from the right ventricle enters the pulmonary circulation, and a smaller proportion of blood enters the systemic circulation through the patent ductus arteriosus. This clinical scenario is often referred to as "pulmonary overcirculation" or "pulmonary steal." Decreasing PVR further exacerbates systemic hypoperfusion and shock that develop with closure of the ductus arteriosus (Fig. 3.2). Moreover, oxygen is a potent pulmonary vasodilator that decreases PVR. A patient with HLHS on supplemental oxygen (like the patient in the vignette) has increased pulmonary steal with reduced systemic blood flow and worse shock.

- As the ductus arteriosus starts to close and pulmonary vascular resistance steadily decreases, cardiac output from the right ventricle flows preferentially to pulmonary vascular bed, causing pulmonary overcirculation and systemic hypoperfusion. The patient will have relatively high oxygen saturations (>85%) and will present in shock.

Diagnosis and Initial Management

The initial diagnostic evaluation and management for a patient with undiagnosed HLHS will be similar to patients with other forms of ductal-dependent systemic blood flow (e.g., critical coarctation of the aorta, interrupted aortic arch). Careful attention must be given to the clinical response to common therapies for shock such as isotonic fluid administration or exogenous oxygen. Infants with undiagnosed ductal-dependent systemic blood flow will respond poorly to these therapies. In these cases, discontinuation of these therapies and initiation of PGE1 is the appropriate next step. The goal for arterial oxygen saturation is 75–85%. Urgent echocardiogram is also imperative. If a pediatric cardiac consultation is not available, emergent transfer to a tertiary care pediatric center must be arranged.

PGE1 infusion is the mainstay of management for ductal-dependent congenital heart disease. If a ductal-dependent lesion is suspected, a PGE1 infusion should be initiated without hesitation. The risks associated with not starting PGE1(e.g., death) outweigh the possible side effects associated with a PGE1 infusion (e.g., apnea, hypotension). These side effects can be managed with endotracheal intubation and vasoactive medications. The recommended starting dose of PGE1 is 0.05 mcg/kg/min. Once ductal patency is established, the dose can be reduced to 0.01–0.02 mcg/kg/min to mitigate its side effects.

Following initiation of PGE1, cautious intravenous volume expansion may be necessary to ameliorate hypotension. In the presence of ventricular dysfunction, excess volume administration may contribute to elevated ventricular end-diastolic pressure, which will compromise coronary perfusion. Inotropic support with dobutamine, epinephrine, and/or milrinone therapy should be considered in these scenarios.

After establishing patency of the ductus arteriosus, it is common for the pulmonary and systemic circulations to remain unbalanced. The increased pulmonary blood flow (Qp) at the expense of the systemic blood flow (Qs) occurs because the pulmonary vascular bed is "the path of least resistance." In the absence of invasive monitoring devices, SpO_2 can be used as a crude measure to estimate Qp:Qs. High SpO_2 (>90%) with clinical signs of systemic hypoperfusion are indicative of Qp:Qs much greater than 1. In these cases, one must employ medical management strategies to minimize systemic vascular resistance and avoid therapies that reduce pulmonary vascular resistance, such as supplemental oxygen, whether via nasal cannula or endotracheal tube. Though counterintuitive for patients presenting in shock, it is common to leave these patients in room air or, in cases of mechanical ventilation, an inspired oxygen concentration of 21%. It is important to remember, however, that the absolute value of the SpO_2 is less important than clinical signs of adequate systemic perfusion, such as warm extremities, strong pulses, adequate urine output (i.e., greater than 1 mL/kg/hr), and absence of metabolic acidosis.

If systemic blood flow remains compromised despite eliminating supplemental oxygen, consider additional therapies. Blood transfusion aimed at increasing the patient's hematocrit to ~40% and sedation to reduce agitation can help to maintain the delicate balance between tissue oxygen supply and demand. In addition, systemic vasodilators such as milrinone (with added benefit of inotropy) or sodium nitroprusside, to reduce systemic vascular resistance, can be helpful, although this remains controversial [9, 10]. Patients with ongoing signs of systemic hypoperfusion in the setting of elevated SpO_2 may require urgent surgery.

- Prior to surgery, patients with HLHS require an unrestrictive atrial septal defect, PGE1 to maintain patency of ductus arteriosus, and careful attention to prevent excessive pulmonary blood flow. Oxygen therapy should be administered cautiously.

Surgical Palliation

The three-staged surgery for patients with HLHS is commonly referred to as staged Fontan *palliation,* rather than *repair*, since an anatomical *repair* is not possible. The goals of the initial surgical palliation, which typically occurs in the first few weeks of life, are as follows: the creation of a nonrestrictive interatrial communication, the creation of an unobstructed systemic outflow tract, and the establishment of a reliable (but not excessive) source for pulmonary blood flow.

Three procedural options are currently offered for the first stage of palliation: the Norwood procedure with a modified Blalock-Taussig shunt, the Norwood procedure with a Sano modification, and the hybrid procedure. The choice of procedure depends upon the patient's underlying anatomy, preoperative clinical condition, and the surgeon's preference.

The traditional Norwood procedure is named after William Norwood, the pediatric cardiac surgeon who first performed this revolutionary surgery. The patent ductus arteriosus is ligated and divided. The pulmonary trunk is divided, and the pulmonary valve is incorporated into the augmented aorta as an unobstructed *neo-aortic* valve (Fig. 3.3) [11, 12]. A reliable source of pulmonary blood flow is created using a Gortex® tube graft to direct blood either from a systemic artery or from the right ventricle to the pulmonary artery. The atrial septum is completely resected to create a common atrium and promote unobstructed flow from the left atrium into the right atrium.

There are two choices for establishing a reliable source for pulmonary blood flow in a Norwood procedure. In a modified Blalock-Taussig shunt (BTS), the Gortex® tube graft is usually inserted between the right subclavian or innominate artery and the right pulmonary artery (Fig. 3.3). More recently, many surgeons have opted to perform the Norwood procedure with a Sano modification, named after Dr. Shinjo Sano (Fig. 3.4) [13]. A right ventricle-to-pulmonary artery Gortex® tube graft replaces the modified BT shunt. The Sano shunt avoids the diastolic runoff into the pulmonary circulation that can occur with the modified BT shunt. Diastolic runoff reduces diastolic blood pressure and adversely affects coronary perfusion, resulting in myocardial dysfunction with low cardiac output. Coronary hypoperfusion is considered to play a major role in mortality in the perioperative period and late after the Norwood procedure [14–16]. The Norwood procedure with Sano modification can provide the advantage of reducing the risk of coronary hypoperfusion.

The first-stage Norwood palliation results in parallel (as opposed to in-series) circulations such that blood ejected from the systemic (right) ventricle flows into the systemic or pulmonary circulations based on their relative resistances. Optimal arterial oxygen saturations continue to be 75–85%. Preoperatively, the pulmonary blood flow relied upon the tenuous and unrestrictive PDA. Postoperatively, the modified BT shunt or the Sano shunt replaces the ductus arteriosus as the source of pulmonary blood flow. In contrast to a large PDA, the BT shunt and the Sano shunt are fixed resistors that help balance flow in both circulations to achieve a more optimal Qp:Qs closer to 1. The resistance in any shunt depends upon its length and diameter. A 3.5 and 5 mm diameter Gortex® shunt is most commonly used for the MBT shunt and for the Sano shunt, respectively. These shunts limit pulmonary blood flow and decrease the risk of systemic and coronary hypoperfusion [17].

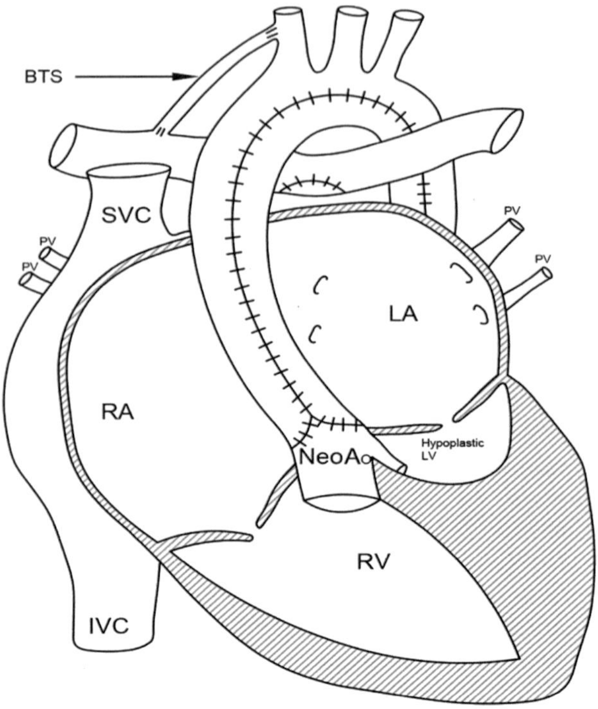

Fig. 3.3 Norwood procedure (classical). A neoaorta is surgically created using the patient's native pulmonary root and a patch to augment the hypoplastic native aorta. A Blalock-Taussig shunt (BTS) is inserted between the right subclavian artery and the pulmonary artery

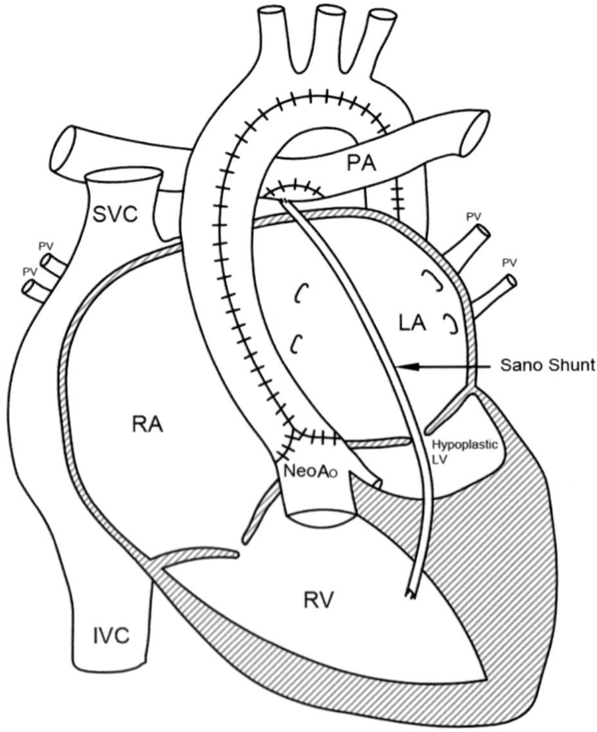

Fig. 3.4 Norwood procedure (Sano modification). The aortic reconstruction is similar to the classical Norwood procedure. However, instead of a modified Blalock-Taussig shunt, a Gortex® conduit is placed between the right ventricle and the pulmonary artery

The hybrid procedure is a cooperative approach utilizing interventional cardiac catheterization and cardiovascular surgical techniques (Fig. 3.5). A stent, placed in the PDA, maintains ductal patency and also serves as the source for systemic blood flow. If restrictive, the atrial septum is dilated by balloon and/or blade atrial septostomy with or without stent placement. Through a limited median sternotomy incision, pulmonary artery bands are surgically placed on both branch pulmonary arteries to act as fixed resistors that control pulmonary blood flow [18, 19]. At the time of surgical placement, the pulmonary artery bands are tightened to maintain oxygen saturations that correspond to a Qp:Qs close to 1. The advantage of the hybrid procedure is that it is more straightforward than the Norwood procedure in that it delays the need for cardiopulmonary bypass, hypothermic total circulatory arrest, and major aortic reconstruction until later in infancy. On the other hand, the disadvantage of the hybrid procedure is that coronary blood flow remains dependent upon retrograde blood flow from the stented ductus arteriosus which can be compromised due to aortic narrowing. Progressive restriction of the interatrial communication can also complicate the hybrid procedure. Both factors are important contributors to post-hybrid morbidity and mortality.

- After stage 1 palliation, irrespective of type of surgical procedure, the systemic and pulmonary circulations remain connected in parallel and compete for their optimal proportion of the cardiac output.

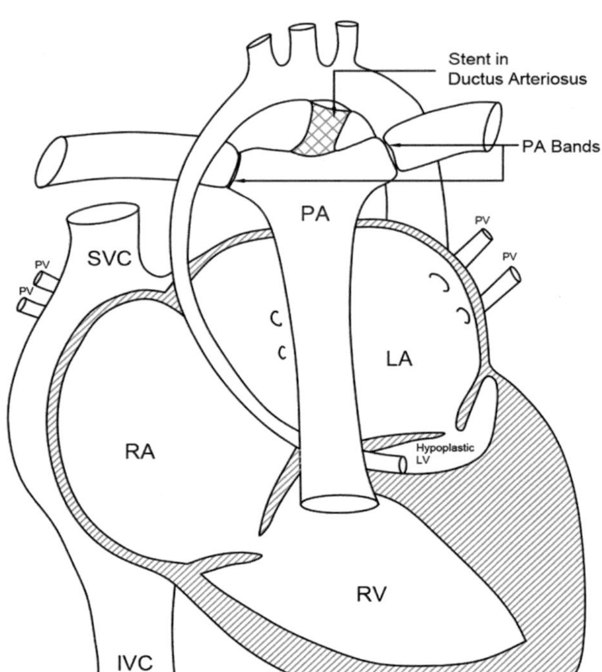

Fig. 3.5 Hybrid procedure. A stent is placed in the ductus arteriosus to maintain patency. Bands are placed around both pulmonary arteries which restrict pulmonary blood flow and allow for a balanced circulation

Interstage Complications

After recovery from stage 1 surgical palliation, most patients are discharged home with close monitoring until their second-stage palliative surgery at 4–8 months of age. During this "interstage period," the right ventricle remains volume overloaded because it receives and ejects twice the cardiac output compared to a normal heart. Despite close monitoring by their primary cardiologist, the volume-overloaded ventricle, in conjunction with inefficient parallel circulation and cyanosis, places the patients with HLHS at risk for sudden and unexpected cardiopulmonary decompensation. Common acquired pediatric illnesses, such gastroenteritis and bronchiolitis, lead to hypovolemia and hypoxemia, and are not well tolerated by these vulnerable infants. Unique complications related to their complex anatomy contribute to high morbidity and mortality in the interstage period. A summary of the presentation and treatment of interstage complications is provided in Table 3.2.

Table 3.2 Interstage presentation of infants with HLHS

Presentation	Differential diagnosis	Management
SaO2 < 75% Dark lung fields No shunt murmur	Hypovolemia Shunt obstruction	1. Volume administration, inotropic support to increase blood pressure and shunt flow 2. If no improvement, endotracheal intubation 3. Echocardiogram (if available) to assess function, anatomy, and shunt flow 4. During the initial evaluation and treatment, prepare for urgent transfer to the patient's congenital heart program for further evaluation and treatment with the need for possible cardiac catheterization and/or surgery
SaO2 < 75% Hazy lung fields Poor perfusion	Arrhythmia Poor cardiac function Atrioventricular valve regurgitation Recurrent arch obstruction If post-hybrid procedure: restrictive atrial septal defect or retrograde arch obstruction Sepsis	1. If arrhythmia present, restore sinus rhythm 2. Consider endotracheal intubation if perfusion poor, regardless of rhythm 3. Inotropic support – Epinephrine 0.05–0.1 mcg/kg/min – Dobutamine 5–10 mcg/kg/min – Milrinone 0.5–0.75 mcg/kg/min 4. Echocardiogram (if available) to assess function, aortic arch anatomy, atrioventricular valve function, and patency of interatrial communication 5. Broad spectrum antibiotics 6. During the emergency room evaluation and treatment, prepare for urgent transfer to the patient's congenital heart program for further evaluation and treatment with the need for possible cardiac catheterization
SaO2 > 90% Hazy lung fields Poor perfusion	Pulmonary overcirculation at the expense of systemic circulation	1. Administer room air (FiO2 0.21) 2. Inotropic support and afterload reduction – Dobutamine 5–10 mcg/kg/min – Milrinone 0.5–0.75 mcg/kg/min – Nitroprusside 0.5–4 mcg/kg/min 3. During the emergency room evaluation and treatment, prepare for urgent transfer to the patient's congenital heart program for further evaluation and treatment

Case Example 2

A 3-month-old baby boy who was born at 39 weeks gestation with a prenatal diagnosis of HLHS underwent the Norwood procedure with a modified BT shunt as his stage-I palliation surgery. The postoperative course was uneventful except for feeding difficulty. He was discharged home with nasogastric tube feeds after 2 months of hospitalization. The echocardiogram at discharge showed normal right ventricular function and mild-to-moderate tricuspid regurgitation. Discharge medications included enalapril and aspirin. One week after discharge, he presented to the primary care physician for a follow-up appointment. In the clinic, the room air SpO_2 was 60%, the heart rate (HR) was 160 beats per minute, and the blood pressure (BP) was normal. He was urgently transferred to the emergency department (ED). There was no history of cough, runny nose, or fever. He had been eating well. The ED physician was unable to hear the shunt murmur. The chest X-ray (CXR) revealed dark lung fields. The capillary blood gas showed a mixed respiratory and metabolic acidosis. Supplemental oxygen was started. The echocardiogram showed minimal blood flow across the BT shunt. The child was taken to interventional cardiology where a partial shunt obstruction was confirmed and stent placement with balloon dilatation was performed.

Acute Shunt Thrombosis

Infants with HLHS after stage 1 palliation tolerate oxygen saturations of 75–85% without significant organ dysfunction but live on the edge with very limited oxygen reserves. A clot formation in the systemic-to-pulmonary artery shunt causes obstruction to pulmonary blood flow and results in clinically significant hypoxia. Because the common atrium receives a minimal amount of oxygenated pulmonary venous blood, the systemic right ventricle ejects this desaturated blood into the systemic circulation. This physiology leads to cyanosis, metabolic acidosis, and potential end-organ damage. The chest X-ray demonstrates dark lung fields (oligemia) due to lack of pulmonary blood flow. The continuous shunt murmur is diminished or absent on chest auscultation. An echocardiogram must be done emergently to evaluate shunt flow, cardiac function, and the status of the interatrial communication. Oxygen supplementation, fluid resuscitation, and mechanical ventilatory support should be undertaken while arrangements are made for transfer of the patient with a thrombosed shunt to a tertiary care center with interventional cardiology and cardiovascular surgical capabilities for definitive management. Minimizing of oxygen consumption with sedation and maximizing oxygen carrying capacity by transfusing blood to a goal hematocrit of 40–45% are also helpful.

Children with a systemic-to-pulmonary artery shunt receive aspirin or other anticoagulant therapy to prevent shunt thrombosis. However, conditions that cause hypovolemia cause sluggish blood flow through the shunt and can promote thrombosis despite antiplatelet or other anticoagulant therapy. Common viral illnesses cause dehydration through vomiting, diarrhea, poor oral intake, or increased insensible losses through fever and tachypnea. In some cases, shunt thrombosis presents acutely without obvious risk factors or prodromal illness.

Hypoxemia, absent shunt murmur, cyanosis, and pulmonary oligemia are suggestive of acute shunt obstruction.

Recurrent Aortic Arch Obstruction

As part of the Norwood procedure, the diminutive ascending aorta is reconstructed to form a neoaorta which is responsible for supplying blood to the systemic circulation. However, due to inherent anatomy, residual ductal tissue, and technical factors, recurrent distal aortic arch narrowing can occur after the Norwood procedure [20–22]. Recurrent aortic arch obstruction creates increased afterload on the already volume-overloaded systemic right ventricle. Right ventricular function deteriorates, and the patient presents in cardiogenic shock with poor perfusion and feeble pulses. Oxygen desaturation may occur due to pulmonary edema. Endotracheal intubation and inotropic support allows for temporary improvement until the obstruction can be relieved. Balloon dilatation or stent placement by the interventional cardiologist is often successful. However surgical revision may be necessary.

Case Example 3

A 7-week-old girl with HLHS who had a hybrid procedure performed at 9 days of life presented with 3 days of cough and 1 day of difficulty breathing. In the ER, she was diaphoretic, tachycardic, and hypoxic with SpO_2 *of 70% on supplemental oxygen. She had severe respiratory distress with subcostal retractions, head bobbing, and accessory muscle use. She was peripherally cold with delayed capillary refill. A capillary blood gas revealed mixed respiratory and metabolic acidosis with an elevation of serum lactate. The CXR demonstrated increased pulmonary vascular congestion* (Fig. 3.6).

She was given fluid resuscitation, endotracheally intubated, and placed on positive pressure ventilation. Intravenous milrinone therapy was also initiated. An urgent echocardiogram showed severe restriction of the interatrial septum with a mean gradient of 18 mmHg. The right ventricular function was normal. She was taken to the cardiac catheterization lab emergently where a stent was placed to dilate the interatrial septum. She was extubated one day later with stable hemodynamics.

Restrictive Atrial Septal Defect

As part of the Norwood procedure, an atrial septectomy is performed to create a common atrium. This procedure allows for oxygenated pulmonary venous blood to cross the interatrial septum to mix freely with the systemic venous blood. This blood is then ejected by the systemic right ventricle. In the hybrid procedure, an

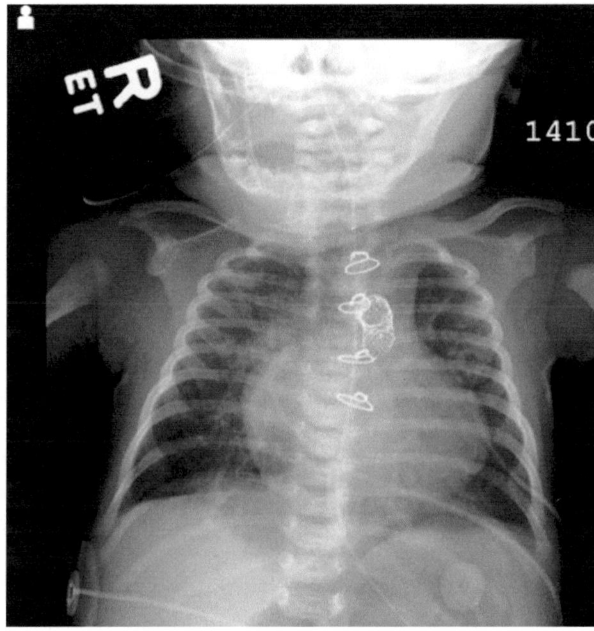

Fig. 3.6 CXR of a 7-week-old patient with HLHS and hybrid anatomy, who presented to the emergency department with acute respiratory failure. CXR shows pulmonary congestion following a hybrid procedure. The ductal stent can be seen within the anterior mediastinum

atrial septostomy, with or without stent placement, is performed in the cardiac catheterization lab either at the time of the hybrid procedure or as a separate procedure at some interval after the hybrid procedure if there is clinically important restriction at the level of the interatrial communication. Over time, after either a Norwood procedure or a hybrid procedure, the atrial septum can become restrictive. The decreased blood flow across a restrictive interatrial communication results in a decreased volume of oxygenated pulmonary venous blood mixing with the deoxygenated systemic venous blood in the right atrium, resulting in increased cyanosis and pulmonary venous hypertension with resultant pulmonary edema. The patient becomes tachypneic and cyanotic. The CXR will show pulmonary vascular congestion. The echocardiogram will reveal an increased pressure gradient across the atrial septum. Endotracheal intubation may be required to improve oxygenation, decrease the work of breathing, and minimize oxygen consumption.

Case Example 4

A 4-month-old boy who was born at 39 weeks gestation with a prenatal diagnosis of HLHS underwent the Norwood procedure with a modified BT shunt as stage 1 palliative surgery. After a prolonged and complicated postoperative course, he was discharged home at 3 months of age. The echocardiogram at discharge showed normal right ventricular function and mild-to-moderate tricuspid regurgitation. He had not been feeding well for 2 days but had no cough, no runny nose, and no fever. His mother called EMS since he didn't "look right." EMS noted the child was pale, lethargic, cold, and cyanotic. Bag and mask ventilation with oxygen at 15 liters per minute was initiated, and he was taken to the closest community emergency department.

Upon arrival to the emergency department, he had agonal breathing, a distended abdomen, and weak pulses. He was afebrile, his heart rate was 170 beats per minute, and his blood pressure could not be obtained. The pulse oximeter was intermittently reading oxygen saturations of 85–90% which were thought to be unreliable due to poor perfusion. Intraosseous access was established, and he was orally endotracheally intubated and placed on mechanical ventilatory support with an inspired oxygen concentration of 60%. Capillary blood gas analysis showed a severe metabolic acidosis with pH 6.9, PCO2 65 torr, PO2 59 torr, bicarbonate 13 mg/dL, base deficit 20, and serum lactate 15 mg/dL. The CXR showed congested lungs and free air under the diaphragm. With PO2 of 59 torr (which roughly corresponded to an oxygen saturation of 90%) on the capillary blood gas, combined with poor cardiac output, the child was thought to have pulmonary overcirculation, systemic undercirculation, and necrotizing enterocolitis. The oxygen concentration was quickly lowered to 21%. A fluid bolus was given and inotropic infusions were ordered. While arrangements were being made to transfer to a tertiary care facility, he experienced a bradycardic arrest. There was no spontaneous return of circulation after 40 min of resuscitation efforts and the patient expired.

Pulmonary Overcirculation

After stage 1 palliation, patients with HLHS remain vulnerable because the systemic and pulmonary circulations are competing in a parallel circuit. The systemic-to-pulmonary artery shunt that is placed during the Norwood procedure and the bilateral pulmonary artery bands that are placed during the hybrid procedure act as fixed resistors to control pulmonary blood flow. However, due to variations in the patient's weight in relation to the shunt size, variations in the pulmonary artery resistance and anatomy and the generally subjective method of bilateral pulmonary artery band adjustment, the pulmonary and systemic circulations can become unbalanced [23, 24]. An SpO_2 >90% is generally indicative of excess pulmonary blood flow at the expense of systemic blood flow. In this circumstance, the patient will have tachypnea, lethargy, a pale or ashen-gray appearance, cool extremities, poor peripheral pulses, poor urine output, and metabolic acidosis. These patients can also present with signs of end-organ damage due to compromised perfusion. In this clinical vignette, the patient developed necrotizing enterocolitis due to gut ischemia.

Pulmonary overcirculation, resulting in systemic hypoperfusion, is postulated to be one cause of sudden cardiac death in babies after Norwood stage 1 palliation. A patient with HLHS who presents relatively high oxygen saturations (i.e., >90%) and evidence of systemic hypoperfusion requires urgent evaluation. The administration of supplemental oxygen can be detrimental due to pulmonary vasodilation that lowers the pulmonary vascular resistance and further increases the pulmonary circulation at the expense of systemic perfusion. Therapy should be geared toward measures that lower the arterial oxygen saturations (75–85%) and that improve systemic perfusion. Careful fluid resuscitation, the administration of room air, systemic afterload reduction, and inotropic support will improve cardiac output. If mechanical ventilation is required, it is important to start with an inspired O_2 concentration of 21%.

Patients with HLHS remain vulnerable due to the parallel systemic and pulmonary circulations, with their competing blood flows, until they can be separated during stage 2 surgical palliation.

Sudden Unexplained Death

The most feared outcome during the interstage period (between stage 1 and stage 2) is sudden unexplained cardiac death. In such cases, infants may not show overt, prodromal clinical signs or symptoms and may suddenly be found lifeless by parents or caregivers. Myocardial ischemia due to multiple causes or relative hypoxemia are postulated mechanisms.

Case Example 5

A 3-month-old girl who was born at 38 weeks gestation with prenatal diagnosis of HLHS underwent the Norwood/Sano palliation procedure. The postoperative course was uneventful except for supraventricular tachycardia. She was eating well and gaining weight adequately. She was discharged home on aspirin after 1 month of hospitalization. The discharge echocardiogram showed normal right ventricular function and mild tricuspid regurgitation. She developed diarrhea 2 days prior to presentation to the emergency department (ED). On the day of presentation, the diarrhea worsened, and she had two episodes of emesis and fever of 100.8 F. The mother was not able to comment on the urine output as all diapers were soiled with diarrhea. A 15-month-old sibling who is behind on vaccinations has also been sick. In the ED, the vital signs showed the following: HR 190 beats per minute, BP 59/35 mmHg, RR 60 breaths per minute, SpO_2 62% in room air. The anterior fontanelle was sunken, and the capillary refill was 5 s. The abdomen was soft with no organomegaly. The capillary blood gas revealed metabolic acidosis with appropriate compensation; sodium was 160 meq/L and serum lactate was 4 mg/dL. The echocardiogram remained unchanged from the discharge study. A clinical diagnosis of gastroenteritis causing dehydration and hypovolemic shock was made, and peripheral venous access was obtained. The laboratory investigations including basic metabolic panel, urine and blood cultures, and stool for rotavirus testing were sent. Ceftriaxone was administered. Supplemental oxygen to achieve goal SpO_2 of 75–85%, and careful fluid resuscitation were initiated. After three fluid boluses of 10 mL/kg of 5% albumin each, the HR dropped to 170 bpm and the BP improved to 70/40 mmHg. Another fluid bolus of 10 mL/kg 5% albumin was given. Dehydration was estimated to be 15%. The child was admitted to the intensive care unit for further management.

In addition to complications inherent to the anatomy and palliative procedures, children with HLHS are fragile and vulnerable to common pediatric illnesses. Gastroenteritis and respiratory tract infections are implicated in increased interstage mortality [25]. Due to poor cardiac reserve, they are more likely to have quick deterioration and hemodynamic compromise from an otherwise benign illnesses. Some clinicians are apprehensive of resuscitating with intravenous fluid in patients with cardiac disease. However, dehydration and hypovolemia are as problematic as volume overload and should be treated appropriately. A hypovolemic state causes sluggish blood flow across the systemic-to-pulmonary artery shunt and increases the risk of thrombus formation with ensuing life-threatening acute shunt obstruction. Hypotension can compromise the vulnerable coronary artery perfusion and can increase the risk of sudden cardiac death. The systemic right ventricle poorly tolerates acid-base imbalance. In the absence of evidence for congestive heart failure, volume resuscitation should be given judiciously in the right clinical scenario in patients with HLHS.

Stage 2 and Stage 3 Palliation

The goal of the stage 2 and 3 palliations is to convert the in-parallel pulmonary and systemic circulations into an in-series circuit. This anatomy decreases the volume load on the right ventricle and alleviates cyanosis. This pathway is undertaken after the pulmonary vascular resistance has decreased enough to permit passive blood flow to the lungs.

Stage 2 palliation is performed at 4–9 months of age, after the pulmonary vascular resistance has dropped to the normal range, and consists of exchanging a pulsatile form of pulmonary blood flow for a passive form mediated by an anastomosis between the superior caval vein(s) and the pulmonary circulation. The two surgical techniques that are employed to accomplish this include the bidirectional Glenn and hemi-Fontan procedures. Although there are technical differences between these two surgical procedures, the physiological results are the same in creating the passive flow of systemic venous blood from the superior caval vein(s) into the pulmonary arterial circulation.

Stage 3 Fontan palliation is performed at 1.5–4 years of age. In this procedure, a total cavopulmonary connection is completed by connecting the inferior vena cava and/or hepatic veins to the pulmonary circulation using a fenestrated or nonfenestrated intracardiac lateral tunnel or an extracardiac conduit.

References

1. Norwood WI Jr. Hypoplastic left heart syndrome. Ann Thorac Surg. 1991;52(3):688–95.
2. Fyler DC. Report of the New England regional infant cardiac program. Pediatrics. 1980;65(2 Pt 2):375–461.
3. Lewin MB, McBride KL, Pignatelli R, et al. Echocardiographic evaluation of asymptomatic parental and sibling cardiovascular anomalies associated with congenital left ventricular outflow tract lesions. Pediatrics. 2004;114:691–6.

4. Hinton RB, Martin LJ, Rame-Gowda S, et al. Hypoplastic left heart syndrome links to chromosomes 10q and 6q and is genetically related to bicuspid aortic valve. J Am Coll Cardiol. 2009;53(12):1065–71.
5. Grossfeld P, Ye M, Harvey R. Hypoplastic left heart syndrome: new genetic insights. J Am Coll Cardiol. 2009;53(12):1072–4.
6. McBride KL, Zender GA, Fitzgerald-Butt SM, et al. Linkage analysis of left ventricular outflow tract malformations (aortic valve stenosis, coarctation of aorta, and hypoplastic left heart syndrome). Eur J Hum Genet. 2009;17:1397–405.
7. Fay FS, Cooke PH. Guinea pig ductus arteriosus. II. Irreversible closure after birth. Am J Physiol. 1972;222:841–9.
8. Morin FC III, Egan E. Pulmonary hemodynamics in fetal lambs during development at normal and increased oxygen tension. J Appl Physiol. 1992;73:213–8.
9. Wessel DL. Commentary. Simple gases and complex single ventricles. J Thorac Cardiovasc Surg. 1996;112:655–7.
10. Liske MR, Aschner JL. Counterpoint: hypoxia is not the optimal means of reducing pulmonary blood flow in the preoperative single ventricle heart. J Appl Physiol. 2008;104(6):1836–8; discussion 1838–9.
11. Norwood WI, Kirklin JK, Sanders SP. Hypoplastic left heart syndrome: experience with palliative surgery. Am J Cardiol. 1980;45:87–91.
12. Norwood WI, Lang P, Hansen DD. Physiologic repair of aortic atresia-hypoplastic left heart syndrome. N Engl J Med. 1983;308:23–6.
13. Sano S, Ishino K, Kawada M, et al. Right ventricle-pulmonary artery shunt in first-stage palliation of hypoplastic left heart syndrome. J Thorac Cardiovasc Surg. 2003;126:504–9.
14. Bartram U, Grunenfelder J, Van Praagh R. Causes of death after the modified Norwood Procedure: a study of 122 postmortem cases. Ann Thorac Surg. 1997;64:1795–802.
15. Malec E, Januszewska K, Klolcz J, et al. Right ventricle to pulmonary artery shunt versus modified Blalock-Taussig shunt in the Norwood procedure for hypoplastic left heart syndrome: influence on early and late hemodynamic status. Eur J Cardiothorac Surg. 2003;23:728–34.
16. Pizzaro C, Malec E, Maher KO, et al. Right ventricle to pulmonary artery conduit improves outcome after stage 1 Norwood for hypoplastic left heart syndrome. Circulation. 2003;108:II155–60.
17. Migliavacca F, Pennati G, Dubini G, et al. Modeling of the Norwood circulation: effects of shunt size, vascular resistances and heart rate. Am J Physiol. 2001;290:H2076–86.
18. Gibbs JL, Wren C, Watterson KG, et al. Stenting of the arterial duct combined with banding of the pulmonary arteries and atrial septectomy or septostomy: a new approach to palliation for the hypoplastic left heart syndrome. Br Heart J. 1993;69:551–5.
19. Ruiz CE, Gamra H, Zhang HP, et al. Brief report: stenting of the ductus arteriosus as a bridge to cardiac transplantation in infants with hypoplastic left heart syndrome. N Engl J Med. 1993;328:1605–8.
20. Lamberti JJ. Editorial comment. Aortic arch obstruction after the Norwood procedure for hypoplastic left heart syndrome. Is it inevitable? Is it preventable? J Am Coll Cardiol. 2011;58(8):877–9.
21. Chessa M, Dindar A, Vettukattil JJ, et al. Balloon angioplasty in infants with aortic obstruction after the modified stage I Norwood procedure. Am Heart J. 2000;140:227–31.
22. Burkhart HM, Ashburn DA, Konstantinov IE, et al. Interdigitating arch reconstruction eliminates recurrent coarctation after the Norwood procedure. J Thorac Cardiovasc Surg. 2005;130(1):61–5.
23. Mastropietro CW, Tourner S. Parallel circulations: managing the neonate with single ventricle physiology. NeoReviews. 2009;10:e239.
24. Li J, Zhang G, Benson L, et al. Comparison of the profiles of post-operative systemic hemodynamics and oxygen transport in neonates after the hybrid or the Norwood procedure: a pilot study. Circulation. 2007;116(11 Suppl):I179–87.
25. Ghanayem NS, Allen KR, Tabutt S, et al. Interstage mortality after the Norwood procedure: results of the multicenter single ventricle reconstruction trial. J Thorac Cardiovasc Surg. 2012;144(4):896–906.

Check for updates

Functionally Univentricular Heart with Right Heart Hypoplasia (Tricuspid Atresia with Normally Related Great Arteries and Pulmonary Atresia with Intact Ventricular Septum)

4

James M. Galas, Deemah R. Mahadin, and Ralph E. Delius

Introduction

Functionally univentricular heart physiology can result from a number of pathological variants in heart structure. This chapter will discuss those which involve hypoplasia of the right heart, namely, tricuspid atresia with normally related great arteries and pulmonary atresia with an intact ventricular septum. As the right ventricle is severely underdeveloped in these two entities, the systemic ventricle is of left ventricular morphology. Tricuspid atresia with malposition of the great arteries and pulmonary atresia with an adequate tricuspid valve will not be addressed in this chapter due to their physiological differences, namely, possible systemic outflow obstruction and the frequent ability to undergo two ventricle palliations, respectively.

Tricuspid atresia is a relatively rare defect with a prevalence of 0.056 per 1000 live births [1]. By definition, there is an absence of a true tricuspid valve, with no direct communication between the right atrium and the right ventricle (Fig. 4.1). An obligatory right-to-left shunt exists at the atrial level, whereby desaturated blood from the systemic venous circulation crosses the interatrial communication into the left atrium and then mixes with oxygenated blood from the pulmonary venous circulation. From the left ventricle, blood is either ejected into the systemic circulation through the aorta, or it crosses into a hypoplastic right ventricle through an interventricular communication and is ejected into the pulmonary circulation through the pulmonary artery. The amount of pulmonary blood flow is controlled by the amount of

J. M. Galas, M.D. (✉) • D. R. Mahadin, M.D.
Division of Cardiology, Children's Hospital of Michigan, Wayne State University School of Medicine, Detroit, MI, USA
e-mail: jgalas@dmc.org; DMahadin@dmc.org

R. E. Delius, M.D.
Division of Pediatric Cardiovascular Surgery, Children's Hospital of Michigan, Wayne State University School of Medicine, Detroit, MI, USA

© Springer International Publishing AG, part of Springer Nature 2018

A. P. Sarnaik et al. (eds.), *Cardiac Emergencies in Children*,
https://doi.org/10.1007/978-3-319-73754-6_4

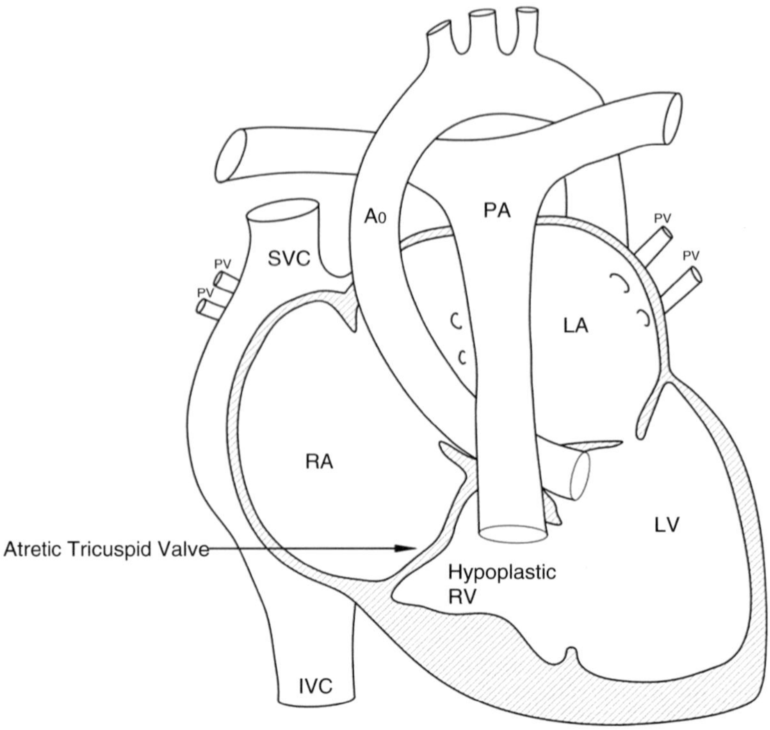

Fig. 4.1 Tricuspid atresia with normally related great arteries, no pulmonary stenosis. In this setting, pulmonary blood flow is unrestricted. Left as is, excessive pulmonary blood flow will result in congestive heart failure. *SVC* superior vena cava, *IVC* inferior vena cava, *RA* right atrium, *LA* left atrium, *RV* right ventricle, *LV* left ventricle, *Ao* aorta, *PA* pulmonary artery, *PV* pulmonary vein

restriction at the level of the interventricular communication, the hypoplastic right ventricle, the pulmonary valve, and the area above and below the pulmonary valve. When these anatomical constraints produce inadequate pulmonary blood flow, the pulmonary circulation becomes reliant on the patency of the ductus arteriosus. In this scenario, the lesion is termed "ductal dependant," and institution of prostaglandin therapy is necessary to maintain adequate arterial saturations shortly after birth. In general, an arterial saturation in excess of 75% is acceptable in a patient with tricuspid atresia who has not undergone any form of surgical palliation.

The surgical palliation of tricuspid atresia involves a staged approach. If insufficient pulmonary blood flow exists at birth or prior to 4 months of age, a systemic-to-pulmonary shunt, typically a modified Blalock-Taussig shunt (MBTS), which is a Gore-Tex® tube graft from a systemic artery to a pulmonary artery, is placed to establish controlled pulmonary blood flow (Fig. 4.2).

In some instances, the pulmonary circulation is unrestricted and excessive, leading to pulmonary congestion. In these cases, palliation requires restriction of

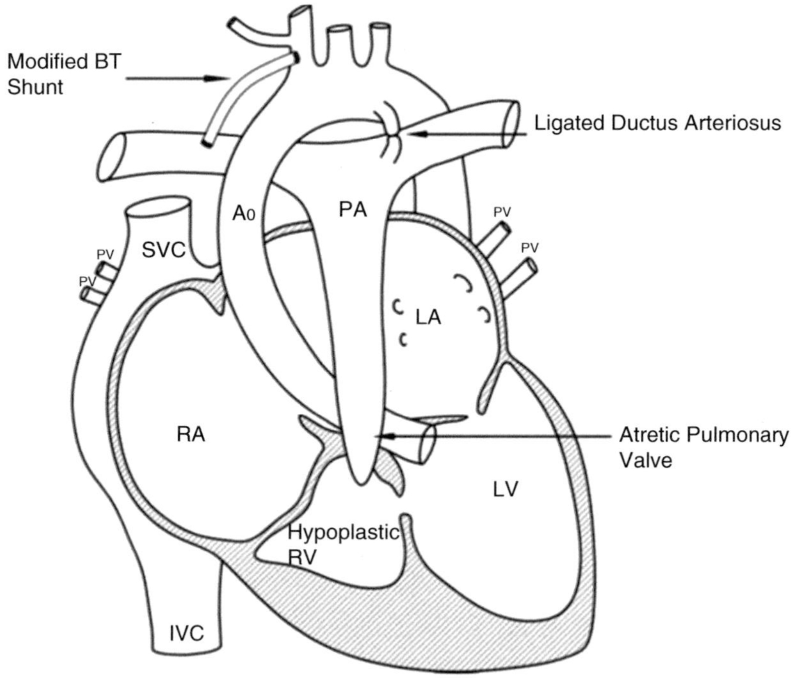

Fig. 4.2 Tricuspid atresia with normally related great arteries and pulmonary atresia, status post-placement of a modified Blalock-Taussig (BT) Shunt. In this setting, pulmonary blood flow is dependant on patency of shunt once the patent ductus arteriosus has been ligated

pulmonary blood flow by placing a constricting band on the main pulmonary artery, referred to as pulmonary artery banding (Fig. 4.3).

Finally, in some cases, the pulmonary and systemic blood flow can be perfectly balanced, with neither pulmonary undercirculation nor overcirculation. In this instance, the patient can be observed, without an initial palliative procedure.

Further palliation typically occurs after 4 months of age, at which time a superior cavopulmonary connection is performed with removal of the systemic-to-pulmonary shunt or the pulmonary artery band. If an initial palliative procedure was not required, the superior cavopulmonary connection becomes the patient's first palliative procedure. This procedure takes the form of either a bidirectional superior cavopulmonary connection or a hemi-Fontan procedure, depending largely on surgeon preference since both procedures accomplish the same physiological result (Fig. 4.4). In both procedures, the systemic venous blood flow from the head and upper extremities is directly connected to the pulmonary arterial circulation. In so doing, the left ventricular volume load is decreased and arterial saturations typically rise into the high 70s to mid-80s.

The final palliative procedure is the total cavopulmonary connection or completion Fontan procedure wherein the inferior caval vein and/or the hepatic veins are connected to the pulmonary circulation. The two most common variants of this

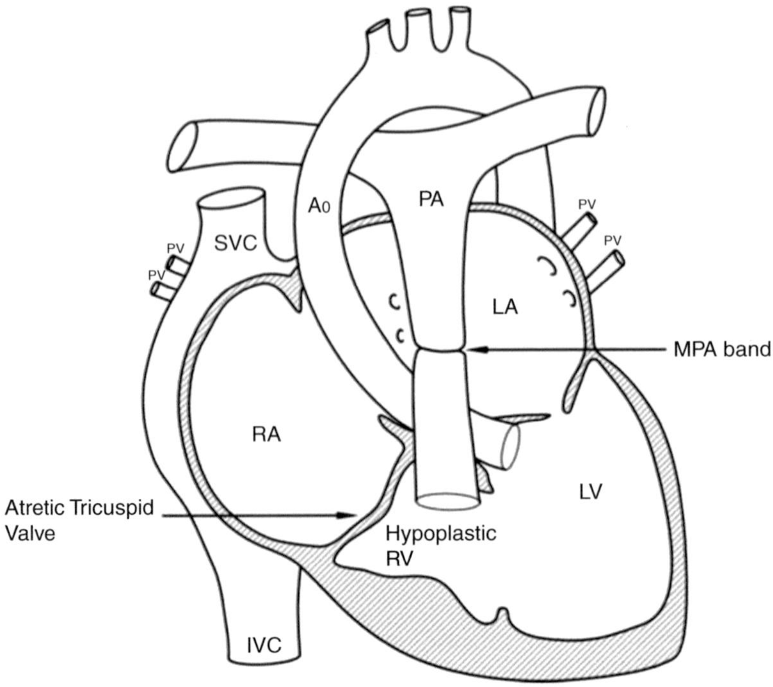

Fig. 4.3 Tricuspid atresia with normally related great arteries, no pulmonary stenosis status post-placement of a pulmonary artery band. Pulmonary blood flow is regulated by the constriction of the main pulmonary artery (MPA) by the band

procedure are the extracardiac Fontan or the lateral tunnel Fontan (Fig. 4.5). Regardless of the exact surgery performed, the goal is separation of the systemic and pulmonary circulations to eliminate mixing of systemic venous blood with pulmonary venous blood. This separation results in more fully saturated arterial blood. In some instances, a small communication between the Fontan circuit and the right atrium called a *fenestration* is established to serve as a pressure pop-off. Under these circumstances, the arterial saturations run primarily in the low 90s, as a small right-to-left shunt remains.

While undergoing serial palliative procedures can greatly improve the patient's hemodynamics, it is important to acknowledge that these surgeries are not reparative, only palliative. Complications of the Fontan procedure include arrhythmias, systolic and/or diastolic cardiac dysfunction, atrioventricular valve regurgitation, protein-losing enteropathy, neurocognitive delay, hepatic failure, and renal failure [2]. As a result, those who survive long enough with a Fontan may ultimately become heart transplant candidates. Encouragingly though, patients have survived several decades with Fontan physiology and continue to push these boundaries as medical advancements take place.

Pulmonary atresia with an intact ventricular septum, like tricuspid atresia, results in hypoplasia of the right heart structures. The prevalence of this disease is 0.083

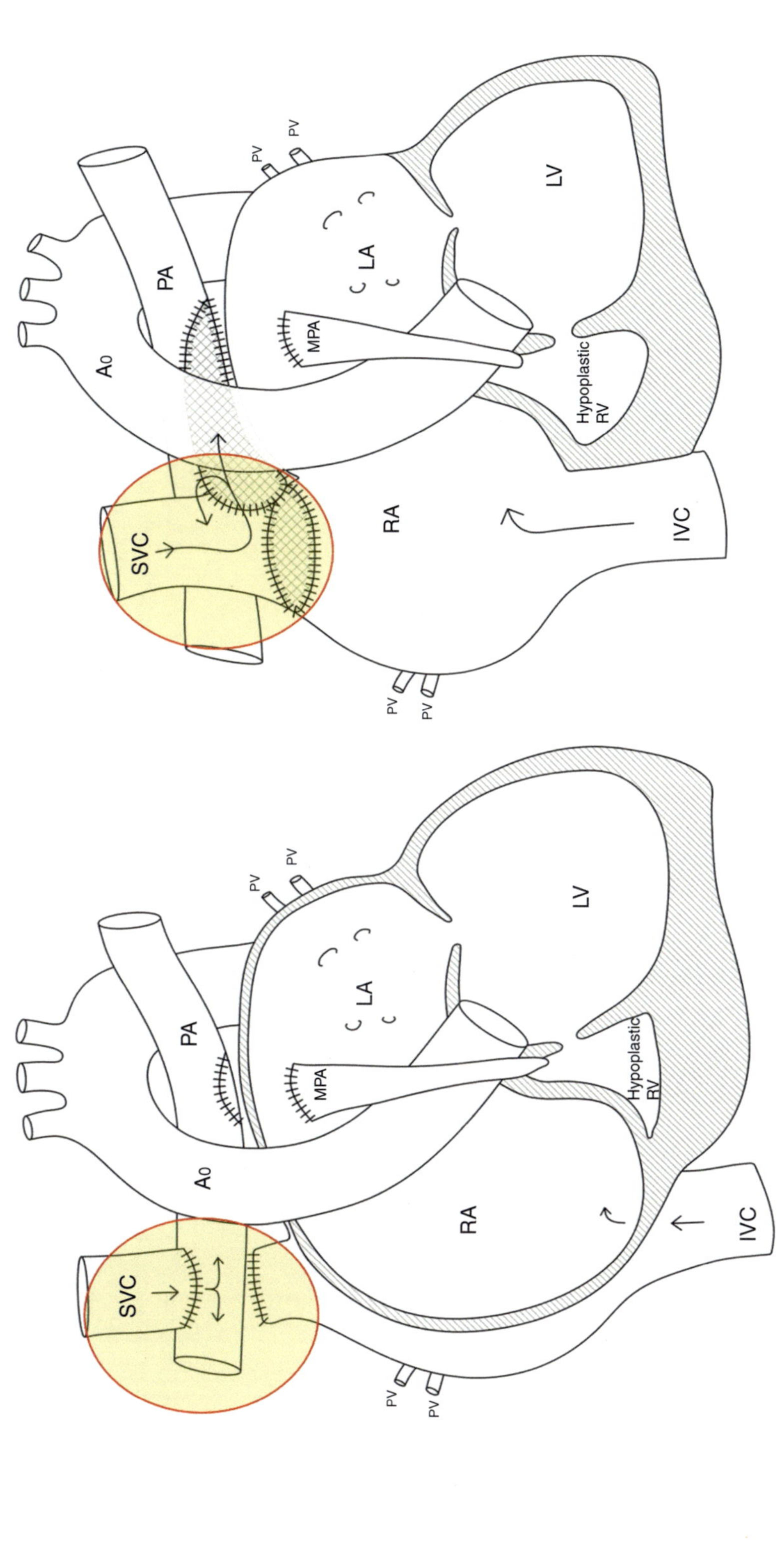

Fig. 4.4 Contrast of the bidirectional Glenn (left) vs. hemi-Fontan (right), both forms of a cavopulmonary anastomosis. Note the direct anastomosis of the superior caval vein to the right pulmonary artery in the bidirectional Glenn in contrast to baffle placement and patch angioplasty of the hemi-Fontan. Both operations serve to redirect venous blood from the head and upper extremities directly into the pulmonary arteries without passing through an intervening ventricle

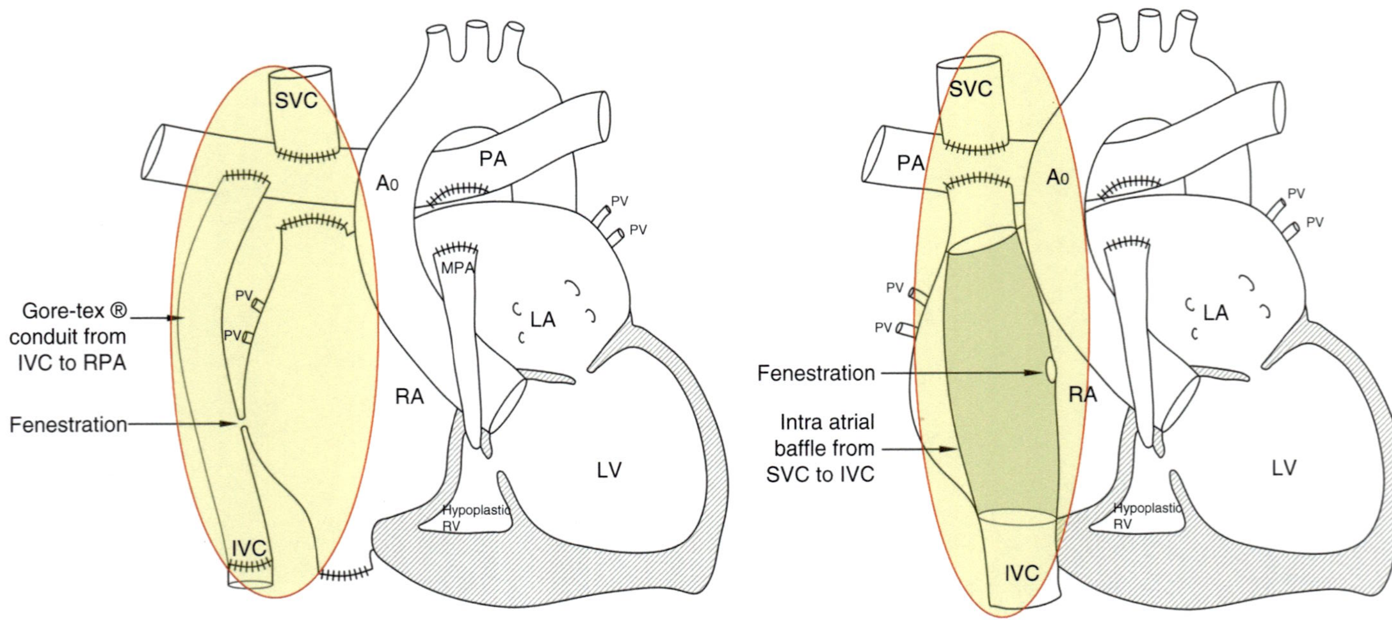

Fig. 4.5 Contrast of the extracardiac Fontan (left) vs. lateral tunnel Fontan (right), both forms of Fontan completion. Note the fixed dimensions of the Gore-Tex® tube outside of the heart in the extracardiac Fontan. This finding is in contrast to use of the right atrial wall in combination with Gore-Tex® or bovine pericardium to construct an intracardiac lateral tunnel from the inferior vena cava to the right pulmonary artery (RPA) in the lateral tunnel Fontan. Both operations serve to direct systemic venous blood into the pulmonary arteries. A fenestration, allowing for a small right-to-left shunt, can be performed in both operations in order to allow for a pressure pop-off from the Fontan circuit into the right atrium

per 1000 live births [3]. The physiology of this lesion is like that of tricuspid atresia, with the main difference being that the pulmonary blood flow is always dependant upon patency of the ductus arteriosus. As a result, prostaglandins should be initiated at birth, and the patient must usually undergo a neonatal systemic-to-pulmonary artery shunt before hospital discharge. The patient with pulmonary atresia with an intact ventricular septum would usually undergo the same serial palliative surgeries as the patient with tricuspid atresia, consisting of a MBTS, followed by a bidirectional Glenn or hemi-Fontan procedure and then followed by a completion Fontan procedure. In some patients, with less severe right ventricular hypoplasia, a transannular patch is placed across the pulmonary valve annulus (in addition to performing a neonatal systemic-to-pulmonary artery shunt) in the hopes that this will promote enough right ventricular growth to avoid the need for Fontan palliation.

Some patients with pulmonary atresia with an intact ventricular septum suffer from right ventricular-dependant coronary artery circulation, due to lack of proper development of the coronary circulation [4]. In this scenario, decompressing the severely elevated right ventricular pressures by placing a transannular patch or creating lower diastolic pressures by placing a systemic-to-pulmonary artery shunt may place the patient at high risk for myocardial ischemia [5]. These patients are considered, by some, to be high risk for functionally univentricular heart palliation, and some centers will elect to list them for cardiac transplantation following rather than offer Fontan palliation [5].

Evaluation

The evaluation of the functionally univentricular heart patient with right heart hypoplasia centers around the presentation, namely, profound cyanosis, shock, arrhythmia, or heart failure. Once the principal concern is determined in the patient, the diagnostic evaluation can be tailored to help the provider work through the differential diagnosis for the presenting issue. Knowledge of the patient's stage of palliation (unoperated, MBTS, superior cavopulmonary connection, or completion Fontan) is essential to correctly interpret the patient's signs and symptoms. Identifying the pathophysiologic process, along with an understanding of cardiac anatomy and physiology unique to that patient, allows the provider to employ the appropriate management.

Cardiac History

In general, a concise, yet complete, history should be obtained. Information germane to the patient known to have functionally univentricular heart physiology with right heart hypoplasia includes:

- Color changes: While the functionally univentricular heart patient may be cyanotic at baseline, noting any progression of cyanosis or episodic hypercyanosis is paramount to detecting issues resulting from inadequate pulmonary blood flow. It is important to determine whether the cyanosis is central (involving the face and body) rather than peripheral (acrocyanosis involving the hands and feet). Acrocyanosis is a normal finding seen in patients with structurally normal hearts, usually after exposure to cold.

- Shortness of breath/tachypnea: Often this history is a symptom of pulmonary edema due to excessive blood flow. Care should be taken to inquire about additional lung-related signs and symptoms to exclude other pulmonary processes, such as infection.
- Racing heart rate/tachycardia: Attention should be given to whether the heart rate is regular or irregular. This may help to determine whether the elevated heart rate is due to an arrhythmia or is a physiologic response to anemia, myocardial dysfunction, dehydration, or metabolic derangements. In older patients who have undergone Fontan palliation, there should be concern for an intra-atrial tachycardia or "slow atrial flutter."
- Feeding history: This history includes the amount and frequency of feeds taken and the time required for an infant to complete the feed. In addition, the associated symptoms of diaphoresis and pallor with feeding may accompany low cardiac output physiology. History of poor oral intake is essential to establishing concern for dehydration as well.
- Syncope: Any history of loss of consciousness in an infant or toddler with functionally univentricular heart physiology should raise concern for obstruction to systemic outflow, inadequate filling of the systemic ventricle, or arrhythmia.
- Lethargy/easy fatigue: Determining if the patient has been abnormally inactive or less responsive than usual raises concern for low cardiac output, metabolic acidosis, or profound hypoxia.
- Irritability/increased fussiness: While patients with functionally univentricular heart physiology are susceptible to infection, just as any other infant/toddler is, patients with pulmonary atresia with intact ventricular septum are at risk of coronary abnormalities that can result in intermittent ischemia [5].
- Recent fevers or illnesses: The well-being of the functionally univentricular heart patient is often in a delicate balance. Even minor febrile illnesses can "tip the patient over" into hemodynamic instability. Fever can also explain an elevated heart rate, to a degree, with particular concern for another etiology of the tachycardia if it is out of proportion to fever.

Physical Examination

Vital Signs

Careful assessment of vital signs are essential to interpreting the physiological state of the patient with functionally univentricular heart physiology. Heart rate, respiratory rate, blood pressure, and pulse oximetry should be obtained in all patients with tricuspid atresia or pulmonary atresia with intact ventricular septum presenting for medical care. Tachypnea and tachycardia should trigger concern for pulmonary overcirculation, though they may also be seen together in other instances. As reviewed in the introduction, arterial saturations are expected to remain within a certain range for a given stage of palliation. Values higher or lower than expected are signs of excessive or too little pulmonary blood flow, respectively.

Chest Wall

At times, it may not be known if a child has congenital heart disease upon presentation to the Emergency Department. The presence of a median sternotomy scar is a sign the patient not only has heart disease but that they have undergone cardiac surgery. Stability of the sternum should be established by gentle palpation with the index and middle finger on either side of the incision, noting any "step off," unevenness, or clicking. Care should be taken to examine the incision for any erythema, warmth, fluctuance, or discharge indicative of infection.

Lungs

Auscultation of the lung fields can lead to the recognition of crackles. While this finding can represent a variety of pathologies, concern for pulmonary overcirculation should arise in a patient with functionally univentricular heart physiology. Bacterial or viral pneumonia should always be considered as well in these patients, depending upon the presence or absence of other signs of infection.

Heart

In patients with tricuspid atresia or pulmonary atresia, a tricuspid valve or pulmonary valve will be essentially absent, respectively. Accordingly, there will be a single first or second heart sound, respectively. A high-frequency, systolic regurgitant murmur at the left lower sternal border is consistent with mitral valve regurgitation. Moderate-to-severe regurgitation is often not well tolerated in functionally univentricular heart physiology. Pulmonary stenosis can be physically manifested by a systolic ejection murmur at the left upper sternal border. As the frequency (pitch) of the murmur increases, the degree of obstruction to pulmonary blood flow increases as well. When the murmur radiates to or is primarily located over the axilla, branch pulmonary artery stenosis may be present. A high-frequency, diastolic decrescendo murmur at the right upper sternal border, radiating to the apex of the heart, is consistent with aortic insufficiency. In a patient who has had a shunt placed, a loud continuous murmur should be audible. In the case of a right MBTS, the murmur should be best heard in the right infraclavicular region. The presence of a fourth heart sound (S4) or gallop can be indicative of myocardial dysfunction.

Abdomen

The presence of hepatomegaly should raise concern for myocardial dysfunction. Ascites may be present in severe cases.

Extremities

Cyanosis can be expected in functionally univentricular heart patients who have not undergone Fontan palliation. Clubbing is routinely seen since these patients have spent a portion of their life with chronic cyanosis. Good peripheral perfusion of the extremities is manifested by strong peripheral pulses, warm extremities, and prompt capillary refill. Cool extremities can be consistent with low cardiac output.

Testing

Electrocardiogram (ECG)

In the era of readily available, high-quality echocardiograms, the ECG is utilized mainly to detect rhythm disturbances or electrical abnormalities such as ventricular preexcitation, prolongation of the QRS duration, or prolongation the QT interval. That said, Fig. 4.6 demonstrates typical features of a resting ECG in a patient with tricuspid atresia and may include right atrial enlargement, leftward and superior QRS axis (S wave greater than R wave in lead aVF) with a predominance of left ventricular forces. These findings are somewhat intuitive, owing to the underdevelopment of the right ventricle. Careful examination of the patient's rhythm,

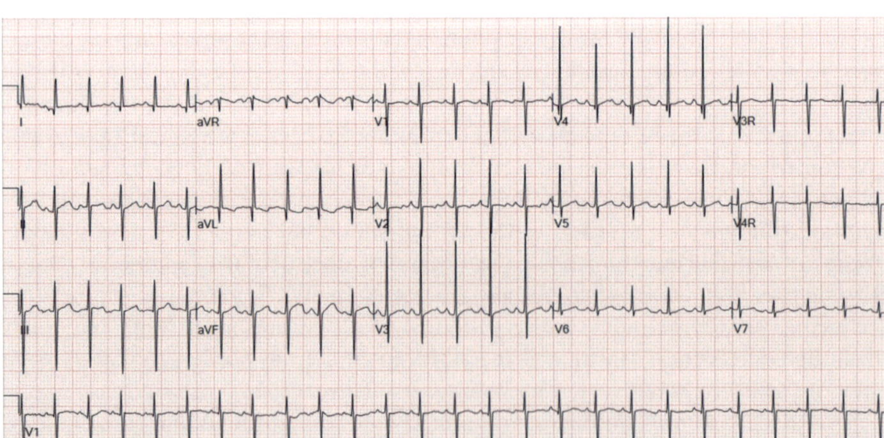

Fig. 4.6 Tricuspid atresia ECG: normal sinus rhythm. Note the left axis deviation and paucity of right ventricular forces

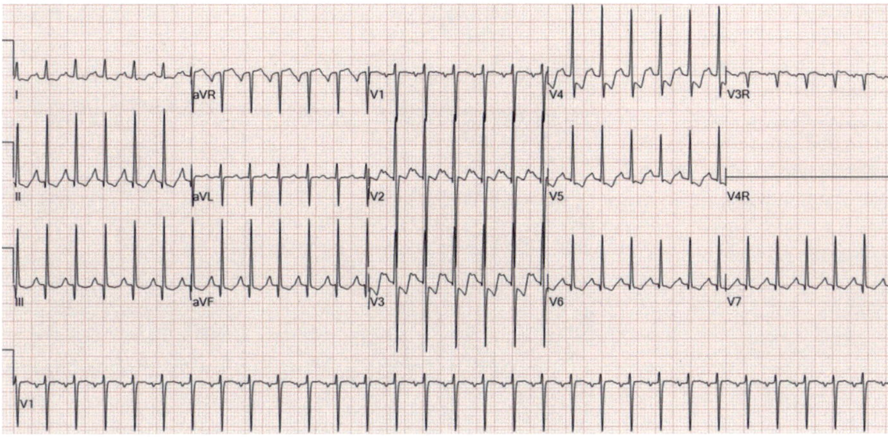

Fig. 4.7 Pulmonary atresia with intact ventricular septum ECG: normal sinus rhythm. Note the predominate left-sided forces and the ST changes in mid-precordial leads

especially after Fontan palliation, is essential, as the risk of intra-atrial reentrant tachycardia (IART), which can be thought of as a slow atrial flutter, is not uncommon in this population [6, 7].

The patient with pulmonary atresia and intact ventricular septum shares the ECG finding of predominant of left ventricular forces over right ventricular forces in common with tricuspid atresia patients (Fig. 4.7). In addition, evidence of subendocardial ischemia due to coronary artery abnormalities may be present in the form of ST segment changes [8].

Chest X-ray (CXR)

The chest X-ray can be helpful in gauging the amount of pulmonary blood flow in both patients with tricuspid atresia and pulmonary atresia. Cardiomegaly, with an increase in pulmonary vascular markings, is seen when blood flow to the lungs is unrestricted (Fig. 4.8). Dark lung fields, with a paucity of pulmonary vascular markings, are indicative of under-perfused lungs.

Echocardiogram

The echocardiogram is the modality of choice in establishing the diagnosis in unpalliated patients with a functionally univentricular heart and right heart hypoplasia. Absence of flow through the tricuspid and pulmonary valves confirms the diagnosis in tricuspid and pulmonary atresia, respectively (Figs. 4.9 and 4.10). In both patient populations, hypoplasia of the morphological right ventricle is observed. Important additional information to be gleaned from the echocardiogram includes establishing that there is unrestricted blood flow at the level of the interatrial communication,

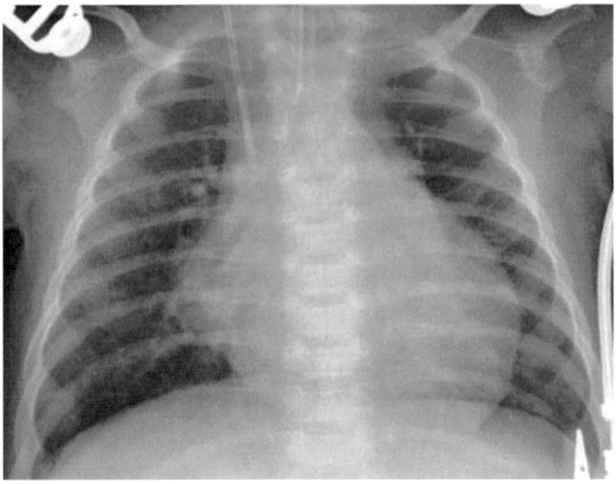

Fig. 4.8 CXR in a patient with tricuspid atresia with normally related great arteries and minimal pulmonary stenosis. Increased pulmonary vascular markings are evident along with cardiomegaly

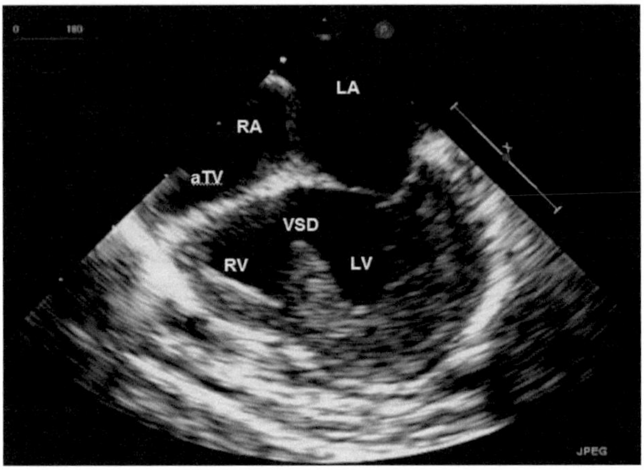

Fig. 4.9 Transesophageal echocardiographic of tricuspid atresia. Note the absence of a connection between the right atrium (RA) and the hypoplastic right-sided ventricle, representing the atretic tricuspid valve (aTV), as well as the interventricular communication (VSD) . *LA* left atrium, *LV* left ventricle, *RV* right ventricle

assessment of the left ventricular systolic function, and delineation of the relationship of the great arteries to each other. In tricuspid atresia, the degree and level of obstruction to pulmonary blood flow, if any, should be noted. In addition, coronary artery fistulae, that could be a harbinger of ventricular ischemia, can be visualized with echocardiography in patients with pulmonary atresia and intact ventricular septum.

Echocardiographic imaging of the various stages of palliation in patients with functionally univentricular hearts and right heart hypoplasia centers around the interrogation of the pulmonary blood supply.

Echocardiography After Initial Palliation

In hypoxic patients who have undergone a systemic arterial-to-pulmonary arterial shunt, most commonly a MBTS, the patient should undergo careful echocardiographic evaluation for shunt obstruction (Fig. 4.11). Not only should flow be

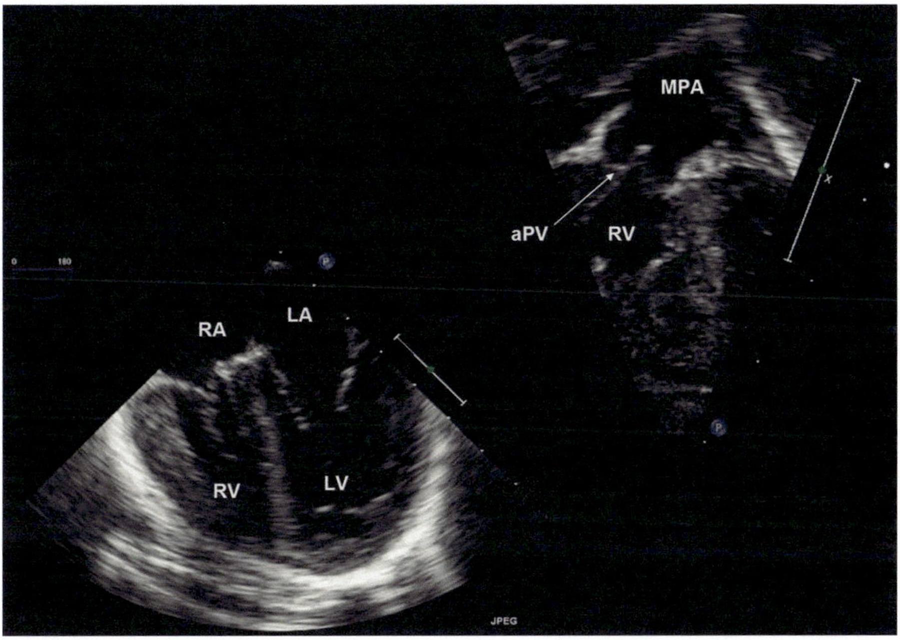

Fig. 4.10 Transesophageal and transthoracic echocardiographic images of pulmonary atresia with intact ventricular septum. Note the relative right ventricular hypoplasia compared to the left ventricle. Tipping the echo probe more anteriorly demonstrates an atretic pulmonary valve (aPV) that does not open, arising from a diminutive right ventricle (RV). *RA* right atrium, *LA* left atrium, *LV* left ventricle, *MPA* main pulmonary artery

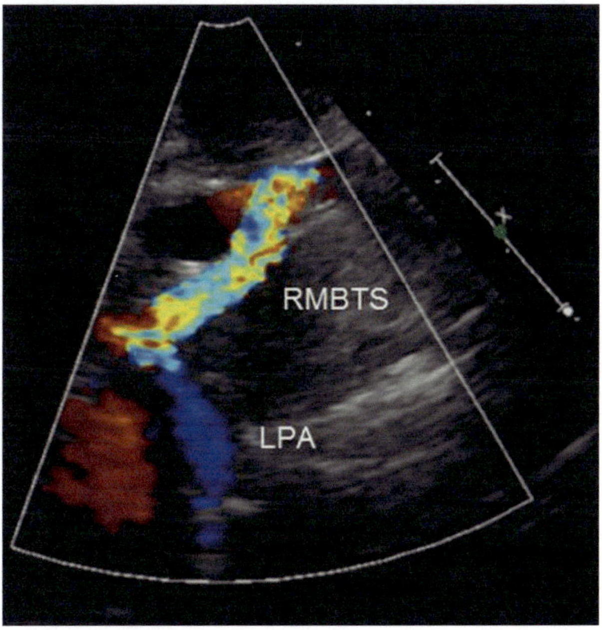

Fig. 4.11 Echocardiogram with color flow mapping demonstrating a right modified Blalock-Taussig Shunt (RMBTS) demonstrated with color flow mapping. *LPA* left pulmonary artery

visualized throughout the shunt and into the pulmonary arteries by color flow mapping, but also attention should be paid to the spectral Doppler pattern on interrogation of the shunt. Both the morphology of the Doppler pattern and the peak velocity, in conjunction with the clinical scenario, can assist in determining if the patient requires emergent angiography. Meticulous two-dimensional interrogation of the shunt can also yield evidence of kinking or thrombosis within the shunt, though these images can be technically more difficult to obtain.

Echocardiography After Superior Cavopulmonary Connection

In patients after a superior cavopulmonary connection, viewing the anastomosis between the systemic venous blood flow from the upper body and the branch pulmonary arteries is imperative. Pulmonary artery stenosis following a MBTS is a known complication. Pulmonary artery stenosis due to congenital stenosis or hypoplasia, causing impaired pulmonary blood flow, can also be visualized echocardiographically.

Due to the passive nature of blood flow from the superior caval vein(s) into the pulmonary vascular bed, there is a potential for thrombus formation in the anastomosis or the branch pulmonary arteries. Therefore low-velocity, phasic flow throughout the proximal pulmonary circuit should be confirmed with color flow mapping, as well as the absence of thrombus by 2D imaging (Fig. 4.12). In patients

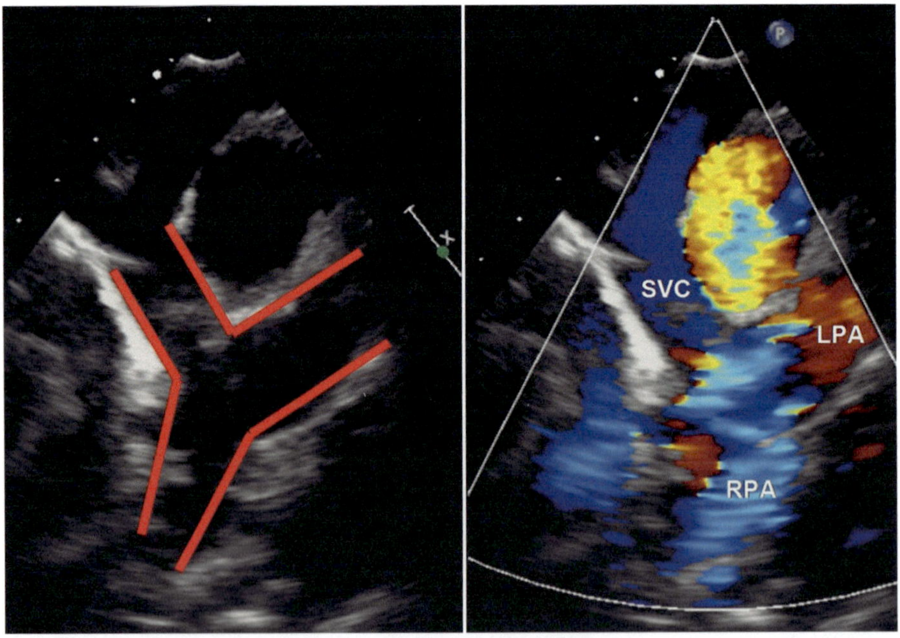

Fig. 4.12 Superior caval to pulmonary artery anastomosis, outlined in red on the two-dimensional echocardiographic image. *SVC* superior vena cava, *LPA* left pulmonary artery, *RPA* right pulmonary artery

with saturations below 80%, right-to-left shunting from a leak in the hemi-Fontan baffle should be excluded as well.

Echocardiography After Completion Fontan

The goals of the echocardiographic imaging of the completion Fontan circuit are similar to those of imaging the superior cavopulmonary connection in terms of examining pulmonary blood flow. In addition to examining the flow of systemic venous blood through the superior caval vein(s) into the pulmonary circulation, systemic venous blood flow from the inferior caval and hepatic vein(s) into the Fontan pathway should be assessed as well. In addition, a transpulmonary gradient (pressure drop over the pulmonary vascular bed) can be obtained via spectral Doppler interrogation of a fenestration gradient, if a fenestration is present (Fig. 4.13). This gradient provides valuable information regarding Fontan hemodynamics.

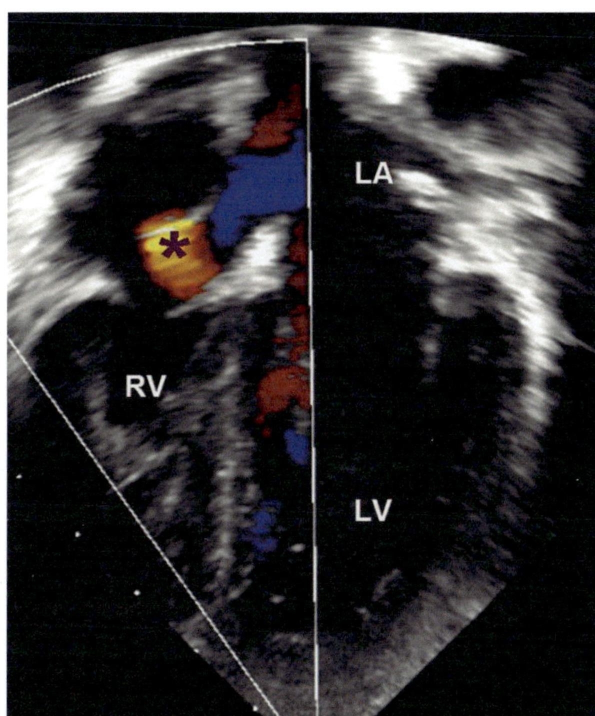

Fig. 4.13 Echocardiogram of a fenestrated Fontan. The fenestration shunts desaturated blood from the Fontan circuit to the right atrium (*). *LA* left atrium, *RV* right ventricle, *LV* left ventricle

Laboratory Evaluation

Chemistry

Patients with ectopy should be evaluated for electrolyte disturbances with a chemistry panel. Also, an abnormally low bicarbonate can signal metabolic acidosis either from impaired cardiac output or dehydration. Older patients benefit from a laboratory assessment of hepatic and renal function, as end-organ damage can be seen as a long-term complication of the Fontan circulation.

Complete Blood Count (CBC)

Anemia impairs oxygen delivery to tissues. Though the anemic patient will appear less cyanotic due to the presence of less deoxyhemoglobin, the effects of anemia in functionally univentricular heart patients can be quite severe. As a result, a normal range hematocrit is often desirable in cyanotic patients who have yet to undergo Fontan palliation. Examination of the white blood cell count and differential can be helpful in raising suspicion for intercurrent illness, which may not be well tolerated in functionally univentricular heart patients.

Arterial Blood Gas

The ABG can establish the etiology of acidosis as metabolic, respiratory, or mixed. The arterial PO_2 is superior to pulse oximetry in reliably assessing severity of hypoxia as pulse oximetry becomes less accurate when oxygen saturations are very less 85–90%. Evidence of CO_2 retention steers the provider toward a pulmonary intervention to improve the patient's ventilation. A low bicarbonate, as well as a base deficit greater than −3 to −5, is unlikely to be tolerated well by the myocardium of a functionally univentricular heart, placing the individual at risk for worsening systolic function and arrhythmia. A steeply rising lactate level is an ominous sign of impending cardiovascular collapse. Lastly, placement of an arterial line is helpful when minute-to-minute monitoring of the systemic blood pressure and frequent assessment of arterial blood gases is desired, such as during the initiation of inotropic or vasodilator support.

Clinical Vignette 1

A 3-month-old female presents to the Emergency Department with "turning blue." She was diagnosed with tricuspid atresia prenatally and has enjoyed excellent somatic growth without any surgeries to date. Her parents give a history of poor oral intake with gastroenteritis-type symptoms over the last 2 days. She is not on any medications at present. Vital signs are temperature 37.5 °C, heart rate (HR) 170 bpm, respiratory rate (RR) 40 breaths per minute, blood pressure (BP) 70/30 mmHg, and

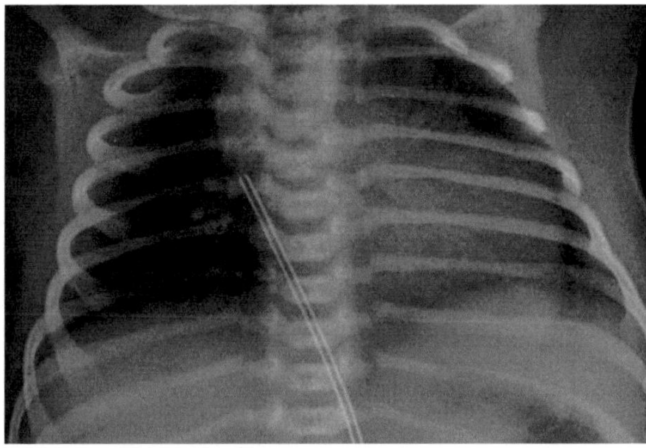

Fig. 4.14 CXR of Tricuspid atresia with normally related great arteries and pulmonary stenosis with reduced pulmonary vascular markings

pulse oximetry 65% on room air. The body weight is at the 50th percentile. The infant appears cyanotic and somnolent with a sunken fontanel. The lung fields are clear to auscultation. A VI/VI, high-frequency systolic ejection murmur is heard at the left upper sternal border, with radiation to the axillae. Diastole is quiet. A thrill is palpable at the left sternal border. The femoral pulses are 1+ with no brachiofemoral delay. The liver edge is not palpable below the right costal margin. The extremities are cyanotic and cool with prolonged capillary refill. A chest X-ray is obtained (Fig. 4.14).

Differential Diagnosis

Differential diagnosis for a patient with tricuspid atresia, presenting with increased cyanosis, includes the following:

1. Worsening obstruction to pulmonary blood flow can be due to restriction below, at, or above the pulmonary valve or restriction at the interventricular communication.
2. Closure of a previously patent ductus arteriosus can make antegrade flow though the stenotic pulmonary outflow tract the only source of pulmonary blood flow.
3. Pulmonary infections can result in an increase in the pulmonary vascular resistance, thereby decreasing pulmonary blood flow.
4. Primary pulmonary hypertension.
5. Shock, or inadequate perfusion of the end organs, can be caused by myocarditis/pericarditis, sepsis, viral systemic inflammatory response, or severely depressed systolic function of any etiology.
6. Pneumothorax.
7. Methemoglobinemia.

Clinical Vignette Comment

The patient has unpalliated tricuspid atresia with worsening restriction to pulmonary blood flow. From the saturation of 65% on room air and the high-frequency systolic ejection murmur, it can be inferred that there is a paucity of pulmonary blood flow. The expected saturation in a patient with unpalliated tricuspid atresia is 75–85%. The abrupt onset of symptoms was most likely triggered by the patient's dehydration.

Regardless of whether the restriction to pulmonary blood flow is at the level of the interventricular communication, at the subpulmonary, pulmonary, or suprapulmonary valve level, or is caused by closure of a previously patent ductus arteriosus, the patent will ultimately benefit from placement of a MBTS to augment pulmonary blood flow.

In the interim, providing supplemental oxygen and aggressive IV fluid resuscitation is essential. If the patient is anemic, a blood transfusion to increase the hematocrit to a normal range will increase the oxygen carrying capacity of the blood. In severely cyanotic patients, intubation, sedation, and paralysis can minimize metabolic demand until a shunt can be placed.

As the patient has no history of excessive pulmonary blood flow, it is unlikely that pulmonary hypertension has developed. The lack of fever, crackles, or radiographic signs of infection makes pneumonia unlikely. The normal lung examination and CXR exclude a pneumothorax. Lastly there was no history of drug exposure to incite methemoglobinemia.

Comments on Evaluation

In the setting of a patient with tricuspid atresia with worsening cyanosis, the following studies may be helpful:

CXR—Findings of a paucity of pulmonary vascular markings supports the diagnosis of obstruction to pulmonary blood flow. Excluding a pulmonary process such as pneumonia, intrathoracic mass, or pneumothorax is also important.

Echocardiogram—Ultimately an echocardiogram should be performed; however, it need not be performed in the Emergency Department where clinical stabilization should be prioritized over determining the level of obstruction to pulmonary blood flow. An echocardiogram will be helpful in confirming the mechanism of obstruction to pulmonary blood flow. It can also confirm closure of a previously patent ductus arteriosus. Profound systolic dysfunction will be evident echocardiographically as well; however this should be clinically obvious if there are physical signs of impaired perfusion.

CBC with differential—A CBC can be used to identify the contribution of anemia to symptoms as well as determination of the white blood cell count to evaluate the possibility of infection.

Arterial blood gas—A blood gas can confirm worsening hypoxia and is appropriate in guiding further interventions in the setting of acute clinical decompensation.

Key Management Principles in a Patient with Unpalliated Tricuspid Atresia

- It is important to know the expected range for saturations in a patient with unpalliated tricuspid atresia since this helps to identify patients who may require augmentation of pulmonary blood flow.
- Any situation that leads to hypotension and/or lower systemic vascular resistance (SVR), such as dehydration or septic shock, can prompt acute decompensation manifested by hypercyanosis in a patient with unpalliated tricuspid atresia.
- Supplemental oxygen, aggressive fluid resuscitation, increasing hematocrit to the normal range, intubation with mechanical ventilation, sedation, and paralysis can all improve saturations in a patient with unpalliated tricuspid atresia.
- A CXR should be obtained in any patient with unpalliated tricuspid atresia whose saturations are lower than expected to exclude a pulmonary etiology for the hypoxia and to search for oligemic lung fields.
- While echocardiography is important in surgical planning, the initial management of cyanosis in a patient with previously diagnosed tricuspid atresia is not contingent on completion of the echocardiogram in the emergency department.

Clinical Vignette 2

A 2-month-old male presents to the Emergency Department with lethargy following 2 weeks of poor feeding. His parents state that it takes him 45 min to complete a feed, with frequent breaks needed to catch his breath. Vital signs include the following: temperature 37.1 °C, HR 170 bpm, RR 80 breaths per minute, pulse BP 90/50 mmHg, and pulse ox 90% on room air. His body weight is at the third percentile. He appears pale, diaphoretic, and tachypneic. Diffuse crackles are heard throughout both lung fields. A II/VI, low-frequency systolic ejection murmur is heard at the left upper sternal border. Diastole is quiet. The femoral pulses are 2+ with no brachiofemoral delay. The liver is palpable 3 cm below the right costal margin. His parents state he was diagnosed with tricuspid atresia at birth and has not had any surgeries performed to date. A chest X-ray is obtained (Fig. 4.15).

Differential Diagnosis

The differential diagnosis for a patient with tricuspid atresia, presenting with tachypnea, and tachycardia includes the following:

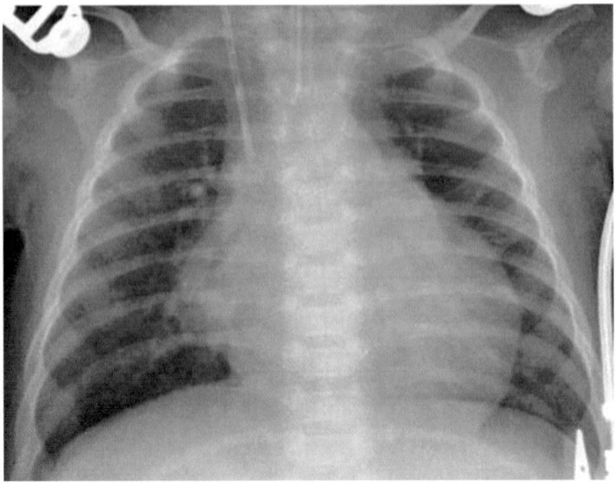

Fig. 4.15 CXR of a 2-month-old male with tricuspid atresia with normally related great arteries (Type Ib) with increased pulmonary vascular markings. The patient has been intubated and a right internal jugular line has been placed

1. Tachypnea, with failure to thrive, is frequently due to pulmonary overcirculation secondary to unrestricted pulmonary blood flow in an unoperated patient with congenital heart disease. The same symptoms can also be caused by moderately to severely depressed systolic function and moderate-to-severe atrioventricular valve regurgitation.
2. Infection in the form of myocarditis, pericarditis, sepsis, or a viral/bacterial infection can change a patient's status from compensated to decompensated heart failure.
3. Anemia.
4. Pericardial effusion.
5. Arrhythmia.
6. Hyperthyroidism/endocrine/metabolic causes.

Clinical Vignette Comment

The patient has tricuspid atresia with minimal restriction to pulmonary blood flow. From the saturation of 90% on room air and the low-frequency systolic ejection murmur, it can be inferred that there is an excess of pulmonary blood flow. The acceptable saturation in a patient with unoperated tricuspid atresia is 75–85%. Since the patient is 2 months old, sufficient time has passed since birth for the pulmonary vascular resistance to fall substantially, resulting in excessive pulmonary blood flow. The high pulmonary to systemic flow ratio (QP:QS) manifests in classic signs of congestive heart failure: tachypnea, tachycardia, and organomegaly (hepatomegaly on examination and cardiomegaly on CXR). Diaphoresis and pallor during feedings occur because of an increased sympathetic response. The history of struggling with feeds and poor weight gain supports this diagnosis as excessive calories are spent on maintaining the elevated heart and respiratory rates.

Pericardial effusion and infection are other disease processes that are in the differential diagnosis for tachycardia and tachypnea in this patient. Treating this patient for dehydration is potentially deleterious and could exacerbate the patient's pulmonary overcirculation.

It would be highly unlikely for this patient to develop a pericardial effusion in the absence of a previous surgery (post-pericardiotomy syndrome), evidence of infection such as fever (pericarditis), or exposure to cardiotoxic mediations (reactive pericarditis from chemotherapy). Therefore, obtaining an echocardiogram to exclude tamponade physiology is extremely low yield in this case. It should be noted that pulmonary overcirculation itself is a clinical diagnosis, and ordering an urgent echocardiogram is seldom necessary when the anatomical cardiac diagnosis is already known. In this case, the clinical picture can dictate the therapy required. The patient will benefit most from administration of diuretic therapy to relieve pulmonary edema. Lastly, increasing the patient's caloric intake to account for increased energy expenditure from tachypnea and tachycardia will help to promote growth and place the patient in a positive nitrogen balance, ultimately making him a more favorable surgical candidate.

The absence of fever or focal infiltrates on chest X-ray make infection less likely, though ordering a CBC to evaluate the white count can assist in excluding an intercurrent illness in the face of heart failure.

Care must be taken to interpret the pulse oximetry reading in the setting of the patient's anatomical diagnosis. Administering supplemental oxygen to the patient is contraindicated, as oxygen saturations in an unoperated patient with tricuspid atresia should be 75–85%. Providing supplemental oxygen could potentially lower the pulmonary vascular resistance further, increasing pulmonary blood flow at the expense of systemic blood flow and exacerbating the patient's pulmonary edema.

Comments on Evaluation

As pulmonary overcirculation is a clinical diagnosis, obtaining an accurate history and physical is paramount. The following additional studies may also be helpful:

CXR—Findings of cardiomegaly and increased pulmonary vascular markings support the diagnosis of pulmonary overcirculation.

ECG—An ECG is useful to confirm normal sinus rhythm or sinus tachycardia and to exclude other arrhythmias.

When the presentation of pulmonary overcirculation is less straight forward, additional testing could be considered.

CBC with differential—This can be used to identify the contribution of anemia to the patient's symptoms and to examine the white count to determine index of suspicion for infection.

Chemistry—This can be useful for the identification of electrolyte abnormalities.

Echocardiogram—An echocardiogram in the ED is only helpful if a new anatomical problem is suspected. It is typically not helpful in the diagnosis of pulmonary overcirculation.

Key Management Principles

- Knowing the expected range for saturations in a patient with tricuspid atresia avoids the pitfall of supplying unnecessary and potentially deleterious oxygen.
- Identify tachycardia, tachypnea, organomegaly, feeding difficulties, diaphoresis and pallor, and poor weight gain as signs and symptoms of pulmonary overcirculation.
- The CXR and pulse oximetry are more diagnostic of excessive pulmonary blood flow in this setting than is the echocardiogram.
- Understand the physiology of unrestricted pulmonary blood flow and the use of diuretics to treat pulmonary congestion.

Clinical Vignette 3

A 2-month-old term male is brought to the ED for worsening cyanosis and increased fussiness. The parents report that a few days previously, he started having a cough, nasal congestion, fever, increased work of breathing, and decreased oral intake. The infant was prenatally diagnosed with pulmonary atresia and intact ventricular septum with a severely hypoplastic tricuspid valve and right ventricle. He underwent a right MBTS placement at 2 weeks of age. His only medication is aspirin. In the ED, he is noted to be tachycardiac with a HR of 180 bpm and tachypneic with a RR of 70 breaths per minute. He appears cyanotic, and pulse oximetry shows an O2 saturation of 50–60%. His peripheral pulses are felt, but are weak, and capillary refill is slightly delayed at 3–5 s. On auscultation, no crackles are heard; however, the shunt murmur is low grade and difficult to ascertain in this irritable child. Shortly after his arrival, as a capillary blood gas is being obtained and an IV is being started, his O_2 saturations drop to 30–40%, and he becomes lethargic.

Differential Diagnosis

Differential diagnosis for an infant with history of MBTS placement presenting with acute and severe desaturation includes the following [8, 9]:

1. A shunt stenosis or occlusion can be acute (in the immediate postoperative period) or chronic. It is most often caused by thrombus formation; however, an anatomical narrowing in the shunt can occur in the immediate postoperative period. A hypercoagulable state, low-flow state secondary to dehydration, intercurrent pulmonary process, sepsis, arrhythmia, or anatomical narrowing can lead to thrombus formation and occlusion of the shunt.

2. A pulmonary process can cause an elevation in the pulmonary vascular resistance leading to decreased pulmonary blood flow. Examples include airway obstruction, reflux, aspiration, infection, pleural effusion, and pneumothorax.
3. Any process that causes a significant decrease in the systemic vascular resistance can incite hypercyanosis by shunting blood flow away from the lungs and toward the peripheral circulation. Hypotension due to vasodilation associated with general anesthesia while undergoing a general surgical procedure is one such example.
4. Anemia.

Clinical Vignette: Continued

The infant is emergently intubated, placed on 100% FiO_2, sedated, a central line placed, and he is given fluid resuscitation and epinephrine. A limited bedside echocardiogram cannot demonstrate shunt patency. He is transferred emergently to the cath lab where angiography, through right femoral arterial access, shows a thrombus and near-complete occlusion of the right MBTS (Fig. 4.16a). *Tissue plasminogen activator* (tPA) is given, and he undergoes balloon angioplasty (Fig. 4.16b) with stent placement. Follow-up angiography shows good flow through the right MBTS and stent and improvement of his arterial saturations to 75–85% (Fig. 4.16c).

Clinical Vignette Comment

This patient has history of a ductal dependant pulmonary circulation, associated with his pulmonary atresia with intact ventricular septum, and a right MBTS was placed to provide a reliable source of pulmonary blood flow. The shunt is the only source of blood flow to the lungs. In this clinical situation, it is important to promptly ascertain the underlying cause for the extreme cyanosis in order to

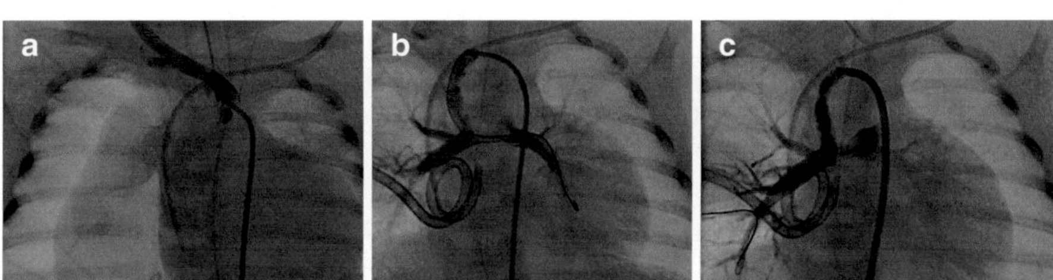

Fig. 4.16 Catheter-based treatment of shunt thrombosis. (**a**) Near-complete thrombosis is evidenced by failure of contrast to enter the branch pulmonary arteries during hand injection of the MBTS. (**b**) After initial administration of tPA, the shunt becomes patent but with some residual obstruction due to thrombosis. (**c**) Following balloon angioplasty and stent placement in the MBTS, the shunt is unobstructed with complete opacification of the shunt and proximal branch pulmonary arteries

achieve a good outcome. If shunt occlusion is responsible for the cyanosis, then the patient will require an emergent intervention, consisting of some combination of ECMO cannulation, catheter-based shunt angioplasty, and/or surgical intervention on the MBTS to reestablish pulmonary blood flow. A prompt diagnosis was made, in this instance, when a robust shunt murmur was not detected in addition to the inability to visualize the shunt on the echocardiogram. Multiple historical factors in this patient place him at risk for shunt thrombosis, including an upper respiratory tract infection causing an elevation in the pulmonary vascular resistance, poor oral intake, and fever, which contribute to dehydration and hypotension. Occlusion or thrombus can additionally be found in one or both branch pulmonary arteries. The management is similar to that of shunt occlusion; however, the presentation might not be as severe if branch pulmonary artery occlusion/stenosis is unilateral.

If a shunt thrombus is not the reason for the presentation, then another pulmonary process needs to be investigated and treated. Other causes, already mentioned in differential diagnosis, include infection, pneumonia, aspiration, airway obstruction, pleural effusion, pneumothorax, dehydration, anemia, and arrhythmia.

Comments on Evaluation

Shunt stenosis or occlusion with decreased pulmonary blood flow will be suspected based upon the clinical presentation, including the history and the physical examination. Additional tests that can help guide the diagnosis include:

CXR—Findings of oligemic lung fields bilaterally will occur with shunt thrombosis. If one branch pulmonary artery is thrombosed, then a unilateral oligemic lung field may be present. Effusion, pneumothorax, infiltration, or atelectasis are other possible causes of hypoxemia that are identifiable on a CXR.

ECG—The confirmation of normal sinus rhythm or sinus tachycardia and the exclusion of arrhythmias are confirmed by the ECG.

CBC with differential—The CBC identifies the contribution of anemia to symptoms, and the white blood cell count assists in determining the index of suspicion for infection.

Chemistry—This identifies electrolyte abnormalities and any evidence for end-organ perfusion deficits.

Echocardiogram—Echocardiography can suggest a diagnosis of shunt occlusion/stenosis or occlusion/stenosis of the branch pulmonary arteries. These echocardiographic findings must be confirmed by angiography.

Key Management Principles

- Prompt recognition of shunt occlusion can facilitate transferring the patient to the catheterization laboratory or to the operating room in a timely manner.

Clinical Vignette 4

A 14-month-old female who has history of tricuspid atresia, type I B (normally related great arteries and pulmonary stenosis), has undergone a superior cavopulmonary connection at 5 months of age. She has been growing well, and her baseline oxygen saturation is in the low to mid 80s. She presents to the ED with a 1-week history of nasal congestion, dry cough, and a low-grade fever. On the day of presentation, she is noted to have tachypnea and increased central cyanosis and was refusing to eat and drink. On arrival to the ED, she appears to be in moderate respiratory distress, 60 breaths per minute with subcostal retractions, HR 160 bpm, BP 80/45, afebrile, and a pulse oximetry reading of 55% on room air. Auscultation reveals wheezing bilaterally. A CXR is obtained (Fig. 4.17).

Differential Diagnosis

Cyanosis in a patient following a superior cavopulmonary connection can be caused by [10]:

1. Veno-venous collaterals are vascular connections that may develop following a superior cavopulmonary connection in a patient with a functionally univentricular heart that can cause progressive cyanosis. These connections are either between a systemic vein and the inferior vena cava (or its tributaries) or between a systemic vein and a pulmonary vein. Both types of types of collaterals can act as a means of decompressing elevated systemic venous pressure. These collaterals create a right-to-left shunt can cause progressive cyanosis.

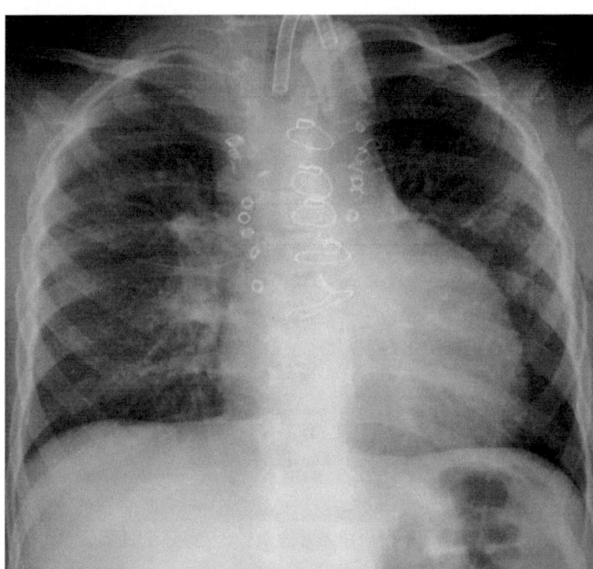

Fig. 4.17 CXR of a patient with a superior cavopulmonary connection and respiratory syncytial virus (RSV) infection. Multiple coils of collateral vessels are noted. Interstitial markings, consistent with an intercurrent respiratory infection, are evident

2. A respiratory process that leads to high pulmonary vascular resistance (PVR) including infection, pleural effusion, pneumothorax, and aspiration can cause cyanosis due to increased resistance to flow from the systemic venous circulation into the pulmonary circulation.
3. An occlusion/thrombosis in the superior vena cava-pulmonary artery (PA) junction or in one or both PAs secondary to any hypercoagulable state.
4. Pulmonary hypertension can lead to profound cyanosis due to increased resistance to flow from the systemic venous circulation into the pulmonary circulation.
5. Anemia
6. "Baffle" leak in a hemi-Fontan.
7. Plastic bronchitis.
8. Dehydration.
9. Fever and infection/sepsis.
10. Arrhythmia.
11. Depressed ventricular function.
12. Worsening atrioventricular valve regurgitation.
13. Methemoglobinemia.

Clinical Vignette Comment

Acceptable oxygen saturations, after a superior cavopulmonary connection, can range from the low 70s to the mid-80s. Knowing the baseline saturations for an individual patient is vital, as this will aid in assessing the severity of the presenting cyanosis. In addition, it is important to ascertain whether the decline in oxygen saturations have been gradual versus an abrupt change is helpful when investigating the cause.

The patient in this clinical vignette has a presentation consistent with a viral upper respiratory tract infection progressing into a viral bronchiolitis. Any pulmonary process that increases pulmonary vascular resistance, which includes a lung infection, pleural effusion, pneumothorax, or aspiration, will lead to decreased pulmonary blood flow and pulmonary venous desaturation, both of which lead to more severe cyanosis [11].

Pleural effusions are common in functionally univentricular heart patients following a superior cavopulmonary connection or a completion Fontan procedure. Patients with pleural effusions present with respiratory symptoms in addition to cyanosis. Prompt recognition and drainage of clinically significant pleural effusions is essential, especially when the effusions lead to an elevation of the pulmonary vascular resistance (PVR). An elevated PVR impedes passive pulmonary blood flow and results in increased cyanosis due to reduced pulmonary blood flow.

Thrombus formation and/or anatomical obstruction in the SVC/PA connection or in one or both pulmonary arteries will present as worsening cyanosis. A variety of things may lead to this complication, including elevation of PVR for any reason, a hypercoagulable state, and/or anatomical obstruction of the superior caval vein or either of the branch pulmonary arteries. The degree and location of the obstruction in the pulmonary circuit will determine the severity of the resultant cyanosis.

Veno-venous collaterals are vascular connections that can develop following a superior cavopulmonary connection in a patient with a functionally univentricular heart. These connections are either between a systemic vein and the inferior vena cava (or its tributaries) or between a systemic vein and a pulmonary vein. Both types of collaterals can act as a means of decompressing elevated systemic venous pressure. These collaterals create a right-to-left shunt and can cause progressive cyanosis [11].

A baffle leak in a hemi-Fontan (a type of superior cavopulmonary connection) is a right-to-left shunt through an opening in the patch that separates the region of the connection of the superior vena cava to the pulmonary artery from the right atrium. This shunt will lead to progressive cyanosis.

Other etiologies of cyanosis after a superior cavopulmonary connection include anemia, dehydration, sepsis, ventricular dysfunction, AV valve regurgitation, arrhythmia, plastic bronchitis, and methemoglobinemia.

In critically ill patients with a superior cavopulmonary anastomoses who require intubation, there are several unique physiological considerations.

Hypercapnia with acidosis causes cerebral vasodilation. This state increases blood flow to the brain (cerebral blood flow) which, in turn, increases the return flow through the superior caval vein(s). These changes increase pulmonary blood flow after a superior cavopulmonary connection. On the other hand, this same hypercapnia with acidosis causes pulmonary vasoconstriction, with increased PVR, which will lead to reduced pulmonary blood flow after a superior cavopulmonary connection [10]. It seems that, on balance, the increased cerebral blood flow, and hence pulmonary blood flow, mediated by mild acidosis, may outweigh the negative effects of increased PVR. When it is clinically feasible, it is best to avoid hypocapnia and to maintain a mild hypercapnia ($PaCO_2$ ~45). At the same time, it is prudent to avoid the increased PVR associated with hypoxia and metabolic acidosis. This multifaceted approach can help to restore the delicate balance to the cerebral pulmonary interaction and encourage a balance between adequate oxygenation and ventilation. Additionally, ensuring other complicating factors, such as infection, dehydration, or pleural effusions, have been adequately treated is essential to achieving a positive clinical outcome.

Another key point to ventilatory management in functionally univentricular heart patients after a superior cavopulmonary connection is to maintain a physiological PEEP and normal lung functional capacity to prevent an increase in the PVR. Judicious use of PEEP is essential to balancing the need for ventilatory support with avoiding alveolar distension and compression of the pulmonary capillary bed. The passive pulmonary blood flow dynamics after a superior cavopulmonary connection will tend to be intolerant of excessive PEEP levels.

Comments on Evaluation

There are multiple reasons for cyanosis in a patient with a superior cavopulmonary connection. The clinical presentation can help in many instances. For example, a history of URI indicates a pulmonary process is involved, while patients with symptoms of SVC syndrome will have some combination of an anatomical obstruction in the pathway or elevated pulmonary vascular resistance. Additional testing is often essential however in identifying the mechanism responsible for cyanosis.

CXR—Hyperinflation and small airway disease, effusion, pneumothorax, infiltration, and atelectasis are all causes identifiable on a CXR.

ECG—Confirmation of normal sinus rhythm or sinus tachycardia and exclusion of other arrhythmias is important.

CBC with differential—The CBC identifies the potential contribution of anemia to producing the patient's symptoms. The white blood cell count will assist in determining the index of suspicion for infection.

Chemistry—The identification of electrolyte abnormalities and evidence of reduced end-organ perfusion can be helpful.

Echocardiogram—An echocardiogram can be important to look for any obstruction in the cavopulmonary pathway when the diagnosis is not obvious from the clinical presentation or other tests. Ventricular function, atrioventricular or aortic valve insufficiency, and pericardial effusion are other important findings to establish by echocardiography.

Key Management Principles

- Identifying the underlying reason for the progressive cyanosis will be the key for determining the appropriate management. In a respiratory infection, supportive care is important with administration of oxygen, fluids, and antibiotics as needed. Draining a large pleural effusion promptly will improve cyanosis. An anatomical obstruction or thrombus in the cavopulmonary pathway or the presence of veno-venous collaterals will require catheterization or surgical intervention.
- Understanding the cerebral pulmonary interactions and maintaining a physiologic PEEP is essential in terms of the ventilatory management of patients with superior cavopulmonary connections.

Clinical Vignette 5

A 28-year-old male with a history of staged Fontan palliation for tricuspid atresia presents to the ED with shortness of breath, generalized fatigue, dizziness, and nausea for the past 48 h. He has had no other recent illnesses or rhythm issues in the past. The only remote rhythm abnormality is a history of supraventricular tachycardia in the immediate postoperative period following his completion Fontan surgery at 3 years of age. He takes aspirin and Enalapril as his only medications. His last cardiology visit was 9 months previously, when his oxygen saturation was 96%, his ECG showed normal sinus rhythm (Fig. 4.18), his echocardiogram demonstrated

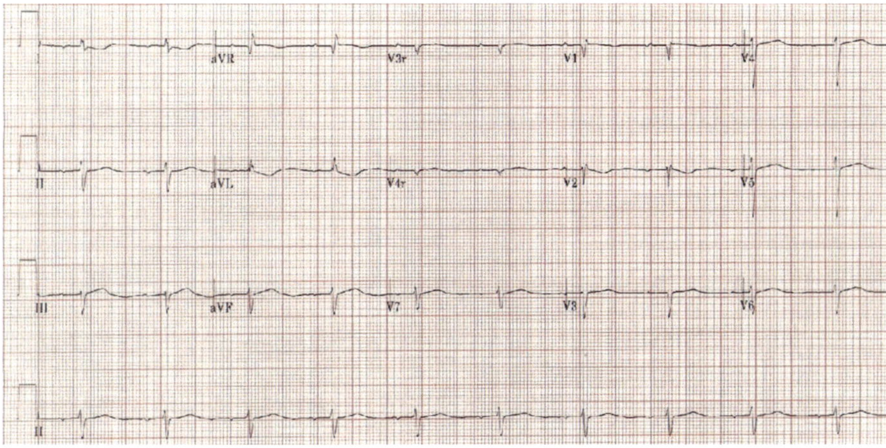

Fig. 4.18 ECG from patient with tricuspid atresia status post-Fontan. Normal sinus rhythm with first-degree heart block

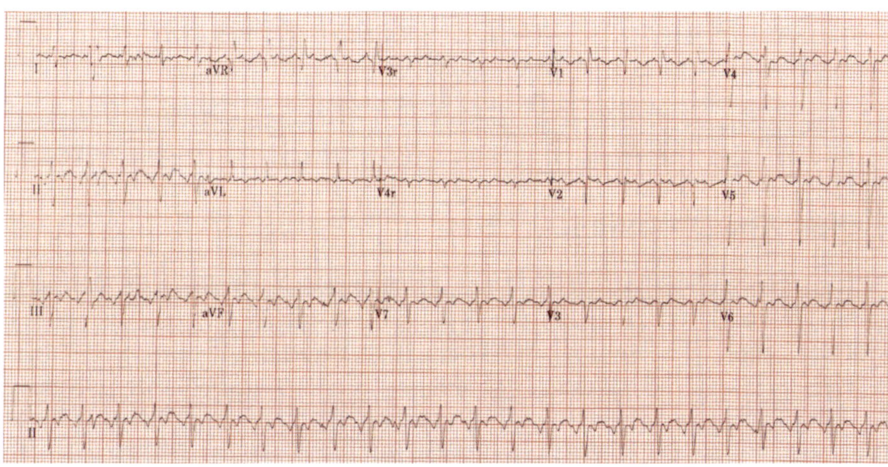

Fig. 4.19 ECG from a patient status post-Fontan palliation with intra-atrial reentrant tachycardia. Note the 2:1 atrioventricular block with a ventricular rate of 145 bpm

low normal morphological left ventricular function with mild/moderate mitral regurgitation and no aortic regurgitation. His last Holter monitor was preformed 2 years ago and showed isolated premature atrial and ventricular contractions. In the ED, his HR is 140 bpm, RR 24 breaths per minute, BP 95/55. The room air oxygen saturation is 90%. The CXR is unremarkable. The ECG demonstrates the rhythm shown in Fig. 4.19.

Differential Diagnosis

The differential diagnosis of an adult patient with a history of Fontan palliation presenting with fatigue, dizziness, and shortness of breath includes:

1. Atrial arrhythmia.
2. Other rhythm disturbance, including sinus node dysfunction, heart block, and ventricular arrhythmia.
3. Ventricular dysfunction.
4. Worsening mitral regurgitation.
5. Obstruction/thrombosis in Fontan pathway, which can be secondary to a hypercoagulable state, anatomical obstruction, or low-flow state.
6. Any pulmonary process that increases PVR, including infection and pleural effusion.
7. Dehydration.
8. Infection/sepsis.
9. Anemia.
10. Protein-losing enteropathy is a failing Fontan state which presents as loss of protein through the intestinal tract [12]. Patients typically present with generalized swelling. This is a very serious and common complication in Fontan patients, however, unlikely the presentation of patient in vignette.
11. Liver dysfunction.

Clinical Vignette Comment

The patient in this clinical vignette has atrial flutter with 2:1 block, with a ventricular rate of 140 bpm. His symptoms are not specific to arrhythmia; however, this type of presentation can be common in patients following a Fontan procedure. Atrial tachycardia is a late complication that affects almost 50% of patients who undergo Fontan palliation, usually 6–11 years post-procedure [13]. The classic or atriopulmonary Fontan operation, which carries a higher risk of rhythm disturbances early on including junctional rhythm, heart block, sinus node dysfunction, and atrial tachycardia, is no longer performed. Lateral tunnel Fontan techniques and extracardiac conduits carry less risk of arrhythmia; however, the late-onset atrial tachycardia remains a common complication. Patients with tricuspid atresia are also thought to have abnormal fibers in the right atrium that can be associated with the additional risk for atrial arrhythmia.

Patients with functionally univentricular heart physiology presenting with arrhythmia and loss of atrioventricular synchrony can become severely symptomatic. The severity of the presentation depends upon the ventricular rate. If 1:1 conduction is present, patients might present with syncope or sudden death. Both ventricular dysfunction and intracardiac or Fontan pathway thrombus formation are complications seen in Fontan patients with atrial arrhythmias. Therefore, the ECG is an essential part of the work-up in any sick patient with a Fontan. The echocardiogram can evaluate for ventricular function, atrioventricular valve regurgitation and the presence of thrombus [14].

Once a patient with a Fontan presents with an atrial arrhythmia, it is very likely the patient will have recurrences. These patients need to be treated in the first 24 h of presentation to prevent adverse outcomes. If a thrombus cannot be ruled out with certainty, the risk of dislodging a potential thrombus during cardioversion versus the benefit of reestablishing sinus rhythm should be weighed. In the acute setting, arrhythmias can be treated with pharmacological cardioversion, transesophageal or intra-atrial pacing, or synchronized cardioversion. If a patient presents with syncope or an aborted sudden death, then invasive hemodynamic assessment with an electrophysiology (EP) study may be appropriate. Chronic treatment and follow-up should ideally be managed by an electrophysiologist specialized in congenital heart disease. The choice of medications and anticoagulation depends on the severity of the presentation, the ventricular function, and the recurrence rate of the arrhythmia, as well as need for further EP studies and/or surgical revision with surgical ablation [15].

Comments on Evaluation

CXR—A CXR will be helpful to rule out any pulmonary processes, especially in a patient presenting with shortness of breath.

ECG—An ECG should be performed in any Fontan presenting for medical care to exclude an arrhythmia.

CBC with differential—A CBC can identify clinically important anemia as well as an elevation of the white blood cell count to determine index of suspicion for infection.

Chemistry—The identification of electrolyte abnormalities is important, and liver function studies with serum protein levels are required to screen for protein-losing enteropathy.

Echocardiogram—As stated in vignette comment, an echocardiogram is important to evaluate ventricular function and atrioventricular valve regurgitation and to assess for intracardiac or in Fontan pathway thrombus.

Key Management Principles

- When evaluating an adult with a Fontan palliation, symptoms of palpitations should raise a high index of suspicion for arrhythmia. Due to the "slow flutter" appearance of intra-atrial tachycardia in Fontan patients, it is important to consider arrhythmia even when very fast heart rates are absent.
- Ventricular function evaluation, assessment of atrioventricular valve regurgitation, and evaluation for thrombus are standard components of arrhythmia management in patients with a Fontan.

- Once an arrhythmia diagnosis has been established, this special group of patients optimally should be managed by an electrophysiologist who has training in adult congenital cardiology.
- Significant pathology can present in an ambiguous fashion in Fontan patients. Evaluation for potential arrhythmias, pulmonary infection, pleural effusion, and protein-losing enteropathy should be routine in all Fontan patients presenting to the Emergency Department.

References

1. Fyler DC, Buckley LP, Hellenbrand WE, et al. Report of the New England Regional Infant Cardiac Program. Pediatrics. 1980;65:388–461.
2. Gewillig M. Congenital heart disease: the Fontan circulation. Heart. 2005;91:839–46.
3. Ferencz C, Rubin JD, McCarter RJ, et al. Congenital heart disease: prevalence at live birth, the Baltimore-Washington infant study. Am J Epidemiol. 1985;121:31–6.
4. Calder AI, Co EE, Sage MD. Coronary arterial abnormalities in pulmonary atresia with intact ventricular septum. Am J Cardiol. 1987;59:436–42.
5. Guleserian KJ, Armsby LB, Thiagarajan RR, et al. Natural history of pulmonary atresia with intact ventricular septum and right-ventricle–dependent coronary circulation managed by the single-ventricle approach. Ann Thorac Surg. 2006;81:2250–8.
6. Weber HS, Hellenbrand WE, Kleinman CS, et al. Predictors of rhythm disturbances and subsequent morbidity after the Fontan operation. Am J Cardiol. 1989;64:762–7.
7. Song MK, Bae EJ, Kwon BS, et al. Intra-atrial reentrant tachycardia in adult patients after Fontan operation. Int J Cardiol. 2015;187:157–63.
8. Guzzetta NA, Foster GS, Mruthinti N, et al. In-hospital shunt occlusion in infants undergoing a modified Blalock-Taussig shunt. Ann Thorac Surg. 2013;96(1):176–82.
9. Kogon BE, Villari CR, Shah N, et al. Occlusion of the modified Blalock–Taussig shunt: unique methods of treatment and review of catheter-based intervention. Congenit Heart Dis. 2007;2:185–90.
10. Allen HD, Driscoll DJ, Shaddy RE, et al. Moss and Adams' heart disease in infants, children, and adolescents: including the fetus and young adults. 7th ed. Philadelphia: Lippincott Williams & Wilkins; 2008. Chapter 20.
11. Heinemann M, Breuer J, Steger V, et al. Incidence and impact of systemic venous collateral development after Glenn and Fontan procedures. Thorac Cardiovasc Surg. 2001;49(3):172–8.
12. Griffiths ER, Kaza AK, Wyler von Ballmoos MC, et al. Evaluating failing Fontans for heart transplantation: predictors of mortality. Ann Thorac Surg. 2009;88(2):558–64.
13. Allen HD, Driscoll DJ, Shaddy RE, et al. Moss and Adams' heart disease in infants, children, and adolescents: including the fetus and young adults. 7th ed. Philadelphia: Lippincott Williams & Wilkins; 2008. Chapter 72.
14. Egbe AC, Connolly HM, Khan AR, et al. Outcomes in adult Fontan patients with atrial tachyarrhythmias. Am Heart J. 2017;186:12–20.
15. Deal BJ, Mavroudis C, Backer CL. Arrhythmia management in the Fontan patient. Pediatr Cardiol. 2007;28(6):448–56.

Check for updates

5 Common Surgical Interventions Resulting in Alterations in Hemodynamics

Kristen Richards, Monika Chauhan, and Ralph E. Delius

Congenital heart disease is the most common birth defect. In the USA approximately 25,000 newborns with congenital heart disease undergo surgical repair every year. In 2010 the CDC estimated that about one million US children were living with CHD who has undergone surgical correction or palliation; about 83% of these children are now surviving long term. It is extremely likely that a clinician will encounter a patient in an Emergency Department (ED) or primary care setting who has undergone a congenital heart operation. The incidence of congenital heart disease is 0.8% of all births and is greater than other more charismatic conditions such as childhood cancers, cystic fibrosis, and juvenile diabetes. In addition, with increasingly successful surgical approaches, there are now more adults with congenital heart disease than children. The relevance of understanding the altered hemodynamics of this patient population was reported in the Journal of Pediatrics by Cashen and colleagues, who interviewed 376 emergency room physicians. A large number (72%) were unsure of the acceptable range of arterial oxygen saturations for infants with single-ventricle physiology, and 58% were uncomfortable about treatment of these infants. A detailed description of all the procedures performed in the field of pediatric cardiovascular surgery is beyond the scope of this chapter. Only the common operations resulting in altered hemodynamics will be discussed.

K. Richards, C.P.N.P.-A.C. (✉)
Pediatric Nurse Practitioner, Department of Pediatric Cardiovascular Surgery,
Children's Hospital of Michigan, Detroit, MI, USA
e-mail: krichard2@dmc.org

M. Chauhan, M.B.B.S.
Division of Critical Care Medicine, Children's Hospital of Michigan, Detroit, MI, USA
e-mail: mchauhan@med.wayne.edu

R. E. Delius, M.D.
Department of Pediatric Cardiovascular Surgery, Children's Hospital of Michigan, Detroit, MI, USA

© Springer International Publishing AG, part of Springer Nature 2018

A. P. Sarnaik et al. (eds.), *Cardiac Emergencies in Children*,
https://doi.org/10.1007/978-3-319-73754-6_5

Case discussion: A 4-month-old male presents to the Emergency Department with a 2-day history of vomiting and diarrhea. Mom has noted the baby to be more irritable than normal and that his extremities are cool to touch. His vitals are as follows: T—36.8 °C, HR—170/min, RR—48/min, BP—83/45 mmHg, and SpO_2 on room air—80%. He exhibits nasal flaring and intercostal retractions. Examination demonstrate a fussy but consolable infant. Extremities are cool with +1 pulses in all limbs. Nail beds are dusky and capillary refill time is 3 s. Chest examination reveals a well-healed midline sternotomy scar and mild retractions. Abdomen is unremarkable. Mother states that her child had a Norwood operation for having only half a heart. Which of the following is the next best step in management?

(a) Administer oxygen by nasal cannula to maintain SpO_2 approximately 95%.
(b) Intubation and positive pressure ventilation.
(c) Administer furosemide intravenously.
(d) Infuse 10 mL/kg 0.9% saline intravenously and reassess circulation.
(e) Initiate intravenous infusion of epinephrine.

Functionally Univentricular Heart Lesions

Functionally univentricular heart also commonly referred to as single-ventricle lesions presents in the neonatal period and requires surgical intervention as a life-saving procedure. In hypoplastic left heart syndrome (HLHS), the right ventricle must bear the responsibility of maintaining both the pulmonary and the systemic circulations. In hypoplastic right heart syndrome (HRHS), the left ventricle serves to maintain the systemic and pulmonary circulations. In HLHS, ductal patency is essential to sustain life to supply both systemic and pulmonary circulation. This is accomplished by emergent and continuous intravenous infusion of alprostadil (prostaglandin E1) until surgical intervention occurs. In HRHS, ductal patency may or may not be essential, depending on whether the pulmonary blood flow is adequate. In some HRHS lesions, such as pulmonary atresia with intact ventricular septum, or tricuspid atresia with a restrictive VSD, ductal patency will need to be maintained. Tricuspid atresia with a nonrestrictive VSD, however, will have an ample pulmonary blood flow, and maintenance of ductal patency is neither needed nor desired. Children with single-ventricle lesions typically follow a pathway of three palliative operations within the first 2–4 years of life. The goals of surgical interventions are to some extent different depending on which ventricle is affected, but in all single-ventricle cases, regardless of which ventricle is serving as the systemic ventricle, the final goal is to have the passive flow of systemic venous return serve as the sole source of pulmonary blood flow.

HLHS Infants with HLHS present either with prenatal diagnosis or with profound circulatory collapse, systemic hypoperfusion, and metabolic acidosis. The patent ductus arteriosus allows for systemic perfusion from the right ventricle through a connection between the pulmonary artery and the aorta. As the ductus arteriosus begins to close, systemic perfusion is compromised. In addition to temporarily maintaining ductal patency with PGE1, the surgical approach is aimed at ultimately making the right ventricle supply systemic blood flow and allowing systemic venous return to passively flow into the pulmonary arteries and subsequently to the lungs. However, the relatively high pulmonary vascular resistance (PVR) present during the first few months of life precludes passive flow of venous return into the pulmonary vasculature in neonates and young infants. A three-stage approach is thus used to accomplish the final physiologic result, with systemic venous return passively supplying the pulmonary circulation. The first stage uses the actively contracting single ventricle to supply forward flow into both pulmonary (Qp) and systemic (Qs) circulations (Norwood operation or Hybrid procedure). The second stage is to first return the superior vena caval blood to passively flow into the pulmonary arteries (Glenn procedure), and the third stage is to also add inferior vena caval blood the pulmonary circulation (modified Fontan procedure).

Norwood procedure In the first stage (Fig. 5.1), an atrial septectomy is performed to allow unrestricted mixing of pulmonary and systemic venous returns in the single atrial chamber. The distal pulmonary artery is transected and separated from right ventricle. The proximal pulmonary artery is then joined with the poorly developed ascending aorta and the aortic arch is augmented with a homograft patch to form a neo-aorta. The ductus arteriosus is ligated. Pulmonary circulation is supplied by either a systemic-to-pulmonary shunt, such as a modified Blalock-Taussig shunt or, more commonly, a Sano shunt, which connects the right ventricle to the pulmonary arteries via a synthetic vascular graft such as a GORE-TEX[R] tube.

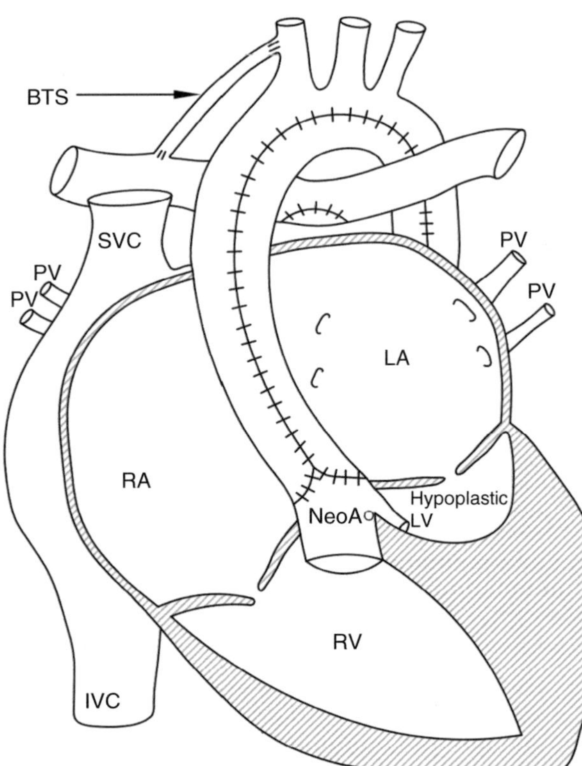

Fig. 5.1 Norwood procedure. An atrial septectomy is performed to provide free communication of the left atrium (LA) and the right atrium (RA) and unrestricted flow of blood from the pulmonary veins into the common chamber. The distal pulmonary artery is transected. The proximal pulmonary artery is used to form the neo-aorta and connected to the aortic arch. A Blalock-Taussig shunt (BTS) connects systemic and pulmonary circulations

Hybrid palliation A hybrid palliation is a procedure performed when comorbidities are present, elevating the risk of cardiopulmonary bypass or the Norwood procedure. For example, low birth weight of <2.5 kg and intracranial hemorrhage are comorbid conditions which may favor the use of the hybrid procedure. This procedure also may be indicated when the size of the left ventricle or the left-sided valves are marginal, and it is unclear if the ventricle is satisfactory to serve the systemic circulation. The hybrid procedure can then allow time to see if the left-sided structures increase in size to the point of where the left ventricle can adequately provide systemic circulation (Fig. 5.2). This procedure is done off cardiopulmonary bypass, with interventional cardiology placing a stent to keep the patent ductus arteriosus open, which can be seen on routine chest radiograph (Fig. 5.3). Bilateral pulmonary artery bands are then surgically placed on the right and the left pulmonary arteries to restrict pulmonary flow and enhance systemic flow.

It is important for clinicians to comprehend the hemodynamics of the functionally univentricular physiology as the management is distinctly different from typical two-ventricle physiology. The crucial aspect is to understand the concept of parallel circulation versus in-series circulation. In normal biventricular circulation, oxygenated blood flows from the left ventricle to the arterial system, and then through the systemic capillary bed. Systemic venous blood returns to the right atrium (RA) and ventricle, which in turns pumps blood through the pulmonary capillary circulation and back to the left atrium and ventricle to start the cycle again. Both systemic and

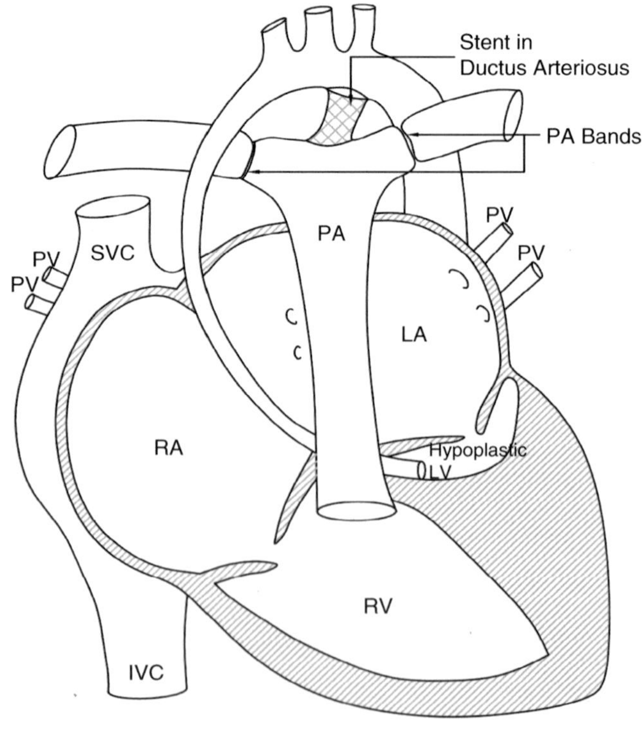

Fig. 5.2 Hybrid procedure. A stent is placed in the ductus arteriosus to maintain systemic-pulmonary communication. Bands are placed around both the right and left pulmonary arteries which restricts pulmonary blood flow and allows for balanced circulation. *RA* right atrium, *LA* left atrium, *RV* right ventricle

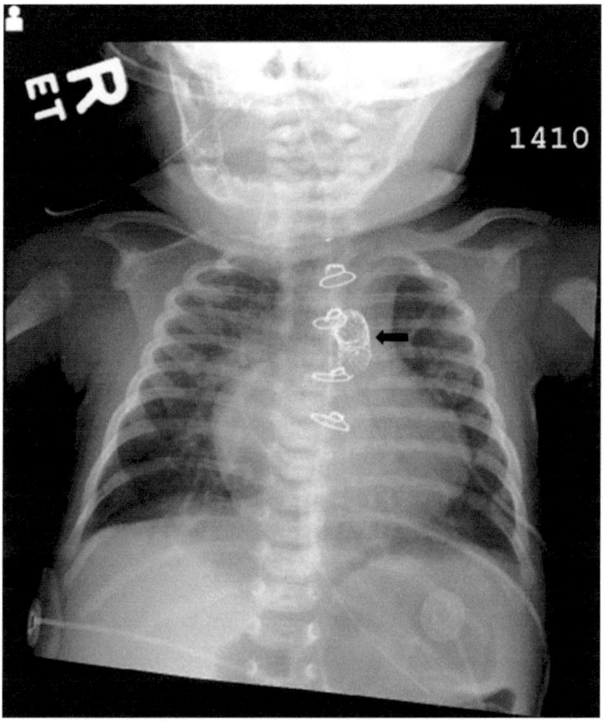

Fig. 5.3 Chest radiograph showing the stent placed in the ductus arteriosus to keep systemic-pulmonary communication open

pulmonary circulation circuits have a designated pumping chamber; this standard circulation is described as being in series (Fig. 5.4).

In contrast, the baby with a single functional systemic ventricle is designed to have parallel pulmonary and systemic circulations, with a single-ventricle supplying both the pulmonary and systemic capillary beds (Fig. 5.5). The relative resistances of the pulmonary and systemic vasculature determine the relative distribution of total ventricular output to pulmonary blood flow (Qp) and to systemic blood flow (Qs). If PVR approximates SVR, Qp and Qs are fairly balanced and equal. This is the most desirable situation.

A fall in the pulmonary vascular resistance or a rise in the systemic vascular resistance will result in excessive pulmonary blood flow at the expense of the systemic flow (Fig. 5.6) manifesting as elevated SpO_2 but systemic hypoperfusion.

In contrast, a rise in pulmonary vascular resistance or a fall in systemic vascular resistance results in enhanced systemic blood flow but also decreased pulmonary blood flow and cyanosis (Fig. 5.7). In functional single-ventricle physiology, optimal systemic oxygen delivery occurs when Qp/Qs equals 1. This occurs with the total ventricular output being twice the normal output of an in-series systemic ventricle, to yield normal values for both Qp and Qs.

The patient in the case discussion had a stage I palliation for HLHS. He has a single ventricle responsible for supplying both the pulmonary and systemic circulations. History and physical examination are consistent with hypovolemia. The

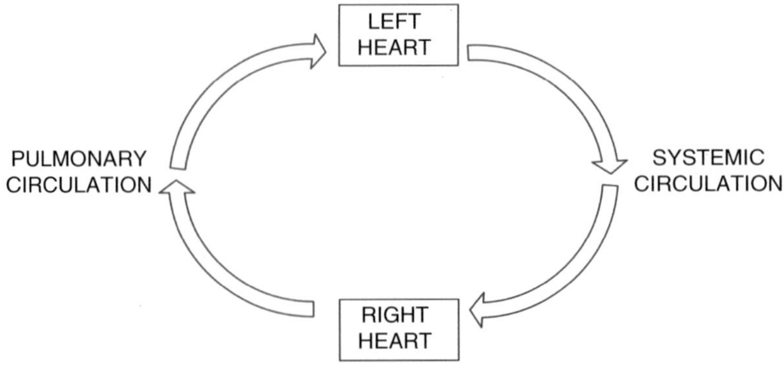

Fig. 5.4 Normal biventricular circulation is in-series with both pulmonary and systemic circulations have their own pumping chamber (RV and LV). Pulmonary and systemic blood flow are separated

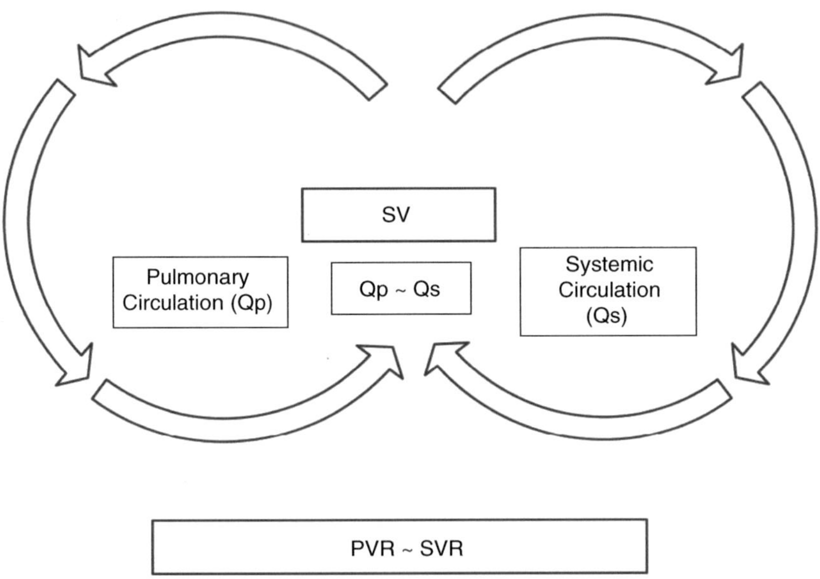

Fig. 5.5 Single ventricle has parallel systemic and pulmonary circulations. Pulmonary blood flow (Qp) and systemic blood flow (Qs) depend on relative resistances in pulmonary and systemic circulations since they both receive blood from the same pumping chamber with the same pressure head. If PVR ~ SVR, Qp ~ Qs

functional single ventricle by definition is volume overloaded since it supplies both pulmonary and systemic circuits. Consequentially, infants with single ventricle are very volume sensitive. Dehydration inscreases the risk of thrombosis of the shunt between systemic and pulmonary circulation. Immediate and appropriate intravascular volume expansion and frequent assessment of his circulatory status are extremely important and first and foremost priority at this time. After Norwood procedure, SpO_2 is normally in the mid-70s. High (> 85%) oxygen saturations

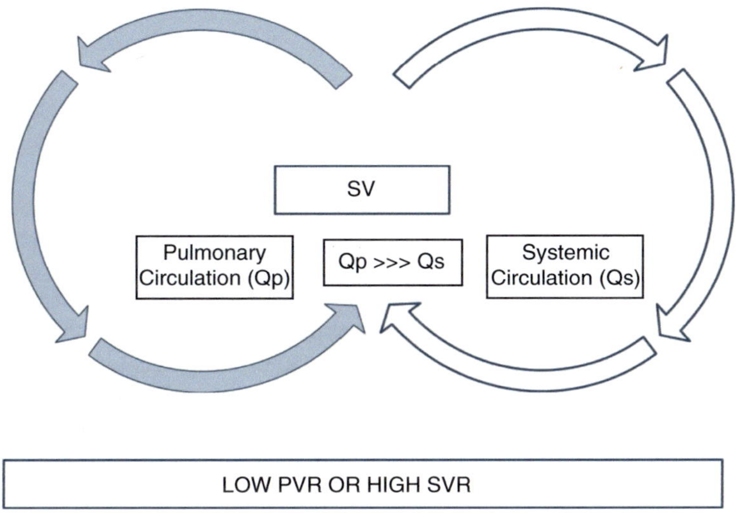

Fig. 5.6 Single-ventricle lesion with PVR ⋘ SVR such as in oxygen administration. Fall in PVR preferentially results in increased pulmonary blood flow at the expense of systemic blood flow. SpO_2 will be increased, but there will be systemic hypoperfusion, lactic acidosis, and multiple organ failure

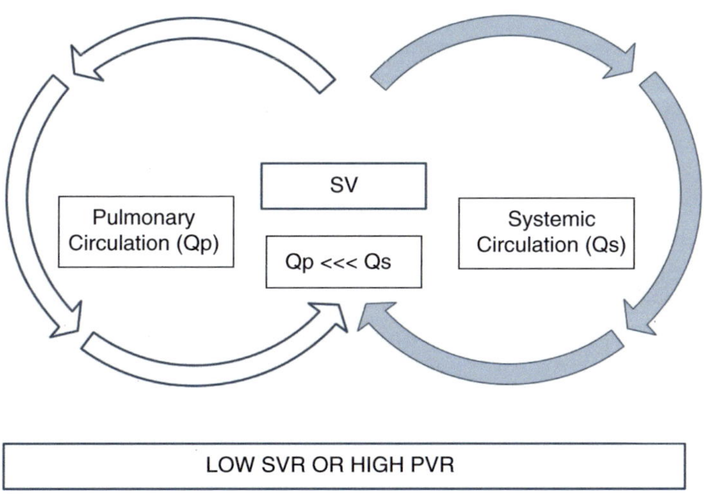

Fig. 5.7 Single-ventricle lesion with PVR ⋙ SVR such as with respiratory infection and dehydration. There is less blood flow into pulmonary circulation compared to systemic circulation, resulting in hypoxemia

suggest that Qp is greater than Qs leading to systemic hypoperfusion and organ dysfunction. The interstage between the first operation, during which a balanced circulation (Qp and Qs) is present, and the subsequent operations, which achieve an in-series circulation, is a high-risk time for infants with single ventricle.

The occurrence of a simple childhood illness such as a respiratory tract infection gastroenteritis, or fever may cause hypovolemia, hypoxemia, and/or increased systemic vascular resistance and may place an infant with minimal cardiovascular reserve at great risk for morbidity and mortality. This interstage period, if not carefully monitored, can carry a mortality risk of approximately 15%. Consequently, infants discharged home following stage I palliation warrant heightened surveillance during this period, and most congenital heart programs have an interstage monitoring program designed to meticulously follow these fragile patients until the next stage can be achieved.

Glenn procedure As the pulmonary vascular resistance continues to fall during infancy, the ultimate goal is to provide passive flow of venous return to the lungs. This reduces the volume load on the singe ventricle and establishes an in-series circulation.

Experience has shown that establishing this physiology is best done in stages to minimize mortality risk. The second-stage procedure is performed by connecting the superior vena cava (SVC) to the pulmonary artery (PA) and disconnecting the aortopulmonary communication or shunt (Fig. 5.8). The communication between the SVC and the PA is termed bidirectional Glenn or hemi-Fontan procedure, depending on the anatomic configuration. However, the physiology of both procedures is identical. Typically this operation is performed in infancy (4–6 months) once pulmonary vascular resistance drops to normal levels. Since the inferior vena cava (IVC) blood still returns to the RA and pumped back into the systemic circulation, there is mixing of oxygenated and unoxygenated blood, and children continue to have a degree of cyanosis, with a SpO_2 in the low 80s. However, an in-series circulation is established with this operation, which takes the volume load off the functionally univentricular heart.

Fontan procedure In early childhood (18 months–4 years), the process of returning most of the systemic venous return directly to pulmonary circulation is completed by redirecting the IVC blood to PA circulation. This is accomplished by one of several techniques available, but the outcome is aimed at having the systemic venous return passively circulate through a relative low-pressure pulmonary circulation and the single-ventricle perform the task of pumping oxygenated blood to the body (Fig. 5.9). Often a small fenestration is made to allow for limited right to left shunting in the event of transient increases in pulmonary vascular resistance. Children are expected to have near normal oxygen saturation after completion of Fontan procedure, although children with a fenestration may have oxygen saturations ranging from approximately 88 to 92%. This is the endpoint for surgical palliation of HLHS.

Even though an in-series circulation is established, the hemodynamics is far from being normal after completion of Fontan procedure. Unlike a normal cardiac cycle, these patients lack a pumping chamber delivering blood flow to the lungs, and instead the systemic venous blood enters passively into pulmonary circulation aided by central venous pressure and negative intrathoracic pressure generated by spontaneous respirations. Any increase in pulmonary vascular resistance will provide impediment to pulmonary blood flow and cardiac output.

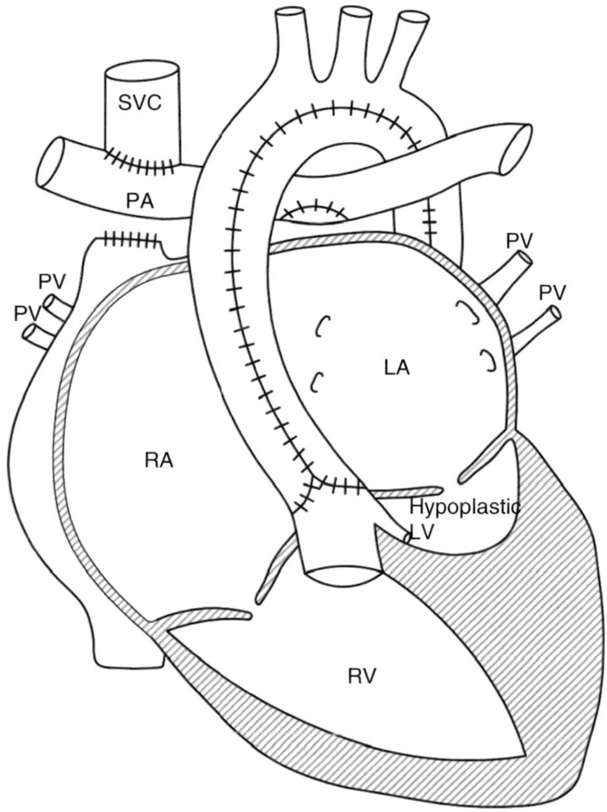

Fig. 5.8 Bidirectional Glenn procedure. Superior vena cava (SVC) is transected from the right atrium (RA) and connected to the pulmonary artery (PA). Blood from the SVC passively flows to the pulmonary arteries serving as the only source of blood flow for the pulmonary circulation. Oxygenated blood from the lungs mixes with deoxygenated blood from the inferior vena cava (IVC) and supplies the systemic circulation via neo-aorta. The Blalock-Taussig shunt that was inserted during the Norwood procedure is removed

HRHS In infants with HRHS, the right-sided structures of the heart (tricuspid valve, right ventricle, pulmonary valve, or pulmonary artery) are underdeveloped to a varying extent. Many variants of HRHS exist, but the clinician mainly needs to understand the abnormal hemodynamics before and after surgical interventions. In HRHS, the left ventricle is the single ventricle which must assume the responsibility of supplying blood flow to the lungs (Qp) and to the systemic circulation (Qs). In a portion of infants with HRHS, pulmonary blood flow is excessive if there is an unrestricted VSD. A PDA can be unnecessary and even counterproductive in these circumstances, as there can be excessive pulmonary blood flow. These patients present with pulmonary overcirculation, congestive heart failure, and decreased systemic perfusion. However, a large number of HRHS present with cyanosis at birth as the pulmonary blood flow is restricted. The degree of cyanosis depends on the extent of reduction in pulmonary blood flow. Cyanotic infants need institution of PGE1 prior to surgical intervention in order to establish sufficient Qp to ameliorate hypoxemia. Much like HLHS, infants with HRHS undergo a series of operations to convert the single-ventricle physiology parallel circulation to in-series circulation.

Pulmonary artery band procedure As mentioned earlier, a portion of patients with HRHS have excessive pulmonary blood flow through the VSD and normal

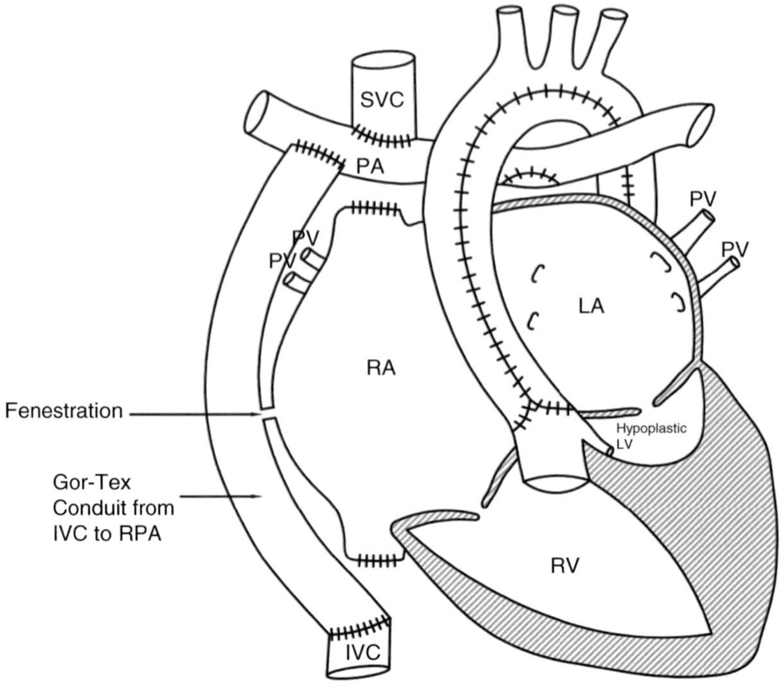

Fig. 5.9 Fontan procedure. Blood from the IVC is directed to enter the pulmonary arteries using a conduit. Blood from both SVC and IVC now passively flow to the pulmonary circulation. The pulmonary and systemic circulations are completely separated, and the circulation is now in-series. Oxygenated blood from lungs enters the atria and is pumped into the systemic circulation via a neo-aorta. A fenestration is sometimes created between the conduit and right atrium (RA) through which some of the deoxygenated blood can enter the RA in the event of elevated systemic venous pressure resulting in oxygen desaturation

pulmonary valve (tricuspid atresia type 1C). This results in excessive Qp at the expense of Qs. These patients are vulnerable to dangerous systemic hypoperfusion with a decrease in PVR which could occur by administration of oxygen. These patients require a pulmonary artery banding to (a) protect pulmonary vasculature from exposure to high systemic pressure and (b) to maintain satisfactory Qs by preventing excessive pulmonary blood flow from the single ventricle (Fig. 5.10).

Blalock-Taussig shunt Some infants with HRHS have reduced pulmonary blood flow and present with limited pulmonary blood flow and cyanosis. In order to maintain a reliable and consistent pulmonary blood flow, during the first few days of life a systemic-to-pulmonary artery (modified Blalock Taussig) shunt is placed, which is a synthetic vascular graft such as a GORE-TEX^{R} tube connecting the innominate artery and the right pulmonary artery, in essence serving as an artificial PDA in the early neonatal period. Infants are maintained on aspirin to prevent clotting of the shunt (Fig. 5.11).

Development of cyanosis and circulatory collapse are complications of a shunt malfunction and must be immediately recognized. It is important to promptly treat

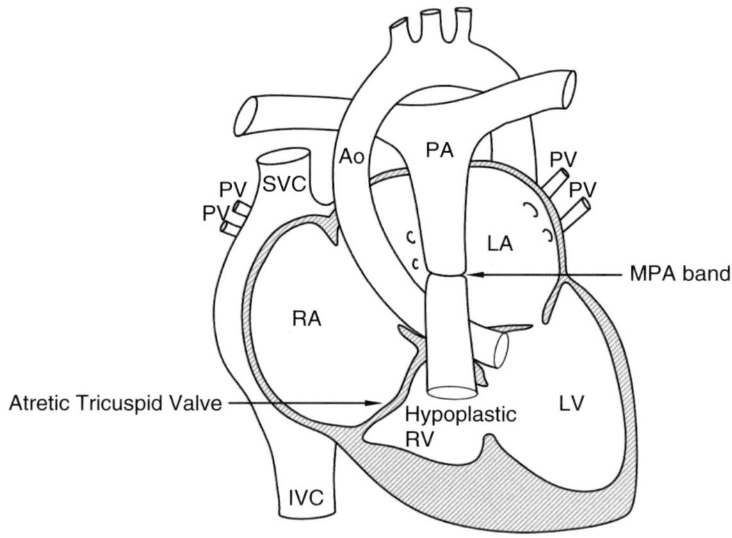

Fig. 5.10 Tricuspid atresia type 1c with a band across main pulmonary artery. A band is placed around main pulmonary artery to restrict pulmonary blood flow in order to have balanced circulations. *RA* right atrium, *LA* left atrium, *RV* right ventricle, *LV* left ventricle, *PA* pulmonary artery, *MPA* main pulmonary artery, *SVC* superior vena cava, *IVC* inferior vena cava, *PV* pulmonary vein, *Ao* aorta

any dehydration that develops as a complication of routine pediatric conditions such as gastroenteritis and febrile illnesses.

Glenn procedure Much like HLHS, in HRHS the pulmonary circulation and systemic circulation are separated by first performing the Glenn procedure which involves anastomosing the superior vena cava and pulmonary artery. This is performed around 4–6 months of age, when the pulmonary vascular resistance has fallen and pulmonary vasculature is able to receive passive flow of systemic venous blood from upper half of the body.

Fontan procedure The separation of pulmonary and systemic circulation is completed by adding the IVC drainage to the pulmonary circulation in early childhood (18 months–3 years) and is identical to that for HLHS patients.

Following Fontan completion, regardless of which ventricle is serving as the systemic ventricle patients are at risk of circulatory compromise when faced with conditions otherwise well tolerated by children with two functioning ventricles. An increase in PVR such as with pulmonary infections, hypoxia, acidosis, and cold stress offers considerable impediment to passive flow of systemic venous blood through the lungs causing decrease in cardiac output. Dehydration and intravascular volume depletion will decrease the central venous pressure necessary to maintain forward flow through the lungs. Even mild anemia can compromise oxygen delivery significantly in these patients. Maintaining normovolemia is always an ongoing priority. Similarly, elevated intrathoracic pressures such as with mechanical ventilation with high-inflation pressures and PEEP increase pulmonary vascular resistance and

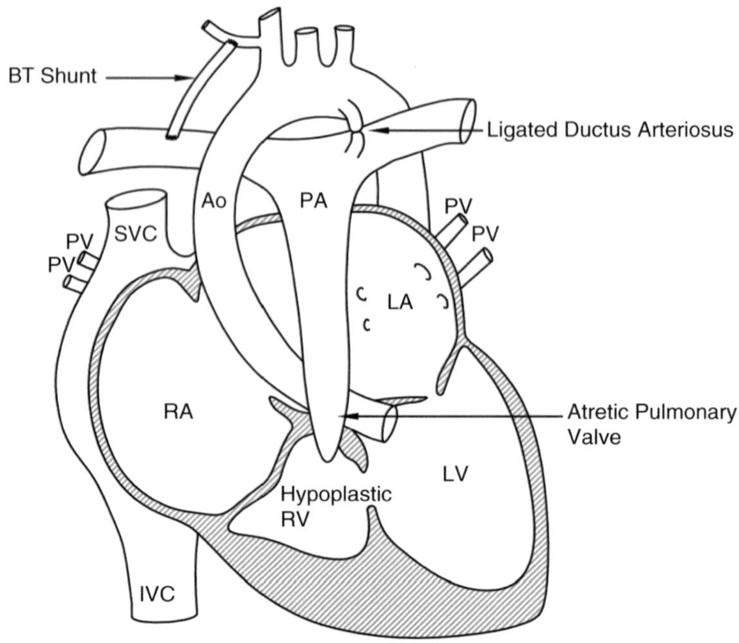

Fig. 5.11 Tricuspid atresia type 1a with Blalock-Taussig shunt. Systemic to pulmonary anastomosis between the right subclavian artery and the pulmonary artery is created to provide pulmonary blood flow. The ductus arteriosus is ligated. *RA* right atrium, *LA* left atrium, *RV* right ventricle, *LV* left ventricle, *PA* pulmonary artery, *SVC* superior vena cava, *IVC* inferior vena cava, *PV* pulmonary vein, *Ao* aorta

are poorly tolerated. If mechanical ventilation is needed, minimum inflation pressures and PEEP should be utilized to maintain minute ventilation and FRC. Oxygen, however, can be used as needed (without risk of dropping pulmonary vascular resistance), as these patients have an in-series circulation following the second-stage Glenn shunt.

Bibliography

1. Bonnet MJ, Lambert V, et al. Catheter-based interventions for modified Blalock-Taussig shunt obstruction. Pediatr Cardiol. 2015;36:835–41.
2. Lawrenson J, et al. Manipulating parallel circuits. Cardiol Young. 2003;13:316–22.
3. Mastropietro CW, Clark JA, Grenalde LM, et al. The patient with a single cardiac ventricle. Curr Pediatr Rev. 2012;8(3):253–76.
4. Cashen K, Gupta P, Lieh-Lai M, et al. Infants with single ventricle physiology in the ED: are physicians prepared? J Pediatr. 2011;159(2):273–7.
5. Jonas R. Comprehensive surgical management of congenital heart disease. New York: CRC Press; 2004.
6. Mavroudis C, Backer C. Pediatric cardiac surgery. 4th ed. Philadelphia: Mosby; 2013.
7. Khonsari S, Sintek CF. Cardiac surgery—safeguards and pitfalls in operative technique. 4th ed. Philadephia: Lipincott Williams & Wilkins; 2008.

6 Management of a Patient with Left-to-Right Shunt

Christian Bauerfeld, Ashok P. Sarnaik, and Kathleen Meert

Clinical Vignette

A 4-month-old girl presents to the emergency department with respiratory distress. Her mother reports that the infant had been well until about 2 weeks ago when she first noticed the infant had rapid breathing. The rapid breathing persists and is present even during sleep. The infant had been previously feeding well but now becomes sweaty and irritable when taking a bottle and takes less than 2 ounces at any one time. The mother is concerned that the infant is losing weight. Physical exam reveals a HR of 140/min, BP 70/45 mmHg, RR 60/min, and T 36.8 °C. There is a prominence of the left precordium and a palpable sternal lift. She has a blowing holosystolic murmur that is best heard along the left sternal border. SpO_2 is 95%. Her chest x-ray shows cardiomegaly and increased pulmonary vascular markings (Fig. 6.1).

Introduction

Acyanotic congenital heart defects with left-to-right shunt are among the most common congenital heart malformations; hence, the basic understanding of the pathology and pathophysiology of these lesions is important for the treating physician. Lesions with predominantly left-to-right shunt include ostium primum atrial septal defect (ASD), ostium secundum ASD, sinus venosus ASD, coronary sinus ASD, ventricular septal defects (VSDs), atrioventricular septal defects (AVSDs), patent ductus arteriosus (PDA), and aortopulmonary window (AP window). VSDs are the most common cardiac defect, accounting for approximately 25–30% of all congenital heart malformations.

C. Bauerfeld, M.D. (✉) • A. P. Sarnaik, M.D., F.A.A.P., F.C.C.M. • K. Meert, M.D.
Division of Pediatric Critical Care Medicine, Department of Pediatrics, Children's Hospital of Michigan, Wayne State University, Detroit, MI, USA
e-mail: cbauerfe@med.wayne.edu; asarnaik@med.wayne.edu; kmeert@med.wayne.edu

© Springer International Publishing AG, part of Springer Nature 2018

A. P. Sarnaik et al. (eds.), *Cardiac Emergencies in Children*,
https://doi.org/10.1007/978-3-319-73754-6_6

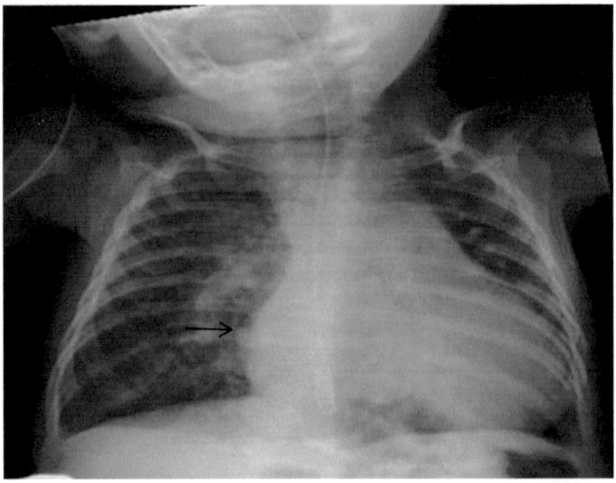

Fig. 6.1 A 4-month-old infant with cardiomegaly, right atrial bulge (shown by the arrow), and increased pulmonary vascularity that extends into upper lobes ("cephalization" of pulmonary vascularity)

Pathophysiology

The general pathophysiologic principle in these defects is the communication of the systemic and pulmonary circulation and the return of oxygenated blood into the lungs leading to volume loading of the right heart and lungs. The amount of shunting depends on several factors, including the size of the defect and the resistance and pressure properties of the pulmonary and systemic circulation. In general, the pressure and vascular resistance is lower, and the vascular compliance is higher in the pulmonary circulation. In small lesions, the flow across the defect will simply be restricted by the size of the communication, and the patients will not develop symptoms and signs of congestive heart failure. Small VSDs, for example, will spontaneously close in up to 80% of cases within the first 2 years of life.

If the lesions are nonrestrictive such as large VSDs, PDAs, or AP windows, significant left-to-right shunting may develop. Nevertheless, even with large defects, the degree of shunting can be highly variable and may increase or decrease with time depending on changes in size of the communication, changes in relative vascular resistance, or therapeutic interventions. The most dramatic change in pulmonary blood flow happens during the newborn period with a drastic decrease in pulmonary vascular resistance (PVR) when transitioning from the fetal to the postnatal circulation. Immediately after birth, the right ventricular (RV) wall is relatively thick and non-compliant, and the mean pulmonary artery pressures (MPAP) are close to the mean systemic pressures or even higher. Within the first 24–72 h of life, MPAP decreases to approximately 50% of systemic pressure. MPAP approximates adult levels (~15–18% of mean systemic artery pressure) at about 6 weeks of age. As a result, significant left-to-right shunting across the lesion may manifest only after the PVR has fallen sufficiently by 6–8 weeks of age or later.

Once the PVR falls, the left-to-right shunting increases substantially leading to increased pulmonary blood flow and pulmonary over-circulation. The initial effect on the right ventricle depends on the lesion. In large atrial septal defects, the left-to-right shunt at the atrial level occurs predominantly during diastole. This results in a diastolic volume overload and right atrium (RA) and RV enlargement. In a large VSD, however, left-to-right shunting occurs during systole. The RV is exposed to systemic pressures first leading to pressure overload. Only when PVR rises in response to increased pulmonary blood flow and pressures, RV dilatation occurs. Pulmonary over-circulation leads to increased pulmonary artery pressures, increased volume load on the left side of the heart, and increased left ventricular end-diastolic pressures, left atrial pressures, and eventually high pulmonary venous pressures. Pulmonary edema results from transudation of fluid into the interstitial and alveolar space from elevated pulmonary artery and pulmonary venous pressures. This can cause restrictive lung disease leading to respiratory failure. Systemic left ventricular output is diminished despite increased stroke volume and heart rate and increased total left ventricular output, as the ejected blood volume to the right side of the heart and the pulmonary circulation may exceed that entering the aorta by severalfold. The low systemic output leads to an increase in plasma catecholamine levels and to the activation of the renin-angiotensin system resulting in salt and water retention as well as peripheral vasoconstriction. Pulmonary vasodilators, such as supplemental oxygen or inhaled nitric oxide, will dramatically increase pulmonary blood flow and worsen congestive heart failure.

If large defects remain unrecognized and unrepaired, the increased pulmonary blood flow will eventually lead to pulmonary vascular disease with various degrees of medial, intimal, and adventitial vascular hypertrophy and fibrosis. The resulting increase in vascular resistance and pulmonary hypertension is generally fixed and unresponsive to pulmonary vasodilators such as supplemental oxygen or inhaled nitric oxide and will lead to reversal of the shunt resulting in cyanosis and progressive right ventricular failure (Eisenmenger syndrome). At this stage, surgical or interventional closure of the defect is contraindicated.

Determinants of Pulmonary Blood Flow (Qp) and Systemic Blood Flow (Qs)

In a normal heart, without any communication between right-sided and left-sided circulations, the circulation is referred to as being in-series. The entire systemic venous return to the right side of the heart must pass through the lungs, and the same amount must come back to the left side of the heart to be pumped to the body. Thus Qp is equal to Qs (Fig. 6.2).

When there is a connection between the left- and the right-sided circulations such as in an unrestricted VSD, the respective vascular resistances of systemic and pulmonary circulations determine the amount of blood flow going to the right side (Qp) and to the left side (Qs). Since the pulmonary vascular resistance (PVR) is lower than the systemic vascular resistance (SVR), some blood will be shunted from the left-sided to the right-sided circulation, and Qp will be greater than Qs (Fig. 6.3).

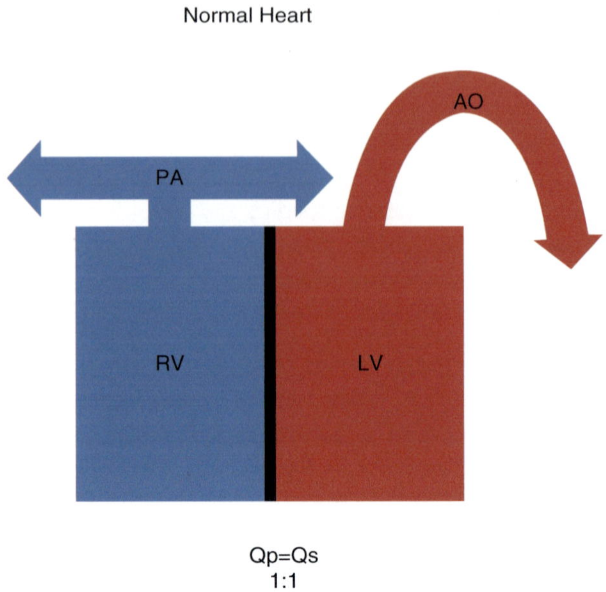

Fig. 6.2 In a normal heart with in-series circulation, Qp is equal to Qs since there is no communication between the right-sided and left-sided circulations

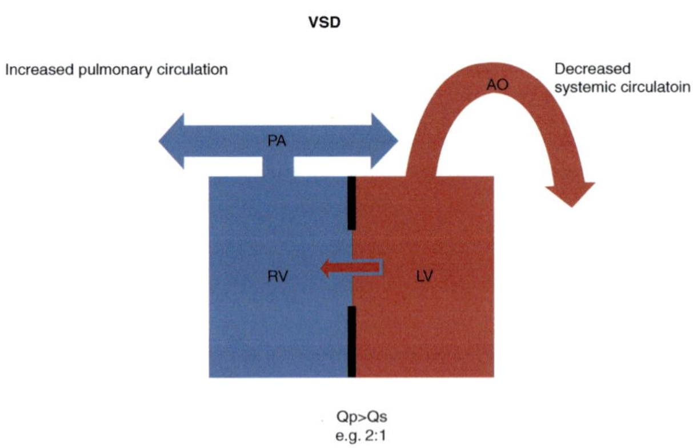

Fig. 6.3 With left-to-right shunt such as with a VSD, a portion of left ventricular stroke volume will be shunted to a lower resistance pulmonary circulation. Qp will therefore be greater than Qs

In a patient with an established left-to-right shunt, the Qp/Qs relationship may be affected by changing conditions such as intercurrent infection or therapeutic maneuvers.

A patient who is placed on supplemental oxygen or inhaled nitric oxide will have pulmonary vasodilatation and a decrease in PVR. Similarly, a patient who has had systemic vasoconstriction either due to dehydration or an administration of a vasoconstrictor will have an increase in SVR. In both these situations, Qp/Qs relationship may change acutely in favor of Qp and at the expense of Qs resulting in worsening pulmonary edema and systemic hypoperfusion (Fig. 6.4). Maintaining SpO_2 in the high 80s or low 90s should be sufficient for oxygenation without compromising systemic perfusion.

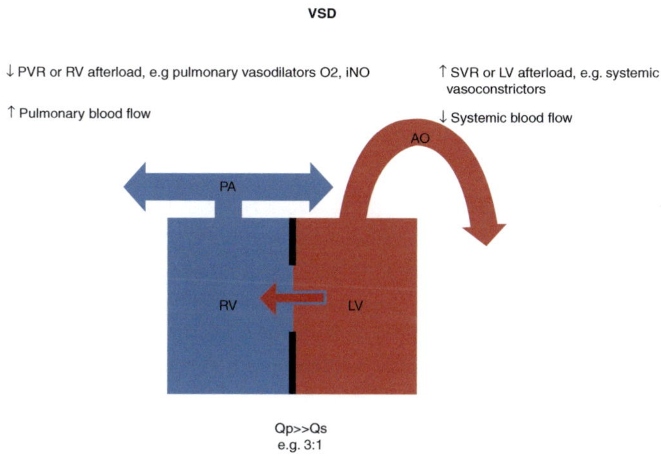

Fig. 6.4 Qp/Qs relationship in situation with decreased PVR and/or increased SVR

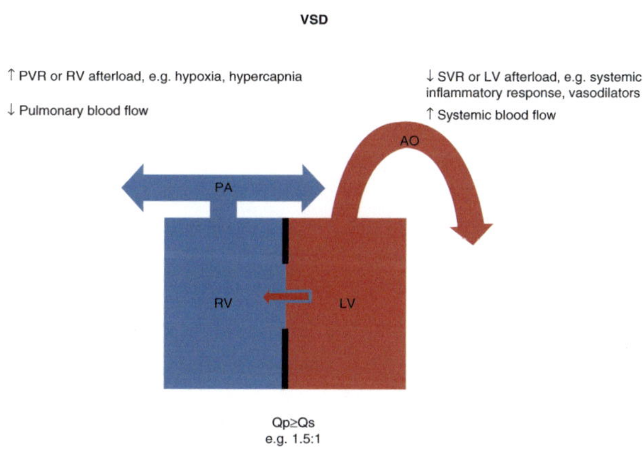

Fig. 6.5 Qp/Qs relationship in situation with increased PVR and/or decreased SVR

On the other hand, conditions resulting in increased PVR (respiratory infections, hypoxia, acidosis, hypothermia) and decreased SVR (systemic inflammatory response syndrome, vasodilators) will decrease Qp in favor of Qs (Fig. 6.5).

In some situations, the left-to-right shunt could change into being bidirectional and worsen hypoxemia. When taking care of children with significant left-to-right shunts, it is important for the clinician to be cognizant of changes in Qp/Qs brought about not only by the intercurrent illness but also by therapeutic interventions. Institution of positive end-expiratory pressure (PEEP) could decrease left-to-right shunt by increasing PVR, thereby improving systemic perfusion.

Calculation of Qp/Qs Ratio

In patients with left-to-right shunts such as with ASD or VSD, the proportion of cardiac output entering the pulmonary circulation (Qp) and the systemic circulation (Qs) can be estimated by application of the modified Fick equation.

Cardiac output (CO) = Oxygen consumption (VO_2) ÷ (C_AO_2 − C_VO_2), where C_AO_2 is content of oxygen in arterial blood and C_VO_2 is content of oxygen in mixed venous blood. Since most of the oxygen present in the blood is accounted for by saturation of hemoglobin at physiologic levels of FiO_2 (≤0.3), oxygen content may be replaced by % of hemoglobin saturated with O_2. Therefore, CO or blood flow (Q) is inversely proportional to the difference in hemoglobin-O_2 saturations in arterial and venous blood, respectively. Therefore, Qp/Qs = (S_AO_2 − S_VO_2) ÷ ($S_{PV}O_2$ − $S_{PA}O_2$) where S_AO_2, S_VO_2, $S_{PV}O_2$, and $S_{PA}O_2$ are hemoglobin-O_2 saturations in arterial, mixed venous, pulmonary venous, and pulmonary arterial blood, respectively. S_VO_2 is often determined in the superior vena cava, and $S_{PV}O_2$ is assumed to be 98% when breathing $FiO_2 \leq 0.3$.

Qp/Qs can be calculated by data obtained during cardiac catheterization. In a child with a VSD, if S_VO_2 is 72%, $S_{PA}O_2$ is 88%, and S_AO_2 is 97%, the Qp/Qs can be estimated as (97 − 72) ÷ (98–88) = 25 ÷ 10 = 2.5, and Qp/Qs = 2.5:1.

Clinical Presentation

The clinical presentation of left-to-right shunt largely depends on the type and size of the defect. Symptoms usually occur earlier in life in patients with high-pressure communications such as VSDs and much later in life in patients with low-pressure communications such as ASDs. Infants with a large VSD or PDA can develop symptoms in the first weeks of life, once PVR falls and pulmonary blood flow increases. Symptoms of heart failure include tachycardia, tachypnea, increased work of breathing, and wheezing (cardiac asthma) resulting from pulmonary edema and peribronchial cuffing. These symptoms can lead to misdiagnosis as respiratory conditions such as asthma, bronchiolitis, or pneumonia. Sweating, poor feeding, poor weight gain, as well as recurrent pulmonary infections are other signs of significant congestive heart failure. Chest x-ray often shows signs of pulmonary edema and cardiomegaly.

Specific Lesions

VSD

Patients with a small VSD are usually asymptomatic and may present during a regular physical exam with a loud, harsh holosystolic murmur at the left sternal border. These defects do not lead to increased pulmonary blood flow as they only allow minimal blood flow across the septum due to their restrictive nature. They have a high rate of spontaneous closure; up to 30–50% will close by 2 years of age, with small muscular VSDs showing a closure rate up to 80%.

Patients with large VSDs may present with feeding difficulties, diaphoresis during feeding, sweaty and clammy skin, poor weight gain, and failure to thrive. Tachypnea and dyspnea as well as tachycardia as signs of left-sided ventricular failure and pulmonary venous congestion may develop. Wheezing (cardiac asthma) as a result of pulmonary edema and peribronchial cuffing may result in misdiagnosis as asthma, reactive airway disease, or bronchiolitis. Patients may have a prominence of the left precordial thorax (voussure cardiaque) and a leftward-displaced apical impulse. The systolic murmur of a large defect is usually not very prominent or may be entirely absent. Long-standing left ventricular failure eventually may involve the right ventricle as well with signs of an enlarged liver and peripheral edema. If large defects remain unrecognized and unrepaired, pulmonary hypertension will eventually become fixed and lead to reversal of the shunt and progressive cyanosis.

Chest x-ray findings in patients with VSD and significant left-to-right shunt typically show biventricular and left atrial enlargement. There may be an enlarged pulmonary artery segment and increased pulmonary vascular markings. In severe cases with congestive heart failure, pulmonary edema and bilateral pleural effusions may be present (Fig. 6.1). An ECG may show signs of biventricular hypertrophy (Fig. 6.6).

Ostium Secundum ASD

Patients rarely present early in life with congestive heart failure or may be entirely asymptomatic throughout their life. In older children, a mild degree of exercise intolerance might be present. Auscultation reveals a systolic murmur at the left sternal border. This murmur is not caused by the defect but by an increased flow through

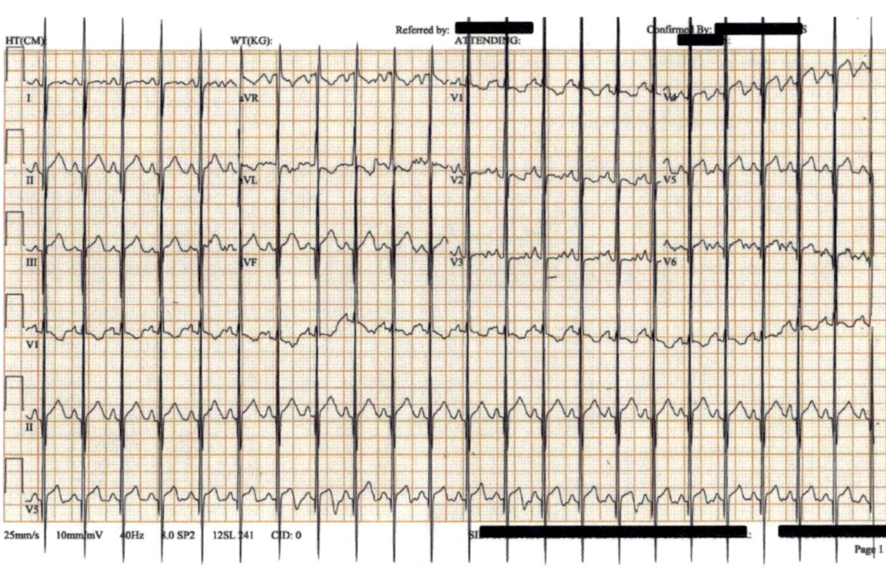

Fig. 6.6 ECG from a child with large VSD showing a normal sinus rhythm and biventricular hypertrophy

a normal pulmonary valve leading to a relative pulmonary stenosis. The second heart sound is split and often fixed.

Chest x-ray in patients with ostium secundum ASD may be normal or show signs of right atrial and ventricular enlargement best appreciated in the lateral view. The pulmonary artery segment can be enlarged, and an increase in pulmonary vascularity may be seen.

AVSD

AVSDs comprise a spectrum of anatomic defects including ostium primum ASD with or without mitral valve cleft and complete AV canal defects with contiguous atrial and ventricular defects accompanied usually by AV valve abnormalities. As many as 25% of patients with Trisomy 21 have an AV canal defect. Patients with ostium primum defects are generally asymptomatic; those with larger shunts have a similar presentation as patients with ostium secundum defects. If there is an additional mitral valve cleft with a leak, there is an apical holosystolic murmur caused by the mitral valve insufficiency.

Patients with complete AV canal may have a degree of right-to-left shunting, especially in the newborn period when pulmonary vascular resistance is high and may present with mild cyanosis. Large shunts can rapidly lead to congestive heart failure, failure to thrive, recurrent pulmonary infections, and hepatomegaly. Heart sounds are characterized by a fixed split second heart sound, a diastolic murmur at the left sternal border secondary to an increased flow across the AV valves and a systolic murmur at the apex if mitral valve insufficiency is present.

Chest x-ray findings in patients with AVSD typically show cardiomegaly, large pulmonary artery, and increased pulmonary vascular markings (Fig. 6.7).

An ECG of a complete AV canal defect typically shows a left axis deviation, a right ventricular conduction delay, and signs of biventricular or isolated right ventricular hypertrophy (Fig. 6.8).

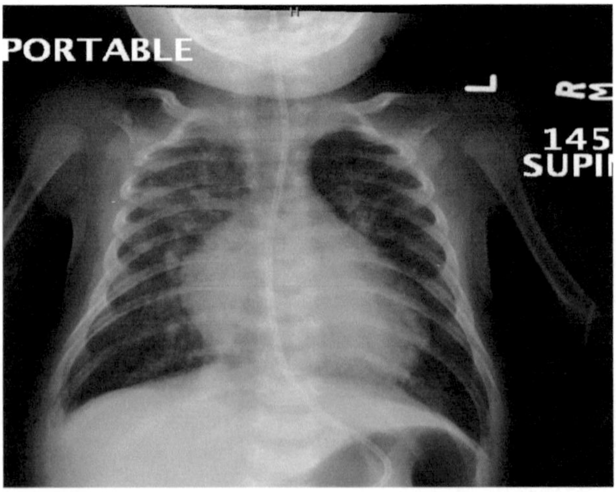

Fig. 6.7 A 1-month-old infant with complete atrioventricular canal. Note bulging right heart border (right atrium), cardiomegaly, increased pulmonary vascularity, and hyperinflated lungs

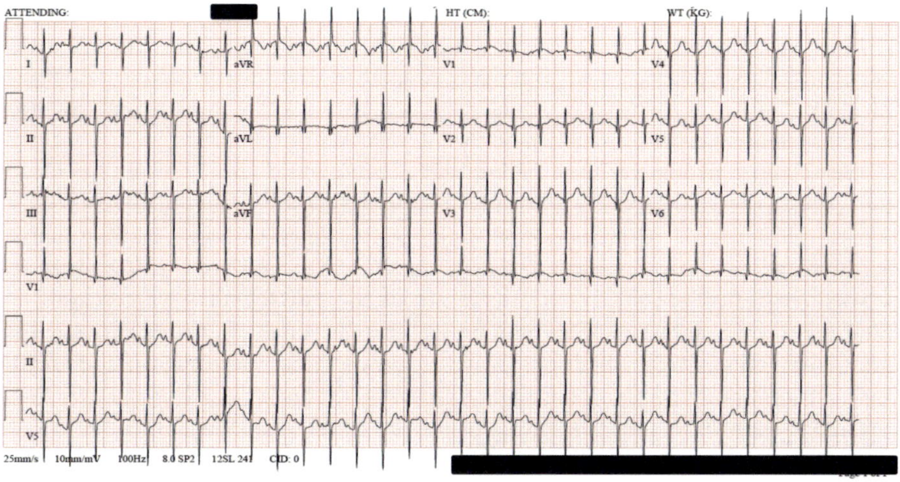

Fig. 6.8 ECG from a child with complete atrioventricular canal showing sinus tachycardia, left axis deviation, and right ventricular hypertrophy

PDA

Small PDAs are usually asymptomatic. A large PDA will present with congestive heart failure similar to a large VSD. The peripheral arterial pulses are bounding with a wide pulse pressure secondary to runoff of blood in diastole into the pulmonary artery. The typical murmur is a continuous systolic-diastolic, machinelike murmur in the left second intercostal space.

Chest x-ray in patients with small PDA may be normal. With large PDA shunts, cardiomegaly and increased pulmonary vascular markings may be seen.

Treatment

Many patients with left-to-right shunts present with symptoms such as tachypnea, dyspnea, and wheezing (cardiac asthma) leading to misdiagnosis as a respiratory illness, especially during winter months when respiratory illnesses peak. It is important to consider a congenital heart defect in these patients to avoid potentially harmful interventions although it is not uncommon that intercurrent viral infections such as RSV can complicate an underlying cardiac condition.

Excessive fluid resuscitation should be avoided in patients with left-to-right shunts, especially those that have signs of congestive heart failure, pulmonary edema, or pleural effusions on chest radiograph. Some patients with left-to-right shunt may have a degree of intravascular volume depletion secondary to poor enteral intake and increased insensible fluid losses from tachypnea and sweating. These patients may benefit from an increase in preload, but initial fluid boluses should not exceed 5–10 mL/kg, after which the patient should be carefully reassessed.

Indiscriminate oxygen therapy should also be avoided. Oxygen is a potent pulmonary vasodilator and may lead to a decrease in pulmonary vascular resistance hence increasing shunting and pulmonary blood flow. This will result in an increase in pulmonary over-circulation, worsening congestive heart failure, and compromised systemic perfusion. Such patients are pink and in shock.

Severe decompensated heart failure will require admission to an intensive care unit and advanced monitoring. Positive pressure ventilation, either invasive or noninvasive, is beneficial in patients with pulmonary edema and low cardiac output. Positive end-expiratory pressure (PEEP), ideally with a FiO2 of 0.21 (to avoid the vasodilatory effect of oxygen), will decrease pulmonary circulation by increasing the afterload on the right ventricle, limiting left-to-right shunting, and improving systemic circulation. PEEP will also improve lung compliance, decrease work of breathing and total body oxygen consumption, causing improvement in respiratory and metabolic acidosis. In addition, positive pressure ventilation reduces the afterload on the left ventricle, hence improving left ventricular systemic output. The ideal transcutaneous oxygen saturation in these patients ranges between 88 and 94%.

Inotropic and/or vasoactive agents may be indicated based on the physical examination and can be used to improve systemic perfusion or hypotension. Most commonly, catecholamines, phosphodiesterase inhibitors, and nitric oxide donors such as nitroprusside as well as diuretics are used.

Catecholamines have a quick onset of action. They are easy to titrate due to their rapid elimination rate. Catecholamines increase myocardial oxygen consumption and carry the risk for significant tachyarrhythmias.

Dopamine is an endogenous catecholamine and acts in a dose-dependent fashion on dopaminergic, β-adrenergic, and α-adrenergic receptors. At low to moderate doses (3–10 mcg/kg/min), it stimulates β-adrenergic receptors; at doses >10 mcg/kg/min, α-adrenergic stimulation increases with peripheral vasoconstriction and increased systemic vascular resistance.

Dobutamine is a synthetic catecholamine with β_1 and β_2 receptor activity leading to an increase in heart rate, positive inotropy, and vasodilation of systemic arterial resistance vessels resulting in an increase in stroke volume and cardiac output.

Epinephrine is an endogenous catecholamine that stimulates β_1 and β_2 receptor as well as α-adrenergic receptors in a dose-dependent fashion. At low doses, epinephrine increases heart rate and contractility and reduces afterload on the left ventricle through β_2 receptor stimulation and systemic vasodilation. At higher doses α-receptor stimulation predominates.

Milrinone is a phosphodiesterase III inhibitor (PDE III). It increases intracellular cAMP by inhibiting its breakdown through PDE III. This increases myocardial contractility and lusitropy (myocardial relaxation during diastole) as well as vasodilation in the pulmonary and systemic arteries. It has significantly longer half-life than catecholamines and is mainly cleared by the kidneys making a dose adjustment necessary in renal failure. Milrinone needs to be used with caution in the setting of large left-to-right shunts, as it may worsen pulmonary overcirculation due to its pulmonary vasodilatory effect.

Table 6.1 Commonly used drugs in congestive heart failure

Agent	Dose range
Dopamine	3–10–(20) mcg/kg/min
Dobutamine	3–20 mcg/kg/min
Epinephrine	0.03–0.2 mcg/kg/min
Milrinone	0.25–1 mcg/kg/min
Nitroprusside	0.5–10 mcg/kg/min
Nitroglycerine	0.25–20 mcg/kg/min
Furosemide	0.5–1 mg/kg/dose
Aldactone	1–3 mg/kg/day PO divided twice daily

Nitroprusside and nitroglycerin are both nitric oxide donors and have a dose-dependent dilatory effect on venous capacitance and arterial resistance vessels. If there is congestive heart failure in the context of arterial hypertension and high systemic vascular resistance, the patient may benefit from afterload reduction through these drugs. Their half-life is very short, and they are easy to titrate. Prolonged use and high doses of nitroprusside are associated with cyanide toxicity, especially in the presence of renal failure.

Diuretics are a mainstay of treatment in patients with heart failure and signs of fluid overload. Usually fast-acting loop diuretics are used if acute and rapid diuresis is required. Electrolyte abnormalities with diuretic use are very common and include hyponatremia, hypokalemia, hypomagnesemia, and hypocalcemia.

Furosemide is the most commonly used loop diuretic. Its fast onset of action results in a rapid reduction of circulating blood volume, a decrease in cardiac preload and ventricular filling pressures, as well as a decrease in pulmonary fluid overload. *Thiazide diuretics* are slower in onset and are less potent than loop diuretics. They are usually used together with loop diuretics and significantly increase their effect. *Spironolactone* is an aldosterone inhibitor and weak diuretic. It is usually used in combination with furosemide or thiazide diuretics for its potassium sparing effect. Commonly used drugs and their dose range are summarized in Table 6.1.

Pearls and Pitfalls

- Large left-to-right shunts can quickly lead to congestive heart failure.
- Congestive heart failure can mimic respiratory disease.
- Inappropriate fluid therapy can lead to worsening of congestive heart failure.
- Inappropriate oxygen therapy can lead to worsening left-to-right shunt, decrease in systemic cardiac output, and worsening heart failure.
- Undetected and untreated large left-to-right shunts lead to pulmonary hypertension and irreversible pulmonary vascular disease (Eisenmenger syndrome).

Multiple-Choice Questions

1. A 2-month-old girl presents to the emergency department with respiratory distress. Her mother reports that the infant had been well until about 2 weeks ago when she first noticed the infant had rapid breathing. The rapid breathing persists and is present during sleep. The infant had previously fed well but now becomes sweaty and irritable when taking a bottle and takes less than 2 ounces at any one time. The mother is concerned that the infant is losing weight. Physical examination reveals a HR of 140/min, BP 80/45 mmHg, RR 60/min, and temperature 36.8 °C. There is a prominence of the left precordium and a palpable sternal lift. She has a blowing holosystolic murmur that is best heard along the left sternal border. SpO_2 is 95%. Her chest x-ray shows cardiomegaly and increased pulmonary vascular markings. Which of the following is the most likely explanation for this child's symptoms?
   (A) Right-to-left shunt
   (B) Left-to-right shunt
   (C) Left ventricular outflow tract obstruction
   (D) Right ventricular outflow tract obstruction
   (E) Intermittent supraventricular tachycardia
   Answer: B
2. A 13-year-old girl presents with a complaint of fatigue and shortness of breath with moderate exercise. She has no significant past medical history. Her exercise intolerance was only recently noted after joining a neighborhood volleyball team. Her HR is 110/min, RR 20/min, BP 115/65 mmHg, and T 36.9 °C. On physical exam, her second heart sound is found to be widely split and fixed in all phases of respiration. A systolic ejection murmur is heard at the left middle and upper sternal border. Her chest x-ray shows enlargement of the right atrium and ventricle. Her ECG shows a right axis deviation. Which of the following is the most likely cause of her murmur?
   (A) Turbulent flow across an ASD
   (B) Turbulent flow across a VSD
   (C) Persistent flow through a patent ductus arteriosus
   (D) Increased flow across the aortic valve
   (E) Increased flow across the pulmonary valve
   Answer: E
3. A 12-year-old girl presents to the emergency department with shortness of breath that gets worse with physical activity. She complains of frequent headaches and sometimes feels dizzy. The mother also noted the girl has a progressive swelling of her feet and lower legs, and that at times she has a bluish discoloration of her lips. She was diagnosed with a hole in her heart as an infant but was told it will close on its own. She has not had any follow-up for this condition. Physical examination reveals a well-nourished child, central cyanosis, digital clubbing, and pitting edema of both lower extremities. She is tachypneic, with a HR of 110/min, RR 32/min, BP 110/65 mmHg, and T 37.0 °C. There is no murmur but a loud single second heart sound. The liver is enlarged. Her hemoglobin is 18.2 g/

dL and hematocrit 65%. Her chest x-ray shows an enlarged right ventricle, prominent central pulmonary arteries, and pruning of the peripheral pulmonary arteries. Which of the following best explains this child's symptoms?
(A) Eisenmenger syndrome
(B) Pulmonary atresia
(C) Transposition of the great arteries
(D) Tricuspid atresia
(E) Single ventricle with aortopulmonary collaterals
Answer: A

4. A 2-week-old male infant with history of 36-week gestational age at birth presents to the emergency department with tachypnea. His mother reports that he initially fed well when discharged from the hospital after birth but for the past several days seems to become tired with feeding and takes less than an ounce at any one time. On physical exam he is tachypneic, with a HR of 140/min, RR 60/min, BP 70/45 mmHg, and T 36.8 °C. The infant is noted to have a hyperactive precordium, bounding peripheral arterial pulses, and a continuous machinelike murmur along the left sternal border. His chest x-ray shows a moderately enlarged heart, a prominent pulmonary artery, and increased intrapulmonary vascular markings. Which of the following is the most likely diagnosis?
(A) ASD
(B) Aortic insufficiency
(C) AV canal defect
(D) Patent ductus arteriosus
(E) Pulmonary branch stenosis
Answer: D

5. A 15-month-old male presents to the emergency department with weakness, poor feeding, failure to thrive, tachypnea, and a nonproductive cough. He recently moved as a refugee from a country with poor health care resources and has been living with his mother in the US for 3 months. He has had no fevers or sick contacts. Physical exam reveals a HR of 142/min, BP 95/45 mmHg, RR 60/min, and T 36.8 °C, and SpO_2 is 94%. He is awake and alert and tachypneic with mild wheezing and retractions. He has marked hypotonia, almond-shaped eyes with epicanthal folds, and a large protruding tongue. He has an active precordium and a pulmonary ejection murmur as well as a holosystolic murmur at the apex radiating to the axilla. His liver is enlarged. Pulses are equal on all four extremities. His chest x-ray shows cardiomegaly and increased pulmonary vascular markings. ECG shows a left axis deviation. Which one of the following is the most appropriate therapy?
(A) Inhaled albuterol
(B) Inhaled nitric oxide
(C) Furosemide
(D) Ceftriaxone
(E) Supplemental oxygen
Answer: C

Bibliography

1. Bernstein D. Acyanotic congenital heart disease: left-to-right shunt. In: Nelson textbook of pediatrics. 20th ed. Philadelphia: Elsevier; 2016, p. 2189–99.
2. Bernstein D. Heart failure. In: Nelson textbook of pediatrics. 20th ed. Philadelphia: Elsevier; 2016, p. 2282–7.
3. Rossano JW, Price JF, Nelson DP. Treatment of heart failure: medical management. In: Roger's textbook of pediatric critical care. 5th ed. Philadelphia: Wolters Kluwer; 2016, p. 1170–87.
4. Silberbach M, Hannon D. Presentation of congenital heart disease in the neonate and young infant. Pediatr Rev. 2007;28(4):123–31.
5. van der Linde D, Yap SC, van Dijk AP, Budts W, Pieper PG, van der Burgh PH, Mulder BJ, Witsenburg M, Cuypers JA, Lindemans J, Takkenberg JJ, Roos-Hesselink JW. Birth prevalence of congenital heart disease worldwide. Am J Cardiol. 2011;108(2):265–71.
6. Hoffman JI, Kaplan S. The incidence of congenital heart disease. J Am Coll Cardiol. 2002;39(12):1890–900.
7. Schweigmann U, Meierhofer C. Strategies for the treatment of acute heart failure in children. Minerva Cardioangiol. 2008;56(3):321–33.
8. Tume SC, Goldberg J, Molossi S, Bronicki RA. Pharmacologic approach to heart failure in children. Curr Cardiol Rev. 2016;12(2):117–20.
9. Emmanouilides GC, Moss AJ, Duffie ER Jr, Adams FH. Pulmonary arterial pressure changes in human newborn infants from birth to 3 days of age. J Pediatr. 1964;65:327–33.

Check for updates

Cardiac Pharmacology

7

Jeff Clark and Brad Tilford

Case 1

A previously healthy 14-month-old girl presents to the emergency department with rapid breathing and irritability. She has had several loose stools and poor oral intake for the past 2 days. She began breathing fast and became fussier today. On examination, she is alert but looks fatigued. She does respond to parents but is otherwise listless. Her heart rate is 174 beats/min, blood pressure is 74/55 mmHg, respiratory rate is 58/min, and pulse oximetry is 95%. Her temperature is 37.1°C. She is in moderate respiratory distress with occasional grunting. Her extremities are cool and mottled with 1+ distal pulses. Her mucous membranes are dry with poor skin turgor. Although she is very tachycardic, a gallop rhythm is suspected. Her liver is palpable 2 cm below the right costal margin. Her abdomen is soft and non-tender.

A capillary blood gas and chest radiograph are obtained. The blood gas reveals pH of 7.28, PCO_2 of 25 torr, PO_2 of 55 torr, and bicarbonate of 15 mEq/L. Lactate is 4.9 mmol/L. Chest radiograph shows bilateral mild diffuse interstitial opacities suggestive of interstitial edema, and cardiac size is normal.

The first step in stabilization of this patient is:

A. Initiation of noninvasive ventilation
B. Establishment of IV access
C. Obtaining additional information from an echocardiogram
D. Afterload reduction
E. Diuretic therapy

J. Clark, M.D. (✉) • B. Tilford, M.D.
Division of Critical Care Medicine, Department of Pediatrics, Children's Hospital of Michigan, Detroit, MI, USA

Wayne State University School of Medicine, Detroit, MI, USA
e-mail: jclark@med.wayne.edu; btilford@med.wayne.edu

© Springer International Publishing AG, part of Springer Nature 2018

A. P. Sarnaik et al. (eds.), *Cardiac Emergencies in Children*,
https://doi.org/10.1007/978-3-319-73754-6_7

Principles of Pharmacology for Circulatory Support

One of the primary modes of support for a child with cardiovascular emergency and shock is pharmacologic. Although much data exist regarding pharmacologic support of children, the basis of most pharmacologic decisions rests in our understanding of pediatric cardiovascular physiology. The circulatory system of children undergoes significant evolution from antenatal to postnatal life and maturation to adulthood. Many of the principles of pharmacologic treatment for children with circulatory dysfunction and shock have their basis in developmental circulatory physiology and can be described using this understanding.

Optimization of Cardiovascular Function and Prevention of Shock

Optimum cardiovascular function maximizes oxygen delivery while minimizing cardiac work. This principle holds true for normal as well as abnormal cardiovascular function. In the setting of cardiovascular dysfunction, oxygen delivery is maintained by compensation in one or more of the factors that determine oxygen delivery. These factors are described by the oxygen delivery equation:

$$\textbf{Oxygen delivery}\left(\text{OD}\right) = \text{cardiac output}\left(\text{CO}\right) \times \text{arterial oxygen content}\left(\text{CaO}_2\right).$$

$$\textbf{CO}\left(\textbf{L}/\text{min}\right) = \text{strokevolume} \times \text{heart rate}$$

Stroke volume is proportional to **preload**, **inotropy,** and **afterload**

$$\textbf{CaO}_2\left(\textbf{mL}/\textbf{dL}\right) = \left[\text{hemoglobin concentration}\left(\text{gm}/\text{dL}\right) \times \%\text{saturation} \times 1.34\right] + \left[0.003 \times \text{PaO}_2\right]$$

Each gram of fully saturated Hb carries 1.34 mL of O_2.
$PaO_2 \times 0.003$ = amount (mL) of dissolved O_2 in 100 mL of plasma.
Note that CO is conventionally measured as L/min and CaO_2 is measured as mL/dL. Therefore, OD (mL/min) = CO × (CaO_2 × 10).

The focus of much of our pharmacologic manipulation of cardiac output and oxygen delivery is by targeting preload, inotropy, and afterload.

Preload

Optimum preload is essential for ensuring adequate oxygen delivery in the setting of cardiovascular dysfunction. Preload is defined as the end-diastolic volume of the ventricle. Because this volume is not practical to measure clinically, end-diastolic pressure is used as surrogate marker (e.g., central venous pressure for the right ventricle). The relationship of preload to stroke volume is described by the length-tension relationship curve depicted in Fig. 7.1 (Frank-Starling relationship): if inotropy and

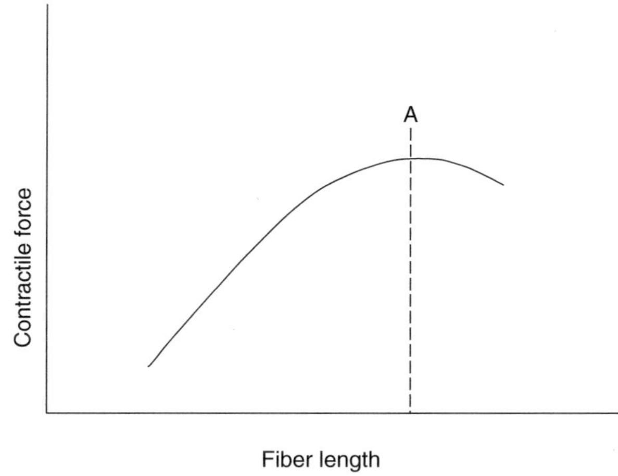

Fig. 7.1 Length-tension relationship. As myofiber length increases during diastole, an increase in force generation during contraction occurs, up to a point (A), beyond which an increase in length results in a decrease force of contraction

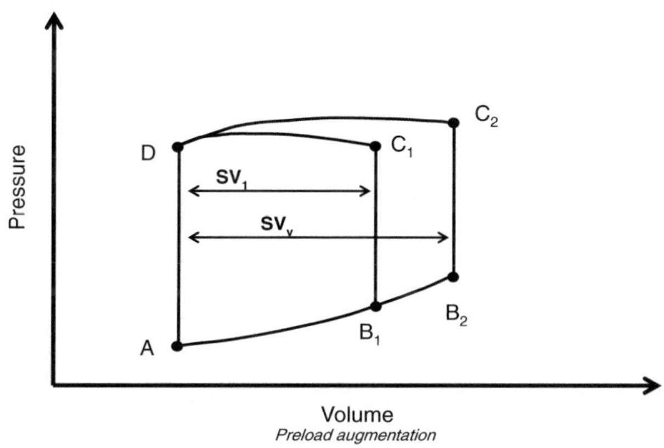

Fig. 7.2 Pressure-volume loop—preload. As end-diastolic volume increases along the *x*-axis from point B_1 to B_2, the tension generated during systole increases such that end-systolic volume returns to the same point, D, thereby increasing stroke volume (SV_2). Increasing diastolic filling further results in increased slope of the diastolic filling curve and results in little additional increase in stroke volume. At significant overfilling, the force of contraction and therefore stroke volume will decrease

afterload are constant, then, as end-diastolic fiber length of the ventricle increases, generation of tension and therefore stroke volume increases, to a point, beyond which it plateaus and then falls [1].

The results of increases in preload are increased end-diastolic fiber length and subsequent increased force of contraction. This leads to increased stroke volume. This is illustrated diagrammatically by the ventricular pressure-volume loop shown in Fig. 7.2.

Manipulation of inadequate preload is relatively straightforward. Increasing circulating volume is usually enough to increase preload. However, pharmacologic manipulation of preload is also possible, specifically by administering vasoactive substances that alter vascular capacitance. The vast majority of vascular volume resides in the venous system, and changes in venous tone can significantly alter preload. In addition, vascular volume is under significant hormonal control by substances such as antidiuretic hormone (ADH), vasopressin, atrial natriuretic peptide (ANP), angiotensin II, and other circulating compounds [2].

The goal of optimizing preload is to maximize diastolic filling without overfilling, thereby maximizing stroke volume. Clinically, optimal preload is difficult to determine with accuracy. Normal CVP is commonly reported as 6–8 mmHg and is associated with adequate ventricular filling in healthy hearts. As CVP increases from low to normal, end-diastolic volume is increasing toward an optimal amount. However, optimal end-diastolic pressure is determined by ventricular compliance, which can be significantly altered with congenital or acquired heart disease. Compliance is the relationship between pressure and volume and is defined as.

$$\textbf{Compliance}(C) = \text{change in volume}(\Delta V) / \text{change in pressure}(\Delta P).$$

In normally functioning ventricles, an increase in volume that is not associated with an increase in pressure is indicative of high (or good) compliance and indicates that the ventricle is on the shallow portion of the pressure-volume relationship curve (Fig. 7.2). The ventricle is accepting more volume without a significant increase in pressure and therefore may not be optimally filled. If CVP is already above normal, the ventricle may be overfilled or may have significantly low compliance. However, abnormal ventricles, which are either thickened or have abnormally low compliance due to ischemia or restrictive physiology, may require abnormally high filling pressures to achieve optimal filling and may have very narrow transition from optimal filling to over-distention [1]. For example, patients with tetralogy of Fallot have abnormally thickened right ventricles and require filling pressures that are often in the 15–20 mmHg range to achieve optimal filling. Because systolic function is usually normal in these patients, overfilling is difficult, and administration of excess fluid is often better tolerated. Patients in acute and chronic heart failure also have increased filling requirements due to diastolic dysfunction. Since systolic function is also commonly abnormal in these patients, overfilling is often poorly tolerated, and it is often challenging to determine what constitutes optimal filling. In addition, patients who have chronic heart failure and are chronically fluid overloaded may already have ventricular over-distention on presentation. This is more common in adults who develop uncompensated heart failure. These patients may benefit primarily from a decrease in preload by decreasing intravascular volume. This may be accomplished using venodilators and diuretics. However, this clinical scenario is much less common in children, and the use of this strategy should be used with caution since many patients with congenital and acquired heart disease rely on adequate intravascular volume to maintain adequate cardiac output.

Answer: B—Establishing adequate intravenous access is a crucial first step to correcting shock or near shock states with the goal of maximizing preload and then adding inotropic agents as needed.

Inotropy

Inotropy is the inherent state of contractility of the ventricle, independent of preload or afterload. The primary contractile element of the muscle is the sarcomere, and methods aimed at improving contractility exert their effects on one or more elements of the sarcomere. It is composed of overlapping thick and thin filaments of actin and myosin, along with modulating proteins such as tropomyosin.

Bundles of actin filaments are attached to each other and extend in opposite directions. They interdigitate with thick myosin filaments. Interaction of the myosin heads with actin is prevented by tropomyosin filament which is wound around the myosin. Contraction occurs when intracellular calcium attaches to the troponin C component of the tropomyosin complex, causing a conformational change that allows the myosin chains to bind to actin [2]. Once binding occurs, a conformation change in the myosin heads causes the actin filament to be pulled along the myosin chain, shortening the sarcomere and causing muscle contraction. Once the conformational change in myosin head occurs, ADP is released and ATP is rebound, allowing disconnection of the myosin head from the actin and subsequent reconnection to actin if enough calcium remains. Once calcium concentrations decline to low enough concentrations, troponin becomes unbound, allowing tropomyosin to again inhibit actin-myosin interaction.

Intracellular calcium therefore is the link between excitation of the muscle cell and contraction and is very tightly regulated. In mature myocytes, intracellular calcium available for excitation-contraction coupling is stored in the sarcoplasmic reticulum. Depolarization of the myocyte results in release of calcium and increase in cytosolic calcium concentration tenfold. Calcium is then re-sequestered in the sarcoplasmic reticulum in an ATP-dependent process. The peak cytosolic calcium concentration and duration of calcium release prior to re-sequestration determine the strength of myocyte contraction. All drugs that increase the force of contraction act by increasing either the concentration or duration of cytosolic calcium during depolarization [3]. The clinical effect of this can be represented by the PV loop in Fig. 7.3.

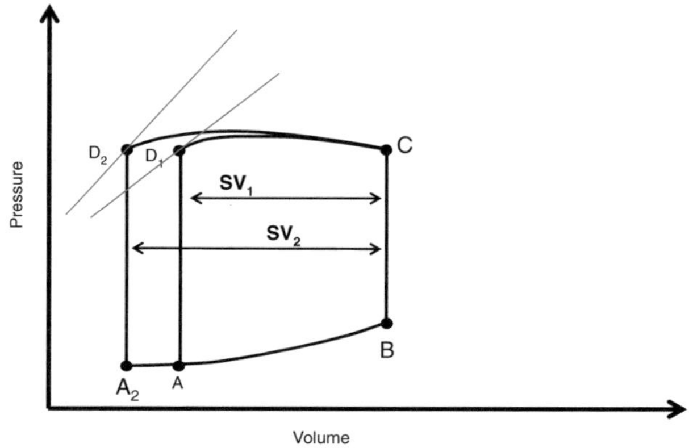

Fig. 7.3 Pressure-volume loop—inotropy. With the same afterload and preload, an increased force of contraction increases the ejection of blood during contraction from D1 to D2, increasing stroke volume. The point at which systole ends is called the end-systolic pressure-volume relationship and is descriptive of the state of contractility. The end-systolic pressure-volume relationship has moved to the left and up, indicating an increase in contractility

Question 2

The primary determinant of afterload in the patient presented in case 1 is:

A. Pleural pressure
B. Central venous pressure
C. Systemic arteriolar vascular tone
D. Pulmonary arteriolar vascular tone
E. Intravascular volume

Afterload

Afterload is defined as the work necessary to open the aortic (or pulmonary) valve and eject blood from the ventricle. It is the cavitary tension the ventricle must generate during isovolumic contraction phase to begin ejection of its stroke volume. As such, the majority of afterload is determined by the resistance and pressure beyond the semilunar valve. Pressure and flow in a hydraulic circuit are linked and described by the equation: **pressure (P) = flow (Q) x resistance (R)**. As flow (cardiac output) increases, pressure will increase in the arterial circulation in the face of unchanged resistance. Conversely, if flow declines, the primary mechanism to return flow to baseline is to decrease resistance. Although this is a simplified relationship of blood flow and resistance, its clinical utility remains. When cardiac output is diminished in the setting of decreased contractility, stroke volume may be improved by decreasing afterload. The effects of alterations in afterload on cardiac output can be seen in Fig. 7.4.

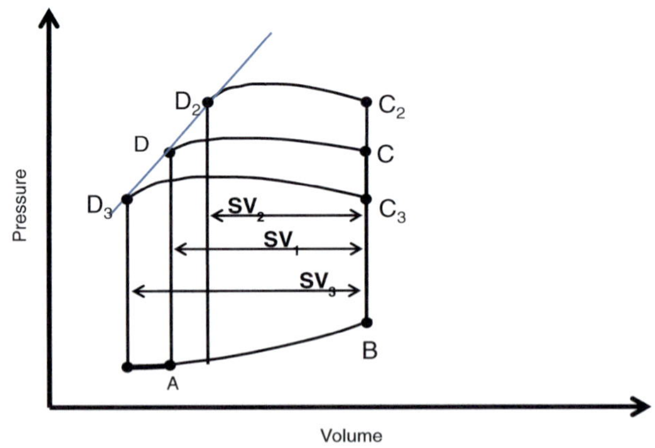

Fig. 7.4 Pressure-volume loop—afterload. As afterload increases and contractility and preload remain unchanged, the pressure required to open the semilunar valve increases from C to C2. Less work is now available to eject blood, and the change in volume that occurs by the end of systole, D2, is less. The alternate is also true. If afterload decreases, less work is required to open the semilunar valve, and more work is available to eject blood, leading to an increase in stroke volume by the end of systole, D3. The end-systolic pressure-volume relationship has not changed, however, as indicated by the blue line connecting all three end-systolic points

Systemic vascular resistance (SVR) is primarily determined by resistance arterioles which are terminal arterioles of 50–100 μm in diameter located in the organs and tissues. The state of tone of these vessels is primarily determined by both local and systemic factors such as sympathetic innervation and hormones [2].

Vascular autoregulation is the mechanism of local control of vascular tone that is determined primarily by the metabolic requirements of the tissue that they supply. This is the mechanism by which blood flow to a vascular bed may remain constant over a wide distribution of perfusion pressure, and much of the innate vascular tone is under local control. Changes in metabolic demands, endothelial derived factors, and red blood cells all may release factors that affect vascular tone and regional blood flow. The endothelium can coordinate information from blood flow, stretch, and metabolic state. In response it produces a number of substance including nitric oxide (NO), prostaglandin I_2 (PGI_2), and adenosine among others. These substances are potent vasodilators, and some, such as nitric oxide production, can be manipulated pharmacologically.

Nearly all systemic arteries are innervated with sympathetic nerve endings which cause vasoconstriction when stimulated. Although some local parasympathetic innervation does exist in certain vascular beds, for the purposes of determining SVR, sympathetic innervation is the primary control. Sympathetic output is regulated primarily in the medulla [4]. Direct sympathetic control of resistance vessels is mediated by release of norepinephrine and regulates vascular tone on a minute to minute basis. Norepinephrine binds to α_1-adrenergic receptors on the vascular smooth muscle and leads to an increased intracellular calcium concentration and vasoconstriction. This is mediated through adenylate cyclase.

Hormonal control over vascular tone is primarily mediated by catecholamines. Vascular smooth muscle contains both α-1 and β_2-receptors. Stimulation of alpha-receptors primarily causes vasoconstriction, and stimulation of beta-receptors primarily causes vasodilation. Norepinephrine is a powerful circulating vasoconstrictor and is secreted by the adrenal medulla. Epinephrine is also secreted by the adrenal gland but, at physiologic concentrations, primarily stimulates β-receptors.

Angiotensin II is a powerful vasoconstrictor. It is converted from angiotensin I by renin, which is secreted by the juxtaglomerular apparatus in the kidney in response to decrease in arterial pressure [5]. It affects the arterial vasculature directly to cause vasoconstriction as well as influences numerous substances from the central nervous system such as vasopressin and others.

Although clinicians tend to focus efforts of afterload reduction on systemic vascular resistance, pulmonary vascular resistance (PVR) may also significantly affect cardiac output if RV function is compromised or PVR is very high. Pulmonary vascular resistance is the primary determinant of right ventricle afterload and is unique in a number of ways. In normal two-ventricle physiology, it is a single vascular bed that receives the entire cardiac output. Pulmonary vascular resistance is high at birth and does not fall to its normal low levels until about 4–6 months of age. Congenital or acquired heart lesions that increase pulmonary blood flow (e.g., left-to-right shunts) may prevent PVR from reaching its nadir.

Although vascular tone and vascular resistance are the major determinants of afterload, additional factors such as viscosity and pleural pressure affect afterload as well. Since blood accelerates during systole, the viscosity of the blood affects its ability to be moved. Therefore higher hematocrits will result in increased afterload. This may present a challenge to clinicians, whose primary means of increasing oxygen delivery in situations where lung function is adequate is to increase hemoglobin concentration. Fortunately, the small increase in afterload associated with an increase in hematocrit is usually outweighed by the increase in oxygen carrying capacity, and clinically significant negative effects of blood transfusion usually only occur in the most poorly contracting ventricles. It is unknown if there are clinical benefits to manipulation of viscosity, such as hemodilution.

Answer: C—The blood vessels mainly responsible for afterload are the distal arterioles in the organs and tissues.

Developmental Differences

A number of key physiologic differences exist between the immature and mature myocardium. The mature myocardium has a myofibrillar arrangement that efficiently generates force during contraction. This optimum arrangement of myofibers is not present at birth, and the inherent ability to generate force and eject blood is limited compared to more mature myocardium [6, 7]. As a result, the immature myocardium relies more heavily on increases in heart rate than stroke volume to increase cardiac output. This in part explains concerns surrounding the administration of beta-blockers to newborns as they rely more heavily on heart rate for maintenance of cardiac output.

At birth, neonates have very poorly developed myocardial sarcoplasmic reticulum and therefore rely heavily on extracellular calcium concentrations for cardiac contraction. As a consequence, serologic hypocalcemia can significantly limit myocardial contractility and ventricular performance. Sarcoplasmic reticulum development occurs rapidly after birth and has progressed significantly by 4 weeks of age. However the response of the myocardium to increases in extracellular calcium concentration remains clinically evident into infancy and likely is determined by additional intracellular factors such as calcium sensitization of contractile and sequestration proteins. This response to extracellular calcium increases is commonly utilized by clinicians to increase cardiac output in situations of shock or postoperative low cardiac output states. In addition, it explains the exaggerated decrease in contractility in young infants when exposed to calcium channel blockers.

Response to Adrenergic Stimulation

Cardiac myocytes contain adrenergic receptors at birth. Both β_1- and β_2-adrenergic receptors are present, although at birth, β_1 predominates [8]. Stimulation of β_1-receptors results in activation of adenylate cyclase and increase in cAMP production and phosphokinase A activity. This results in increased peak intracellular calcium concentration, increased response to calcium by contractile apparatus, and increased force of contraction. β_2 stimulation results in increased automaticity of pacemaker cells in the atria and increased heart rate. Autonomic innervation of the cardiovascular system is incomplete at birth. Parasympathetic innervation at term is nearly complete, but sympathetic innervation is rudimentary. This explains why neonates and young infants manifest bradycardia as a response to stress.

Maintenance of Ductal Patency

Ductus arteriosus-dependent congenital heart lesions are a unique and highly lethal form of congenital cardiac malformations. Therefore the ability to maintain ductal patency in the newborn period may be lifesaving. The ductus arteriosus in utero connects the pulmonary artery and aorta and allows blood from the right ventricle to enter the aorta and systemic circulation. At birth, the drop in PVR and increase in SVR cause blood flow to reverse and the ductus arteriosus to be perfused with well-oxygenated blood from the aorta. The high oxygen tension of this blood is thought to be the stimulus for ductal constriction within the first few hours to days of life [9]. In congenital lesions that include malformation of the proximal aorta or pulmonary arteries, or severe valvular stenosis or atresia, maintenance of ductal patency may be the only significant source of systemic or pulmonary blood flow. Prostaglandin (PGE_1) infusion is effective in establishing and maintaining ductal patency in many children with ductal-dependent congenital heart disease and is the mainstay of therapy in these conditions prior to repair [1].

Determination of Heart Rhythm

Arrhythmias are a common source and complication of cardiovascular dysfunction. Therefore utilizing the appropriate medication for the type of underlying rhythm abnormality is crucial. Cardiac conduction and rhythm generation are determined by the flow of anions and cations across the myocyte membrane. Sodium and calcium ions are primarily sequestered outside the cell, and potassium and calcium ions are primarily sequestered inside the cell. Action potentials are brief changes in membrane polarity that allow propagation of electrical signals responsible for stimulation of the myocytes and subsequent contraction in a coordinated and efficient manner. Normally these depolarizations originate in the sinoatrial (SA) node and propagate through the atria via specialized conduction tissue to the atrioventricular (AV) node and then throughout the ventricles [1]. Propagation of depolarization from atria to ventricles and then in a coordinated fashion throughout the ventricles allows for the most efficient pattern of contraction and maximization of stroke volume and cardiac output.

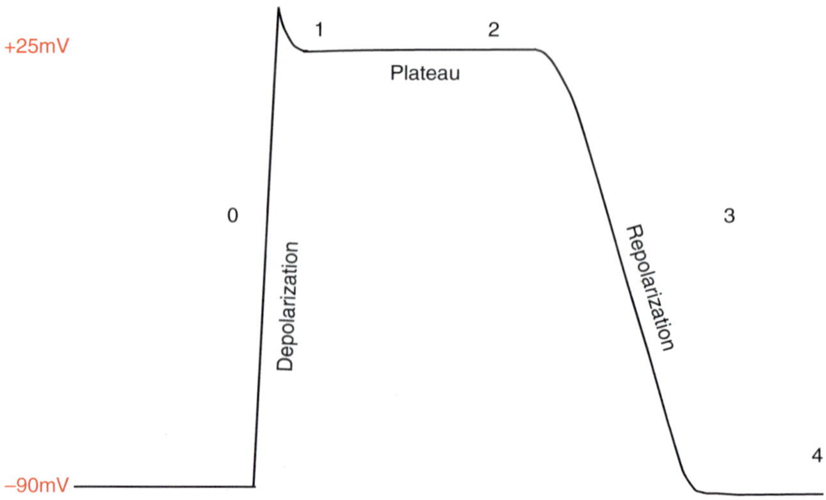

Phase 0 : *rapid depolarization*–controlled by voltage gated Na+ channels that rapidly deactivate.

Phase 1 : *early repolarization*–transient repolarization controlled largely by outward movement of potassium through voltage gated K+ rectifier channels.

Phase 2 : *Plateau*–controlled primarily by influx of calcium through L-type Ca^{2+} channels.

Phase 3 : *Repolarization*–controlled by potassium efflux through K+ rectifier channels

Phase 4 : *Restoration*–largely detremied by potassium influx via inward rectifying channels. The Na^+/K^+ ATPase also helps maintain the resting membrane potential.

Fig. 7.5 Cardiac action potential

The mechanism of depolarization is depicted in Fig. 7.5. Resting membrane potential is maintained at around −90 mV by the sequestration of potassium inside the cell and sodium outside the cell. This gradient is maintained by ATP-dependent ion pumps. When stimulated, rapid influx of sodium ions briefly increases the membrane potential to positive (depolarization), is held for a period (plateau) by the movement of calcium into and potassium out of the cell, and then membrane potential is returned to baseline (repolarization) primarily by movement of potassium out of the cell.

Although all cardiac cells are capable of spontaneous depolarization, pacemaking activity is confined to the specialized tissue in the SA and AV nodes primarily. Pacemaking tissue exhibits natural spontaneous depolarization due primarily to leakage of calcium into the cells during phase 4 and lack of inward potassium influx during phase 1 (Fig. 7.6).

Because maintenance of resting membrane potential requires ATP, states of myocardial energy failure commonly lead to arrhythmias. In addition, primary arrhythmias can be induced by abnormal ion concentrations inside and outside the cell, as well as genetic variability in location and concentration of ion channels as well as genetic mutation of ion channels. These are discussed in Chap. 8.

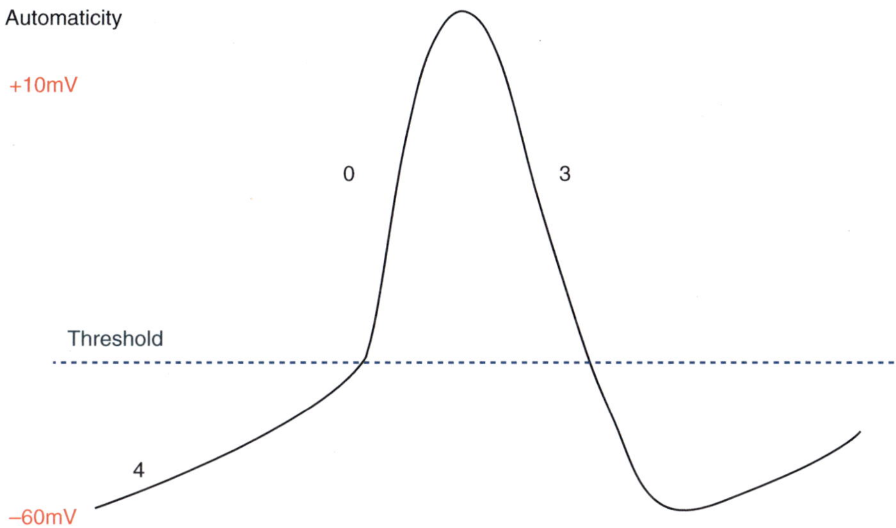

Phase 0 : *rapid depolarization*–controlled by rapid influx of Ca^{2+}

Phase 3 : *Repolarization*–controlled by potassium efflux through K^+ rectifier channels

Phase 4 : *Slow influx of* Na^+

Fig. 7.6 Pacemaker action potential

Question 3

An echocardiogram confirms that this patient has severely decreased systolic function of both her left and right ventricle, with normal ventricular size and mild mitral regurgitation. No structural abnormalities are identified.

Appropriate initial therapy for the case 1 patient is:

A. Norepinephrine infusion at 0.05 mcg/kg/min
B. Sodium nitroprusside infusion at 1 mcg/kg/min
C. Furosemide bolus of 1 mg/kg IV
D. Epinephrine infusion at 0.1 mcg/kg/min
E. Normal saline fluid bolus of 5 ml/kg

Pharmacologic Manipulation of Preload

Optimization of preload in the setting of low cardiac output or shock is often the first and most important step in management and stabilization. This is due to the fact that volume expansion is easy and intravenous solutions are readily available. Many studies in adults, children, and animals have evaluated the efficacy of varying types of volume expansion to determine the optimum type [10]. Results are varied, and to date, no single type of fluid has been determined to be superior to another in the setting of shock from cardiac dysfunction in children.

Volume Expanders

Fluid used for volume expansion should be nearly isotonic to avoid sequelae associated with rapid serum osmotic changes.

Crystalloids

Crystalloid refers to solutions that are primarily sodium based. Distribute throughout the extracellular fluid volume. Under normal circumstances, only about a quarter or less of the initial volume remains intravascular after administration.

0.9% Saline: 0.9% weight/volume sodium chloride solution. 154 mEq/L sodium chloride; total 308 mOs, pH = 5.0–5.5. This is also referred to as isotonic saline or "normal" saline.

Advantages: cheap and easily available in most clinical settings. This is compatible with almost all intravenous fluids and medications.

Disadvantages: has an increased strong ion difference compared to other solutions and may predispose to metabolic acidosis if administered in large quantities. May have a mild vasodilator effect in large quantities and may increase risk of post-resuscitation hyperkalemia.

Lactated Ringer's (LR) solution: 130 mOsm sodium, 109 mEq/L chloride, and 28 mMol/L lactate (or acetate). Potassium 4 mEq/L (as chloride). Calcium 3 mEq/L (as chloride). Total 272 mOsm/L. pH—6.5. Lactate (or acetate) is metabolized to bicarbonate and may help improve metabolic acidosis.

Advantages: readily available in many clinical settings. Less risk of metabolic acidosis or hyperkalemia post-resuscitation compared to 0.9% saline.

Disadvantages: more expensive and potentially less availability than 0.9% saline. Not desirable in setting of hyperkalemia.

Colloids

Colloids refer to large molecular weight substances that do not pass through capillary walls easily. Many colloid solutions exist and are available throughout the world. The use of colloids in the setting of trauma has been extensively studied, but their use in the resuscitation and volume expansion for children with critical heart disease has not been well defined.

Albumin 5%: derived from human plasma, 5% wt/vol albumin. It is buffered with sodium bicarbonate and heat treated for sterilization. It is isoosmotic and isotonic with a sodium concentration of 130–160 mEq/L.

Advantages: as a large oncotic molecule, albumin is more likely to remain intravascular and increase intravascular volume.

Disadvantages: expensive and not readily available in many places. As a human-derived protein, there is a risk of allergic reaction and a small risk of infection transmission. Because it increases serum oncotic pressure much more than crystalloid solutions, it should be used with caution in the setting of chronic congestive heart failure or other situations presenting with pulmonary edema as rapid increasing in serum oncotic pressure may worsen this. In addition, as a negatively charged protein, it binds ionized calcium and decreases serum ionized calcium concentrations. This may have negative inotropic effects in those patients who are reliant on extracellular calcium concentrations for contraction, such as neonates and infants.

Blood Products

Packed red blood cells (PRBCs): obtained from whole human blood with much of the plasma removed. Hematocrit is usually around 60–65%. It is generally not recommended for resuscitation in cardiac disease unless concomitant anemia or blood loss is present. In addition, it may be of benefit in cyanotic heart lesions for increasing systemic arterial saturations.

Venodilators

Another means of altering preload is alteration of vascular capacitance. In the acute setting of low cardiac output, the benefit of venoconstriction has not been proven but may bc of some benefit after administration of fluids. More commonly, venodilation is used to decrease preload in patients who have chronic heart failure and become fluid overloaded. This may significantly improve ventricular function, and the effects are usually more rapid than diuretics.

Nitroglycerin: at low doses, it is a venodilator and has increased vascular capacitance effects. At higher doses, it has more arterial vasodilator effects and may cause hypotension. It has favorable effects on myocardial oxygen consumption, either by decreasing myocardial work or by coronary vasodilation. It has a rapid onset of action and short half-life.

Diuretics

One of the mainstays of treatment of decompensated heart failure is decreasing intravascular volume with diuretics. However, it is important in the acute phase that adequate intravascular volume is maintained and balance between diuretic use and intravenous volume expansion may be challenging. Urgent transfer to a pediatric intensive care unit for hemodynamic monitoring of central venous pressure provides the safest mechanism for providing appropriate fluid balance.

Furosamide—a loop diuretic leading to retention of sodium, potassium, and chloride in the lumen of the ascending loop of Henle and subsequent increase in urine volume. It is the mainstay of diuretic therapy in acute heart failure and fluid overload. It may precipitate or worsen hyponatremia and hypokalemia. Typical starting dose is 1 mg/kg IV or oral. Range is 1–2 mg/kg per dose. Alternately, it can be given as a continuous infusion for those that may not tolerate sudden diuresis. Dose is typically 0.05–0.2 mcg/kg/min.

Onset of action: 30–90 min IV, 2–4 h orally.

Half-life: roughly 6 h.

Elimination: renal. If there is significant renal insufficiency present, this will decrease the response of diuresis and should not only limit dosing interval but prompt consideration of alternative forms of diuresis. Toxicity to the optic nerve has been well documented but likely only with larger doses and prolonged use.

Chlorothiazide—a thiazide diuretic; it is usually adjunctive to furosemide. It causes retention of sodium and chloride, and secondarily potassium in distal tubule lumen, leading to diuresis. Typical dose is 2 mg/kg IV or PO. Side effects include hypokalemia and hyponatremia.

Onset of action: 30 min IV or 2 h oral.

Half-life: 2–3 h.

Elimination: unhanged in the urine.

Metolazone—a thiazide-like diuretic with similar mechanism of action and side effects to chlorothiazide. It is only available orally and may be a good alternative for those patients without IV access. Dose is typically 0.2–0.4 mg/kg/dose.

Onset of action: 1 h.

Half-life: 20 h.

Elimination: mostly renally excreted.

Answer: E—Judicious volume expansion with normal saline is the first step to restore perfusion pressure in a patient in shock who is obviously dehydrated. This is closely followed by administration of inotropes. After appropriate stabilization with adequate preload and inotropy, afterload reduction may be employed with close monitoring of the circulatory status.

Pharmacologic Manipulation of Inotropy

Adrenergic Agents (Table 7.1)

Dopamine—stimulates β_1- and α_1-receptors in the heart and vasculature. It also increases endogenous norepinephrine production. Administration results in increased contractility and vasoconstriction. At lower doses (3–8 mcg/kg/min), it primarily stimulates β-receptors and results in increased contractility and cardiac output. At higher infusion rates (~15 mcg/kg/min), it stimulates α-receptors and results in vasoconstriction. It also stimulates dopamine receptors in renal, splanchnic, and cerebral vasculature at low doses; however the clinical significance of this is still unclear and of significant clinical debate.

Dobutamine—stimulates primarily β_1-receptors, although it also has light β_2 effects. It does not increase endogenous norepinephrine production [11]. Primary effect is increased stroke volume and cardiac output and increased chronotropy at

Table 7.1 Inotropic drugs

Drug	Mechanism	Onset (min)	Dose	Comments
Dopamine	β_1 α_1	2–10	3–8 mcg/kg/min >10 mcg/kg/min	
Dobutamine	β_1,β_2	2–15	3–15 mcg/kg/min	
Epinephrine	β_1 α_1	1–5	0.03–0.01 mcg/kg/min >0.1 mcg/kg/min	
Norepinephrine	α_1, β_1	1–5	0.03–0.2 mcg/kg/min	Increased afterload
Milrinone	PDE_3	5–20	0.375–1.0 mcg/kg/min	Adjust dose in renal failure
Levosimendan	Ca^{2+} sensitizer	10–30	6–12 mcg/kg load (10 min) 0.05–0.2 mcg/kg/min	Not available in the United States

α alpha-adrenergic agonist, *β* beta-adrenergic agonist, PDE_5 phosphodesterase-5 inhibitor

higher infusion rates (above 5 mcg/kg/min). It does not result in systemic vasoconstriction and may result in systemic vasodilation at higher infusion rates (>5 mcg/kg/min) due to β_2 stimulation effect on peripheral arteries.

Epinephrine—stimulates β_1–, β_2– (at lower doses), and α_1-receptors (at higher doses). It increases stroke volume, heart rate, and systemic vascular resistance.

Norepinephrine—stimulates primarily α_1-receptors and β_1 at higher concentrations. This results in increased systemic vascular resistance and increased stroke volume.

Isoproterenol—stimulates primarily β_2-receptors at clinical doses and results in increased heart rate without increased contractility. Its primary use is for symptomatic bradycardia without decreased contractility or coronary insufficiency (e.g., heart block or sinus node dysfunction).

Phosphodiesterase Inhibitors

Milrinone—inhibits phosphodiesterase III, leading to increased cAMP concentrations in cardiac and vascular smooth muscle. Its use leads to increased contractility and stroke volume, with vascular smooth muscle relaxation and decreased SVR [12, 13]. In addition, there is some evidence that milrinone improves diastolic function, possibly by improving sarcoplasmic reticulum calcium flux. It is especially effective in improving cardiac output in setting of diminished contractility and increased SVR. It may also be beneficial in ischemic heart disease. Hypotension is the main side effect. It has been demonstrated to be pro-arrhythmic in adults with heart failure, possibly by shortening AV conduction times. However its arrhythmogenic effect in children is unclear, and milrinone has become the mainstay of treatment in children with acute and chronic heart failure.

Calcium Sensitizers

Levosimendan—increases myofiber sensitivity to calcium by binding to troponin C and improving actin-myosin cross-linking, without increasing myocardial oxygen consumption. It also causes systemic arterial vasodilation by binding to ATP-sensitive potassium channels in the vascular smooth muscle. Its use is primarily in decompensated heart failure in adults [14]. The dose is usually 6–12 μg/kg loading dose over 10 min followed by 0.05–0.2 μg/kg/min as a continuous infusion. The limited data for its use in children suggest similar hemodynamic and tolerance as in adults. This drug is approved for use in Europe and Asia, but not in the United States.

Vasoconstrictors (Table 7.2)

Adrenergic

Norepinephrine—although at lower doses of norepinephrine β_1 effects predominate, at higher doses, α_1-mediated vasoconstriction predominates. It causes an increase in SVR that is usually well tolerated in normally functioning ventricles. It needs to be used with caution in the setting of ventricular systolic dysfunction especially in younger children as the increase in afterload may precipitate acute ventricular failure. Vasoconstriction is more prominent above 0.05–0.1 mcg/kg/min.

Epinephrine—both β_1 and α_1 stimulant. α_1 effects predominate above 0.1 mcg/kg/min. It causes increased SVR that is usually well tolerated due to significant inotropic effects of β_1 stimulation.

Phenylephrine—pure α_1 agonist. It causes dose-dependent vasoconstriction and increased SVR. As it has no β effects, caution should be observed in the setting of ventricular dysfunction as the increase in afterload may precipitate acute ventricular failure especially in younger children. It is commonly used to treat severe hypercyanotic spells of tetralogy of Fallot.

Vasopressin (antidiuretic hormone)—neuropeptide secreted by the posterior pituitary. At low doses it causes water reabsorption form the distal nephron. At higher doses, it acts via the vasopressin V1a receptor in vascular smooth muscle, leading to peripheral arterial vasoconstriction. Vasopressin deficiency has been demonstrated in adults with vasodilatory shock and certain states of cardiac disease

Table 7.2 Vasoconstrictors

Drug	Mechanism	Onset (min)	Dose	Comments
Norepinephrine	α_1, β_1	1–5	0.03–0.2 mcg/kg/min	Some ↑ inotropy
Epinephrine	β_1,α_1	1–5	0.03–0.01 mcg/kg/min >0.1 mcg/kg/min	↑ SVR at higher doses only
Vasopressin	V_1	10–30	0.1–1.0 U/kg/min	
Phenylephrine	α_1	1–4		No inotropic effect

α alpha-adrenergic agonist, *β* beta-adrenergic agonist, V_1 vasopressin receptor 1 agonist (ref). It is unclear if vasopressin deficiency is common in children with cardiac disease, but dose-dependent increase in blood pressure has been demonstrated in children after cardiac surgery. Dose is 0.1–1.0 U/kg/min. Higher doses have been used in vasodilatory shock. As with all pure vasoconstrictors, it should be used with caution in the setting of ventricular dysfunction.

Vasodilators and Antihypertensives (Table 7.3)

Nitrates

Nitroprusside—very commonly used vasodilator because of its rapid onset and easy titratability. It leads directly to smooth muscle relaxation by generation of nitric oxide (NO) [15] and causes more arteriolar than venular dilation. A by-product of its metabolism is cyanide. It is used primarily in hypertensive emergencies and decompensated heart failure. By causing venular dilation, it may improve cardiac output in heart failure. Typical dose is 0.5–5 mcg/kg/min continuous infusion.

Nitroglycerin—converted to NO by aldehyde dehydrogenase in the mitochondria. It is more venous than arterial vasodilator. It is especially effective for treating decompensated heart failure due to its venodilator potency. It also may be helpful in setting of coronary insufficiency by decreasing preload and improving coronary blood flow. It also decreases myocardial work.

Calcium Channel Blockers

Nicardipine—dihydropyridine class of calcium channel blockers. It inhibits transmembrane flux of calcium into smooth muscle, thereby causing vasodilation. It is more selective to cerebral and coronary vessels than other calcium channel blockers. Dose is 0.5–3 mcg/kg/min infusion.

Table 7.3 Vasodilators and antihypertensives

Drug	Mechanism	Onset (min)	Dose	Comments
Nitroprusside	Nitrate	1–3	0.5–5 mcg/kg/min	Adjust for long-term use in renal failure
Nitroglycerine	Nitrate	2–5	0.5–5 mcg/kg/min	Effect wanes after 12–24 h
Nicardipine	CCB	10–20	0.5–3 mcg/kg/min	Efficacy in <6 months unclear
Nifedipine	CCB	10–45	0.25–0.5 mg/kg PO	Oral or transmucosal
Esmolol	β-blocker	1–5	50–500 mcg/kg/min	Negative inotrope
Labetolol	β-blocker α-blocker	30–60	0.4–3 mg/kg/h 0.3–1 mg/kg q 8 h	

CCB calcium channel blocker, *α-blocker* alpha-adrenergic receptor blocker, *β-blocker* beta-adrenergic receptor blocker

Nifedipine—dihydropyridine class of calcium channel blockers. It is used for hypertensive emergencies and long-term hypertension control. It is administered by oral or transmucosal route. It is less selective than nicardipine and must be used with caution in neonates and infants as it may lead to decreased contractility. Dose is 0.25–0.5 mg/kg PO every 6 h.

Beta-Adrenergic Blockers

Esmolol—primarily β_1-selective blocker which decreases the force and rate of cardiac contraction. Its primary use is for hypertension in the setting of normal contractility, and primary benefit is that it is short acting and easily titratable. However, it should be used with extreme caution with impaired contractility. Typical dose is 50–500 mcg/kg/min infusion.

Labetolol—blocks both β_1- and β_2-receptors as well as α_1-receptors (approximately $\beta:\alpha = 4:1$). It causes decrease force and rate of contraction but also has some peripheral vasodilator effects at higher doses. It can be given as a continuous infusion or intermittent IV doses. Typical doses are: IV infusion, 0.4–3 mg/kg/h, or intermittent IV 0.3–1 mg/kg every 6–8 h.

Onset of action: 30–60 min.

Half-life: 5 h.

Elimination: metabolized in the liver.

Antiarrhythmics (Table 7.4)

Case 2

A child who presents in shock has been stabilized with intubation and mechanical ventilation, placement of central venous and arterial lines, and initiation of epinephrine and milrinone infusions. You are called to assess the patient by the bedside nurse due to increasing frequency of premature ventricular contractions. While waiting for a 12-lead EKG to be performed, you witness *monomorphic ventricular tachycardia* on the physiologic monitor, and the patient quickly becomes pulseless. You provide immediate cardiopulmonary resuscitation and prepare for defibrillation. Which of the following medications is most likely to facilitate conversion to a normal sinus rhythm and return of spontaneous circulation in this scenario?

A. Diltiazem
B. Adenosine
C. Esmolol
D. Amiodarone
E. Isoproterenol

Table 7.4 Antiarrhythmics

Drug	Mechanism	Onset (min)	Dose	Comments
Adenosine		5–10 s	0.1–0.2 mg/kg	Must be given rapid push with large flush
Esmolol	β-blocker	1–5	50–500 mcg/kg/min	Negative inotrope
Lidocaine	Na^+ channel blockade	1–2	1 mg/kg bolus 20–50 mcg/kg/min	
Amiodarone	Na^+, K^+ channel blockade		5–15 mg/kg (max 150) 5–15 mcg/kg/min inf.	Negative inotrope
Isoproterenol	β2, β1 agonist	5–10	0.05–2 mcg/kg/min	
Magnesium sulfate			25–50 mg/kg (2 g max)	Hypotension

β1-blocker beta-adrenergic receptor blocker, *β2-blocker* beta-adrenergic receptor blocker, *α-blocker* alpha-adrenergic receptor blocker, *Na^+* sodium, *K^+* potassium

Adenosine is an endogenous nucleoside useful for treatment and diagnosis of many supraventricular arrhythmias. When given intravenously, adenosine causes a transient conduction block in the atrioventricular (AV) node. It will terminate many cases of reentrant tachycardias involving the sinoatrial or AV nodes [16]. It has an extremely short half-life (less than 10 s) due to rapid uptake and metabolism by erythrocytes and the vascular endothelium. Adenosine is included in the 2015 American Heart Association guidelines for management of tachycardia with a pulse and poor perfusion in pediatric patients.

Adenosine should be given by rapid intravenous push followed by a rapid normal saline flush due to its short half-life. The initial dose is 0.1 mg/kg (maximum 6 mg). A subsequent dose of 0.2 mg/kg (maximum 12 mg) may be given within 1–2 min if the initial dose is not successful in terminating the arrhythmia. Adenosine has been rarely associated with atrial fibrillation and wide complex tachyarrhythmias. An external defibrillator and providers experienced in providing pediatric advanced life support should be present when it is administered.

Esmolol is a class II antiarrhythmic medication that acts by selective blockade of β_1-receptors. It has little effect on β_2-receptors except at high doses. Blockade by esmolol prevents catecholamine stimulation of the pacemaker cells of the heart resulting in decreased automaticity [17]. Esmolol also increases the refractory period of the AV node, slowing conduction. These actions result in decreased heart rate. Esmolol is useful for treatment of supraventricular tachycardia and may be used to decrease the ventricular rate response in atrial flutter and atrial fibrillation.

Esmolol is administered by continuous IV infusion due to its extremely short half-life (5–10 min). A loading dose of 100–500 mcg/kg may be administered over 1 min, followed by a continuous infusion at 25–100 mcg/kg/min. Dose can be titrated to clinical effect in 25–50 mcg/kg/min increments. The usual maintenance dose ranges from 50 to 500 mcg/kg/min. Esmolol is metabolized in the blood by red blood cell esterases. Side effects include impaired ventricular function, vasodilation, hypotension, and bradycardia, but its short half-life makes it an attractive option for initiating beta-blocker therapy in critically ill patients.

Lidocaine is a class Ib antiarrhythmic medication that exerts its effects via sodium channel blockade during the phase 0 upstroke of the cardiac action potential. It slows ventricular conduction and raises the threshold for ventricular fibrillation. Lidocaine is included as an alternative to amiodarone in the 2015 American Heart Association guidelines for management of ventricular fibrillation and pulseless ventricular tachycardia in pediatric patients. It is not effective in the treatment of supraventricular arrhythmias.

Lidocaine is administered an IV bolus dose of 1 mg/kg, followed by a continuous infusion of 20–50 mcg/kg/min. An additional 1 mg/kg bolus dose may be given if initiation of the continuous infusion is delayed by 15 min or more. Lidocaine is primarily hepatically metabolized, and elimination may be prolonged in patients with heart failure, liver dysfunction, and shock. Central nervous system toxicity, including seizures, can occur at supratherapeutic blood concentrations.

Amiodarone is a potent class III antiarrhythmic medication that delays repolarization and prolongs the refractory period of myocytes by potassium channel blockade. Amiodarone also exhibits beta-blocking effects and some sodium and calcium channel blocking effects [18]. It is effective for the treatment of a wide variety of atrial and ventricular tachyarrhythmias. Amiodarone is included in the 2015 American Heart Association guidelines for management of ventricular fibrillation and pulseless ventricular tachycardia in pediatric patients.

Amiodarone can be administered by enteral or intravenous routes. It has an extremely long half-life (30–60 days) and may require repeated loading doses. A typical intravenous loading dose of 5 mg/kg (maximum dose 300 mg) is administered over 30–60 min, followed by a continuous infusion at 5–15 mcg/kg/min. The loading dose may be repeated twice for a total of 15 mg/kg. In the setting of ventricular fibrillation or pulseless ventricular tachycardia, the loading doses may be given by intravenous push. Amiodarone is hepatically metabolized and has numerous drug-drug interactions, so dose adjustments may be necessary. Immediate adverse effects of amiodarone include hypotension, bradycardia, and QT prolongation. Long-term side effects include thyroid and hepatic dysfunction, corneal deposits, and pulmonary interstitial fibrosis.

Answer: D—Amiodarone is an effective drug both for treatment and for prevention of ventricular tachycardia.

Isoproterenol is a pure beta-agonist which stimulates β_1- and β_2-receptors, resulting in increased heart rate and contractility. It also causes relaxation of the vascular, bronchial, gastrointestinal, and uterine smooth muscle. Isoproterenol may be indicated for the treatment of symptomatic bradycardia where temporary cardiac pacing (transcutaneous, transvenous, transesophageal) is unavailable or unsuccessful.

Isoproterenol is administered by continuous intravenous infusion at a rate of 0.05–2 mcg/kg/min. The dose is titrated to heart rate response. Isoproterenol has a short half-life (5 min or less), so dose adjustments can be made relatively quickly.

Magnesium sulfate is indicated for the treatment of torsade de pointes (polymorphic ventricular tachycardia). Torsade de pointes is typically associated with QT interval-prolonging medications in hospitalized patients. The QT interval-prolonging medication should be stopped if possible along with administration of magnesium sulfate.

Magnesium sulfate is provided by intravenous infusion of 25–50 mg/kg (maximum dose 2000 mg). Intravenous infusion of magnesium sulfate can cause hypotension, so it should be administered slowly (10–20 min) in patients with hemodynamic instability. In pulseless patients, it should be administered as a bolus dose. Additional antiarrhythmic therapy and cardioversion/defibrillation may be necessary in a patient with torsade de pointes.

References

1. Allen HD. Moss and Adams heart disease in infants, children, and adolescents: including the fetus and young adult, vol. 2. 8th ed. Philadelphia: Wolters Kluwer Health/Lippincott Williams & Wilkins; 2013.
2. Guyton AC, Hall JE. Textbook of medical physiology, vol. xxxv. 11th ed. Philadelphia: Elsevier Saunders; 2006. 1116 p
3. Katz AM, Smith VE. Regulation of myocardial function in the normal and diseased heart. Modification by inotropic drugs. Eur Heart J. 1982;3 Suppl D:11–8.
4. Ghali MGZ. Role of the medullary lateral tegmental field in sympathetic control. J Integr Neurosci. 2017;16(2):189–208.
5. Cody RJ. The integrated effects of angiotensin II. Am J Cardiol. 1997;79(5A):9–11.
6. Takayama Y, Costa KD, Covell JW. Contribution of laminar myofiber architecture to load-dependent changes in mechanics of LV myocardium. Am J Physiol Heart Circ Physiol. 2002; 282(4):H1510–20.
7. Adhyapak SM, Parachuri VR. Architecture of the left ventricle: insights for optimal surgical ventricular restoration. Heart Fail Rev. 2010;15(1):73–83.
8. Robinson RB. Autonomic receptor--effector coupling during post-natal development. Cardiovasc Res. 1996;31 Spec No:E68–76.
9. Clyman RI. Mechanisms regulating the ductus arteriosus. Biol Neonate. 2006;89(4):330–5.
10. Myburgh JA, Mythen MG. Resuscitation fluids. N Engl J Med. 2013;369(25):2462–3.
11. Kho TL, et al. Influence of dobutamine and dopamine on hemodynamics and plasma concentrations of noradrenaline and renin in patients with low cardiac output following acute myocardial infarction. Eur J Clin Pharmacol. 1980;18(3):213–7.
12. Jaski BE, et al. Positive inotropic and vasodilator actions of milrinone in patients with severe congestive heart failure. Dose-response relationships and comparison to nitroprusside. J Clin Invest. 1985;75(2):643–9.
13. Hoffman TM, et al. Efficacy and safety of milrinone in preventing low cardiac output syndrome in infants and children after corrective surgery for congenital heart disease. Circulation. 2003;107(7):996–1002.
14. De Luca L, et al. Evidence-based use of levosimendan in different clinical settings. Eur Heart J. 2006;27(16):1908–20.
15. Ignarro LJ, et al. Mechanism of vascular smooth muscle relaxation by organic nitrates, nitrites, nitroprusside and nitric oxide: evidence for the involvement of S-nitrosothiols as active intermediates. J Pharmacol Exp Ther. 1981;218(3):739–49.
16. Overholt ED, et al. Usefulness of adenosine for arrhythmias in infants and children. Am J Cardiol. 1988;61(4):336–40.
17. Reynolds RD, Gorczynski RJ, Quon CY. Pharmacology and pharmacokinetics of esmolol. J Clin Pharmacol. 1986;26 Suppl A:A3–A14.
18. Singh BN. Amiodarone: historical development and pharmacologic profile. Am Heart J. 1983; 106(4 Pt 2):788–97.

8 Arrhythmia Identification: Stabilization and Treatment

Raya Safa, Chenni Sriram, and Peter P. Karpawich

Introduction

Of the over 25 million yearly pediatric emergency room (ER) visits in the United States, primary cardiac-related issues in children <18 years of age are much less common than seen in adults who frequently present with acute coronary issues [1]. However, heart rate changes and arrhythmias occur not infrequently, and monitoring the rate and rhythm and obtaining an electrocardiogram (ECG) are often useful. Since children are seen in many ER settings from those in a dedicated children's hospital to primarily adult-oriented hospitals, to urgent care facilities, and to rural areas where pediatric specialty services may not be readily available, interpretation of pediatric ECGs often becomes the responsibility of physicians who may have limited experience with the age-related variances of ECG patterns among children with and without congenital heart defects (CHD [2]. In addition, with the increasing numbers of patients with repaired congenital heart defects surviving into adulthood who present to emergency rooms with various complaints, variations of their ECGs associated with their underlying anatomical/structural CHD may mimic ECG findings associated with ischemic coronary disease. In this regard, close examination of the full 15-lead ECG, rather than a single rhythm strip, is often required for proper interpretation. In addition the computer interpretation of ECGs may be erroneous

R. Safa, M.D., F.A.A.P.
Divisions of Cardiology and Critical Care Medicine, Department of Pediatrics, Children's Hospital of Michigan, Detroit, MI, USA

Wayne State University School of Medicine, Detroit, MI, USA
e-mail: RSafa@dmc.org

C. Sriram, M.D., F.A.A.P, F.A.C.C. • P. P. Karpawich, M.Sc., M.D., F.A.A.P., F.A.C.C. (✉)
Division of Cardiology, Department of Pediatrics, Children's Hospital of Michigan, Detroit, MI, USA

Wayne State University School of Medicine, Detroit, MI, USA
e-mail: csriram@med.wayne.edu; PKarpawi@dmc.org

© Springer International Publishing AG, part of Springer Nature 2018
A. P. Sarnaik et al. (eds.), *Cardiac Emergencies in Children*,
https://doi.org/10.1007/978-3-319-73754-6_8

with a reported error rate up to 75% which can result in unnecessary additional testing and costs, as well as patient distress and inappropriate referrals to cardiac specialists [3, 4].

The purpose of this chapter is to enable the reader to identify commonly seen normal and abnormal ECGs and the diverse rhythm disturbances seen in children and adults with various congenital heart defects. In addition, specific pathophysiologies of arrhythmias and appropriate therapies will be presented.

1-Normal Variants

Case 1

An 8-year-old patient presented to the emergency department with a 1-week history of chest pain localized to the left lower chest. The pain is stabbing in nature and occurs at rest with no radiation. No associated symptoms are present except for occasional palpitations. Physical examination is unremarkable except for chest wall tenderness on palpation. He was seen 2 days ago at another facility where an EKG was performed (Fig. 8.1). Repeat EKG at the time of presentation is shown in Fig. 8.3. What is the next appropriate approach?

(A) Place a 24 h Holter monitor.
(B) Order an echocardiogram.
(C) Reassurance of non-cardiac chest pain.
(D) Check electrolytes.
(E) Obtain troponin levels.

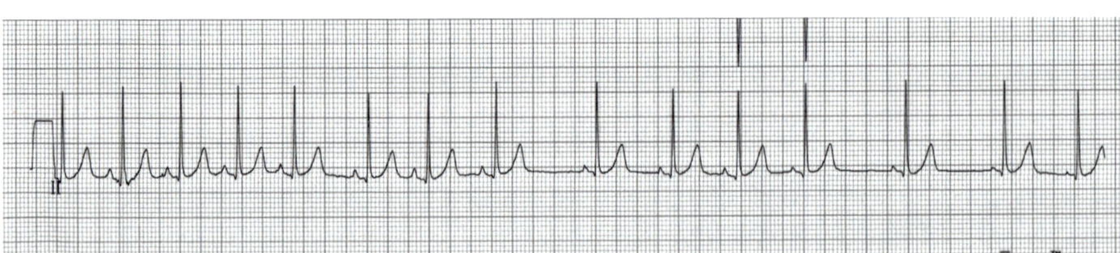

Fig. 8.1 Sinus arrhythmia. Lead II: normal P waves and PR intervals with rate changes

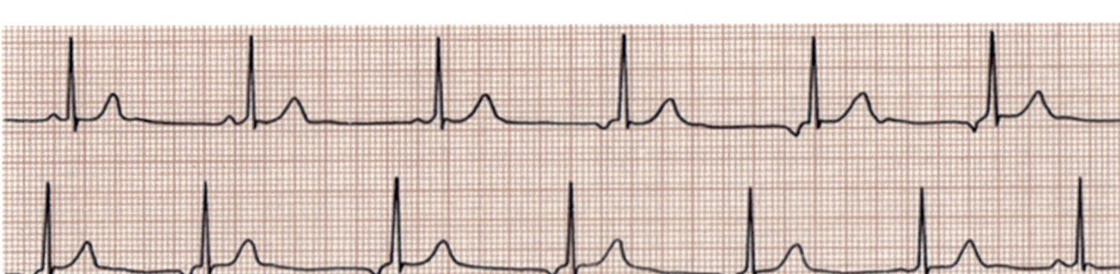

Fig. 8.2 Wandering atrial pacemaker. Lead II: P waves change from upright to inverted and back to upright. The PR interval shortens with the inverted P waves

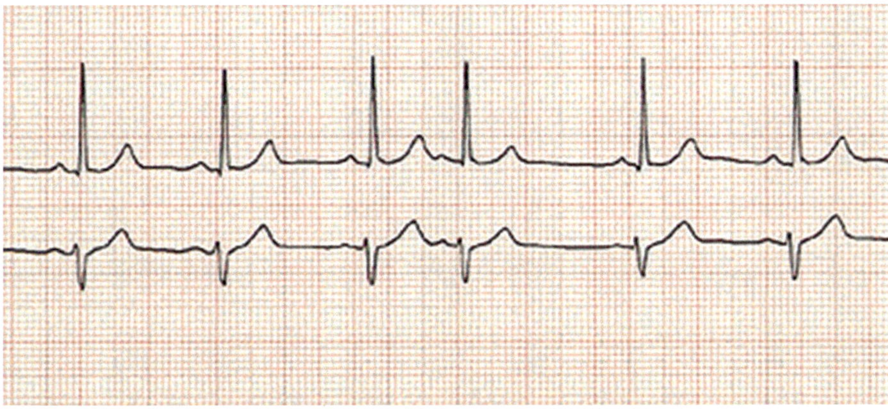

Fig. 8.3 Three sinus complexes (left) are followed by a PAC, which then conducts to the ventricle. This is followed by a compensatory pause before sinus rhythm resumes

Discussion

When interpreting ECGs, it is important to determine if any particular pattern is normal or not. Heart rate variability is normal, and often a child or teenager's complaint of sensed tachycardia or palpitations does not have a primary cardiac etiology. Sinus arrhythmia is normal and is a benign condition. The heart rate varies with respiration, and this is more pronounced in children. It is a normal physiologic finding caused by changes in parasympathetic input of the vagal tone to the heart during respiration. The ECG pattern shows normal P waves and PR intervals with rate variability (Fig. 8.1). Another common finding among children is a wandering atrial pacemaker. This benign variant is characterized by changes in P wave morphology and PR intervals and reflects atrial activation along the preferential conduction pathways (Fig. 8.2).

Premature atrial complexes (PAC) are typically benign and common especially in infants and young children. They can occur throughout childhood [5–7]. No treatment is required. Typically, the P wave morphology of the premature complex is different from sinus rhythm. It may be visible immediately after the T wave or be hidden in and distort the T wave of the preceding QRST complex. Careful examination of preceding T waves will often disclose "humps-n-bumps" distortions of atrial P waves, which may or may not conduct to the ventricles (Figs. 8.3 and 8.4). At times, the single premature atrial impulse (PAC) is conducted through the AV node before the ventricle has recovered electrically from the previous impulse and results in an abnormal QRS morphology (PAC with aberration) mimicking a premature ventricular complex (PVC) (Fig. 8.5).

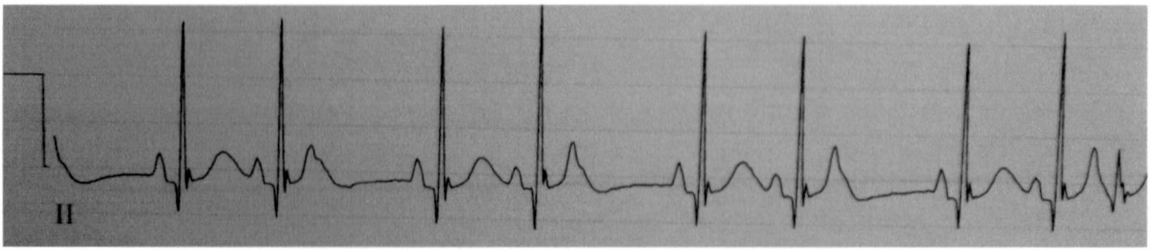

Fig. 8.4 Sinus rhythm with PACs falling on top of the T wave causing distortion. The P wave is blocked from conducting to the ventricle due to refractoriness of the AV node. The last complex conducts with aberrancy

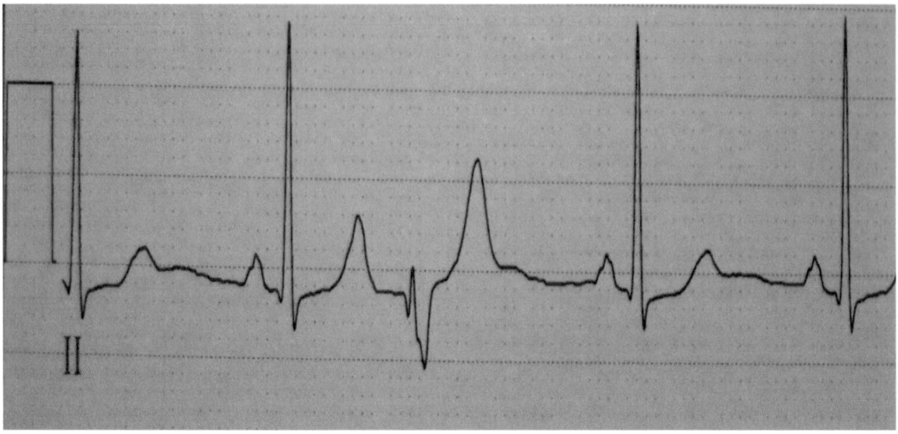

Fig. 8.5 PAC with aberration. The third QRS complex is abnormal and wide as a result of the PAC being conducted before the ventricle has completely recovered from the previous impulse. Note that the T wave of the preceding QRS is peaked and taller than the other sinus complex T waves, indicating distortion by a hidden P wave

Answer: C. The ECG findings of sinus arrhythmia and PACs are benign variants in children, and the localized chest pain that is reproducible is typical of chest wall discomfort and not cardiac in origin.

Case 2

A 10-year-old patient with a past medical history of diabetes mellitus presented to the emergency department and is found to be in diabetic ketoacidosis. His cardiovascular examination is remarkable for tachycardia. His initial lab work-up shows potassium at 6 meq/L.

What is the first EKG finding of hyperkalemia?

(A) Sinus tachycardia
(B) Prolonged QT interval
(C) U waves
(D) Peaked T waves
(E) Inverted T waves

Discussion

1. **Electrolyte Imbalance**

   It must be remembered that the cardiac cellular action potential that initiates electrical activity is electrolyte dependent. Alterations in potassium and calcium currents can have profound effects on the ECG. Thus, non-cardiac etiologies may be responsible for significant ECG changes. A tall, peaked, and symmetrical T wave is the first change seen on the EKG on a patient with hyperkalemia (Fig. 8.6). As the hyperkalemia increases, there is further slowing of conduction through the myocardium, manifested by a prolonged PR interval with eventual absence of P waves, and an increase in QRS duration. Ultimately the QRS complex widens to a severe conduction delay and becomes a "sine wave" mimicking ventricular tachycardia (Fig. 8.7). If untreated, true ventricular tachycardia and fibrillation can result.

   Hypokalemia causes ST segment depression, decrease in the amplitude of the T wave, and increase in the amplitude of the U wave (Fig. 8.8). These changes are best seen in the precordial leads V4–V6. The T and following U waves can merge resulting in the misdiagnosis of prolonged QT interval.

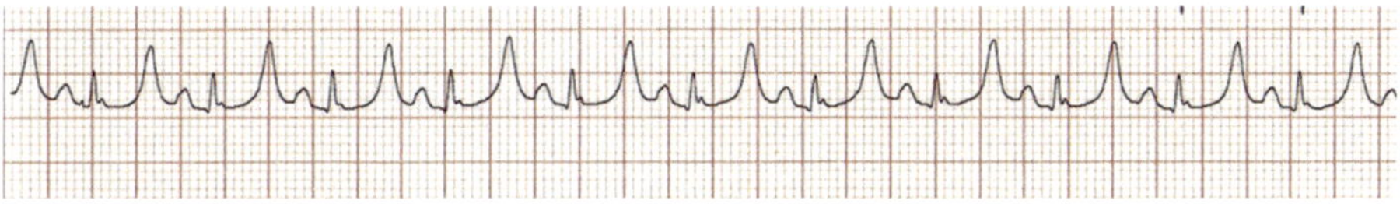

Fig. 8.6 Peaked T waves are very evident

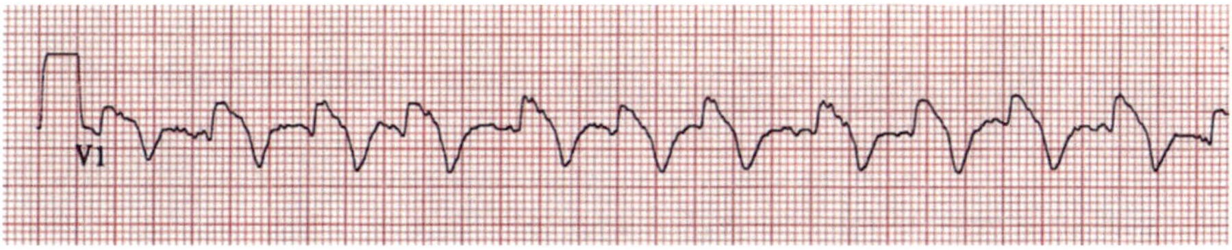

Fig. 8.7 QRS "sine wave" appearance associated with a potassium >8 meq/L

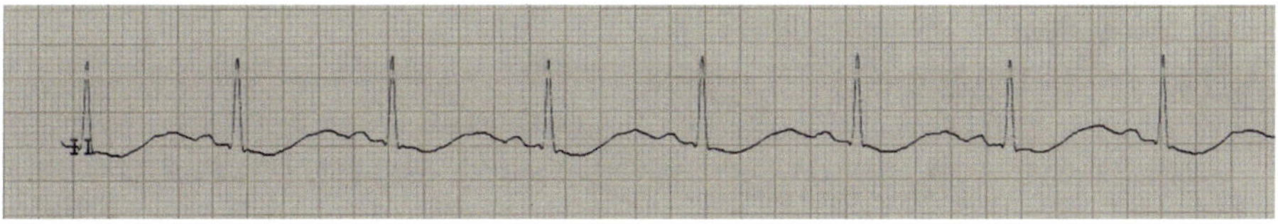

Fig. 8.8 A 5-year-old patient on oral furosemide with a 4-day history of vomiting and diarrhea. His potassium level was 2.5 meq/L. Diffuse ST-T slurring is evident

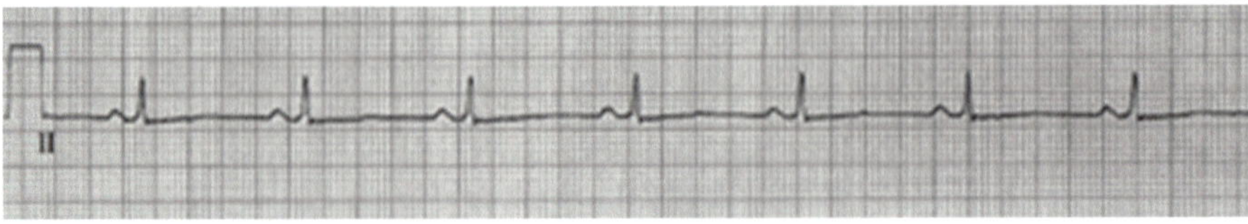

Fig. 8.9 ECG from a child with a calcium of 7.5 mg/dL. The QT interval is prolonged and the T waves are flat

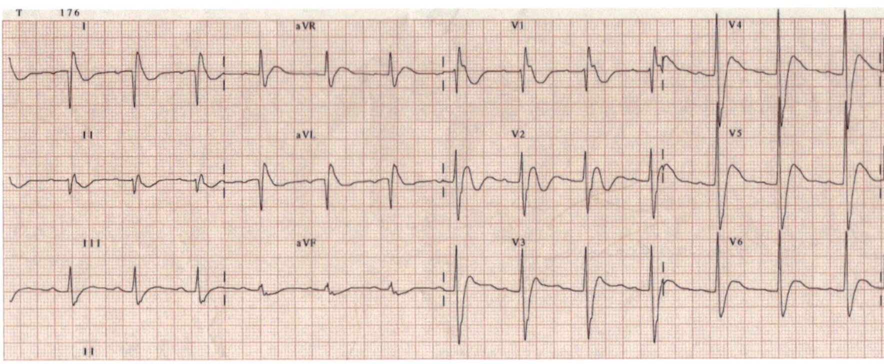

Fig. 8.10 Hypercalcemia results in shortening of the ST and the QT segments. There is rapid upstroke of the initial portion of the T wave. Another finding is the ST segment elevation in V1–V2

Calcium affects the cardiac action potential during phase 2 ("plateau phase"). This is reflected on the surface ECG by changes in the QT interval and the ST segments. Hypocalcemia can cause a lengthening of the QT interval (Fig. 8.9), while hypercalcemia will be associated with the opposite effect and a shortened QT interval (Fig. 8.10).

2. **Drug Related**

The ECG is sensitive to pharmacologic agents that interfere or alter ion transport in cardiac tissue. These agents include antimicrobials, antifungals, antidepressants, antipsychotics, and antiarrhythmics. Listing of these agents can be found elsewhere [8, 9]. Typically, the QT interval can be prolonged (Fig. 8.11) putting patients at risk for ventricular arrhythmias. The measured QT interval is age- and gender-dependent [10] and is thus corrected for heart rate using Bazett's formula: $QTc = QT/\sqrt{RR}$. A corrected QT interval of more than 0.47 s is considered abnormal in males and more than 0.48 s in females. Genetically inherited long QT syndrome is discussed below.

3. **Early Repolarization**

A current controversy exists as to the implications of early repolarization seen on the terminal part of the QRS and any predisposition to potentially serious arrhythmias (Fig. 8.12). This QRST wave variant is characterized by at least a 0.1 mV J elevation at the terminal part of QRS in two contiguous inferior and/or

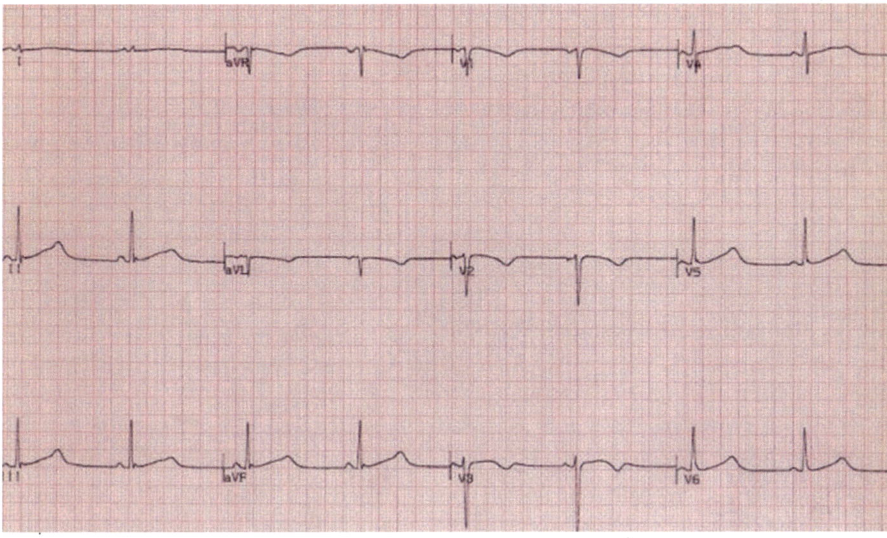

Fig. 8.11 ECG from a 9-year-old patient with pneumonia, treated with a macrolide antibiotic. The QTc interval measures >0.5 s

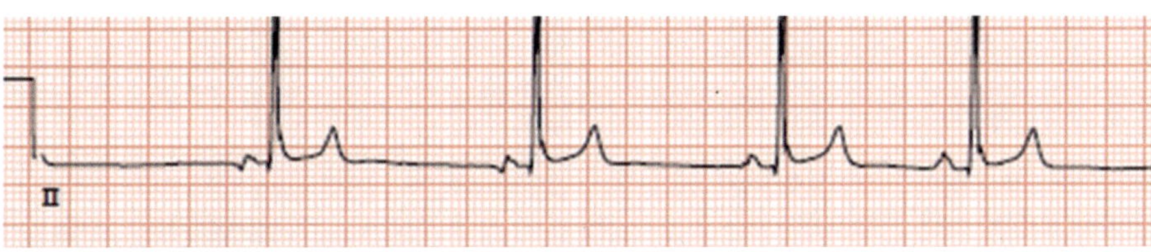

Fig. 8.12 Early repolarization pattern. Note the terminal slurring upstroke of the QRS as it reaches the ST segment

lateral ECG leads. This is in contrast to ST-T wave changes seen with myocardial injury (see below). The prevalence is highly variable between 1 and 13% of children. It is more common in males, young athletes, and those of African-American descent, although it can be seen in any ethnic group. Although there may be an association with arrhythmias among adults with early repolarization, to date, there have been no definitive adverse findings reported in children, and it is thus considered a benign condition [11].

4. **Dextrocardia**

As a result of normal embryologic development, the cardiac silhouette and apex are to the left side of the chest. However, at times, normal heart development occurs but with the cardiac silhouette to the right (mirror image dextrocardia). If this occurs, the position of the sinus node and right atrium is on the left side of the heart, and the resultant P wave axis will be inverted in lead I. In this condition, the right-sided precordial leads (V1–V3) will show increased QRS voltages, and left precordial leads will have diminished voltages (V5–V7) (Fig. 8.13). This can be confirmed by chest radiography. It is important to confirm that the negative p waves in lead I are not due to lead misplacement (see section on "Artifact").

Answer: D. A tall, peaked, and symmetrical T wave is the first change seen on the EKG on a patient with hyperkalemia.

Ventricular Premature Contractions

Ventricular premature contractions (PVCs) are early depolarizations of the ventricles leading to early systolic ventricular contractions. They are usually followed by a pause resulting in an irregular heart rate (Fig. 8.14). They are usually benign in an asymptomatic healthy child and disappear with exercise. In symptomatic patients who present with low cardiac output syndrome, frequent ventricular premature contractions may be associated with depressed ventricular function predisposing to malignant arrhythmias. They will need cardiology consultation with an echocardiogram to assess the function.

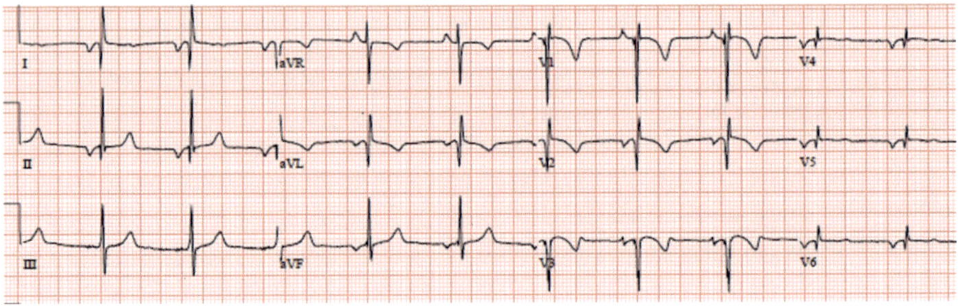

Fig. 8.13 ECG in a child with dextrocardia showing a left sinus node rhythm with negative P waves in leads I, II, and AVL and positive in AVR with low-voltage QRS complexes in the left precordial leads (V5–V6)

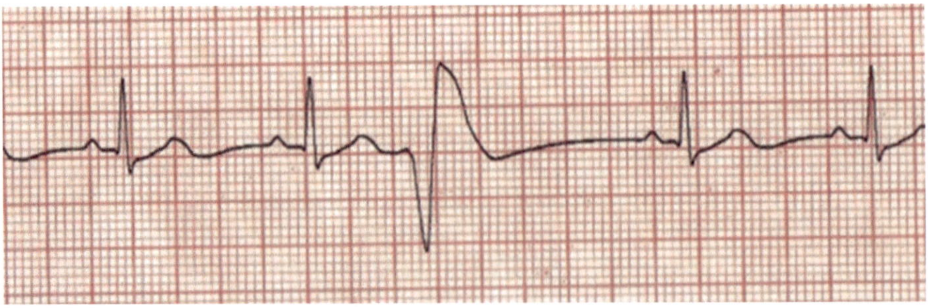

Fig. 8.14 The third QRS complex is wide and occurs earlier than the sinus rate. Depending on location in the respective ventricle, the QRS can exhibit a right, left, or nonspecific bundle branch block pattern

Artifact/Lead Misplacement

A common cause of concern is apparent ECG changes that are artefactual and may lead to unnecessary cardiology consultation and patient and family distress. Limb lead reversal, especially the arm leads, can present a QRS pattern that mimics dextrocardia or a lateral infarct (Fig. 8.15). This may compound anxiety if the patient presents with unrelated nonspecific chest wall pain or costochondritis. This is a common error despite current ECG limb leads that are both color-coded and embossed with letters indicating on which limb to place the electrode (RA, LA, RL, LL). The negative P wave deflection in leads I and AVL indicates that the P wave axis is reversed and should immediately prompt a repeat ECG with proper lead placement.

Everything that appears as an ECG abnormality is not always a real rhythm abnormality. In Fig. 8.16, even the monitor erroneously recorded a wide complex

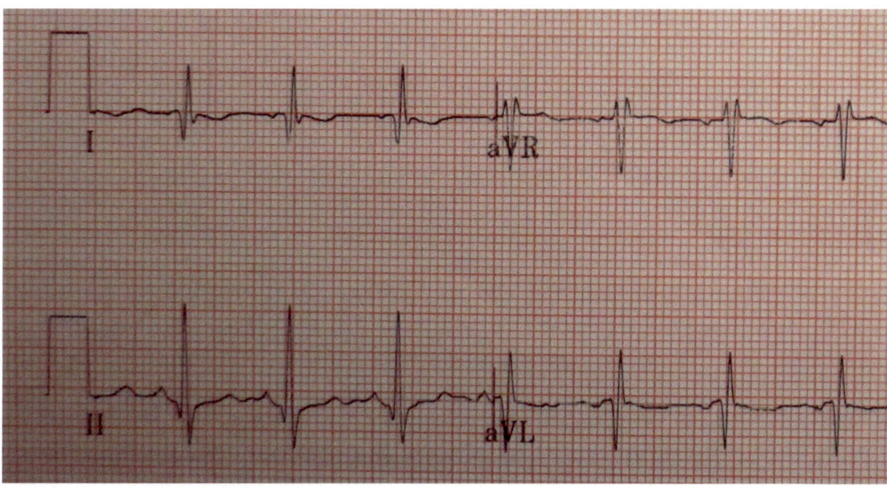

Fig. 8.15 Typical appearance of an arm limb lead reversal. In leads I and AVL, there are negative P waves as well as abnormal Q waves. The appearance of Q waves in these leads is consistent with a lateral infarct. However, the inverted P waves suggest a simple lead placement error

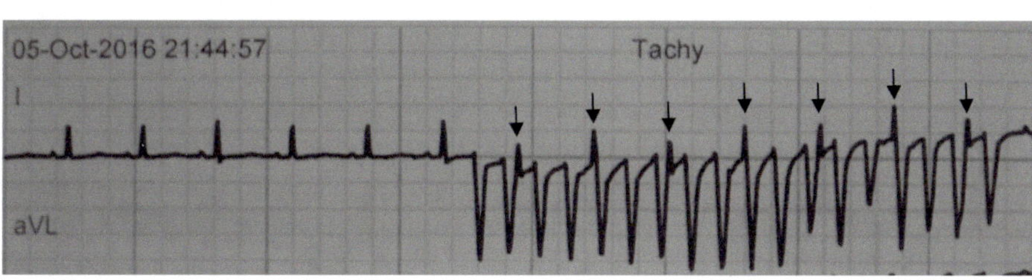

Fig. 8.16 Baseline artifact being detected as an abnormal tachycardia. Close examination shows that the ECG rate is constant as evidenced by the regular upright QRS complexes (arrows) as seen in lead I

tachycardia, when the deep negative deflections are artifactual. This is evidenced by the regular upright QRS complexes which march through at the same rate as the sinus rhythm and are distorted by the artifact.

Case 3
A 1-month-old baby presented to the emergency department with 1-week history of poor feedings and irritability. There are no recent illness, fever, or other associated symptoms. Physical examination: vital signs – afebrile; HR, 290/min; BP, 59/40 mmHg; and RR 40/min. Lungs: clear to auscultation. No murmurs heard. Abdomen: soft and the liver 3 cm below the right costal margin. Peripheral perfusion is decreased with a capillary refill time of 4 s. EKG is performed, and it shows narrow complex tachycardia at a rate of 290/min.
What would be the next appropriate step?

(A) Give adenosine.
(B) B- Synchronized cardioversion.
(C) C- IV antibiotics.
(D) D- Order an echocardiogram.
(E) CXR.

Supraventricular/Atrial Tachycardias

Among children presenting to emergency rooms (ER) with possible rhythm issues, supraventricular tachycardia (SVT) remains the most common etiology presenting at any age. However, the term "SVT" is not in itself a distinct diagnosis but rather a general term simply implying an atrial origin to the arrhythmia.

The atria do not possess a distinct electrical system comparable to the ventricular His-Purkinje system. Therefore, electrical impulse conduction is transmitted via muscle cell- to-cell interaction. Preferential muscle alignments permit rapid conduction to extend from the sinus node, located close to the superior vena caval-atrial junction to the AV node located near the septal leaflet of the tricuspid valve. This electrical impulse propagation can be compared to an ocean wave and is typically uniform. However, when the wave meets an obstacle, it bounces back. As a result of individual anatomy and muscle alignments in otherwise normal heart or due to scar tissue in patients with repaired CHD, atrial tissue conduction at times may not be uniform. This can result in pathways of both "slow" and "fast" conduction. The most common reason for any arrhythmia is "reentry" in which an electrical impulse propagates down one pathway, then backs up another, and circles around to reenter the first. This reentry phenomenon may be confined to the atrial tissue (atrial reentry), has an atrioventricular node (AVN) reentry pathway, or occurs through a direct atrioventricular tissue component as found with pre-excitation conditions such as Wolff-Parkinson-White.

In the current era, correct identification of the reentry site is important as therapeutic options differ based on location. For example, adenosine is commonly administered to attempt termination of SVT but is ineffective in terminating a primary atrial arrhythmia such as atrial flutter. Adenosine may still be useful as it may block the AVN conduction enough to expose the flutter waves to facilitate the proper diagnosis. The QRS morphology during the various forms of SVT is typically narrow or normal unless the patient has preexisting damage to the conduction system, such as following congenital heart surgery, or has any of the pre-excitation syndromes. Immediate therapeutic options will depend on clinical presentations. If there is evidence of impeding shock/heart failure, synchronized D/C cardioversion should be done immediately. However, if the child is hemodynamically stable, adenosine may be an effective first choice of therapy. This is given as a rapid bolus intravenous injection followed by a rapid saline flush as the half-life of adenosine is very short. The dose is 0.05–0.1 mg/kg which can be increased by 0.05–0.1 mg/kg per dose every 1–2 min up to 0.3 mg/kg/dose. For older children >50 kg, start with 6 mg IV, and then try 12 mg rapid IV push.

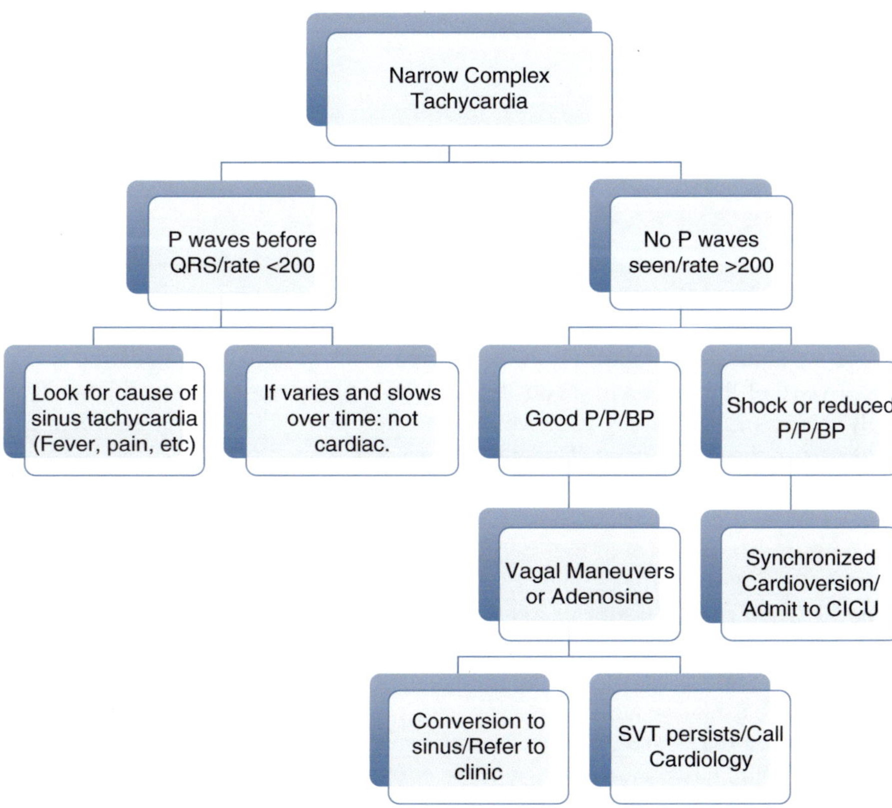

Algorithm for management of narrow complex tachycardia
P/P/BP = perfusion/peripheral pulses/blood pressure

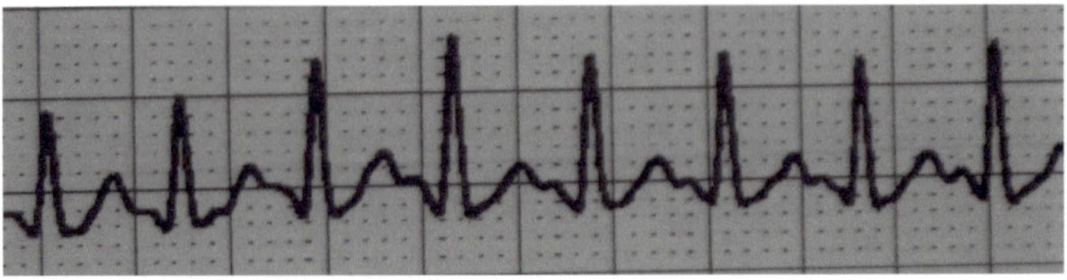

Fig. 8.17 Lead I. Sinus tachycardia. The heart rate is 220 bpm, there are P waves preceding every QRS, and the P axis and morphology are normal

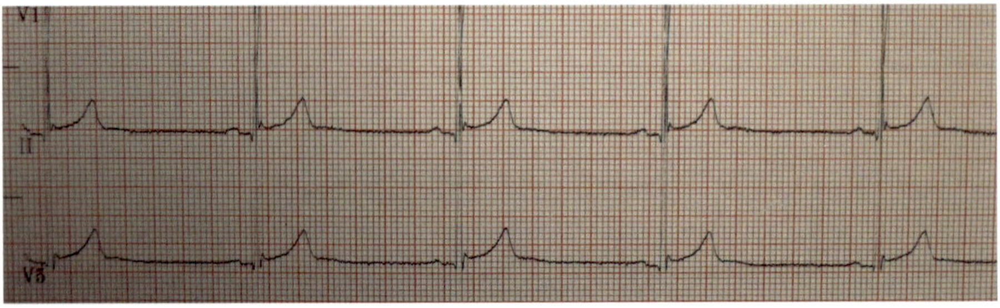

Fig. 8.18 Sinus bradycardia at a rate of about 40 bpm in an asymptomatic 16-year-old who runs varsity cross country and track. Improved physical conditioning results in efficient cardiac performance and slower heart rates. No therapy is required

Primary Atrial Rhythms

Since the sinus node impulse normally travels right to left across the atrial tissue, the P wave of the ECG will be positive in lead I during normal sinus rhythm. This will be irrespective of any changes in rate often up to 230 bpm in an infant and 220 bpm in the young child. The rate is dependent on contributing physical factors and will increase with fever, anxiety, or a high metabolic state [7]. In this regard, sinus tachycardia is associated with a normal P wave axis and morphology and accounts for the majority of narrow QRS tachycardias (Fig. 8.17).

Another frequent area of concern is a slow heart rate or bradycardia (Fig. 8.18). Knowledge of normal heart rate ranges for age is mandatory to be able to recognize heart rates out of ordinary for the child's age. The most common cause of a slow heart rate is sinus bradycardia due to high vagal tone such as seen in adolescents who undergo extensive athletic training which will result in slow resting heart rates. Sinus bradycardia is rarely a cause for concern or need for a referral to a cardiologist unless the child has symptoms of syncope or near syncope.

If the patient has an intrinsic bundle branch block, as is frequently seen following repair of congenital heart defects such as tetralogy of Fallot, the wide complex QRS pattern of right bundle branch block may mimic ventricular tachycardia (Fig. 8.19). Prompt history taking and clinical examination can help to distinguish between SVT and VT.

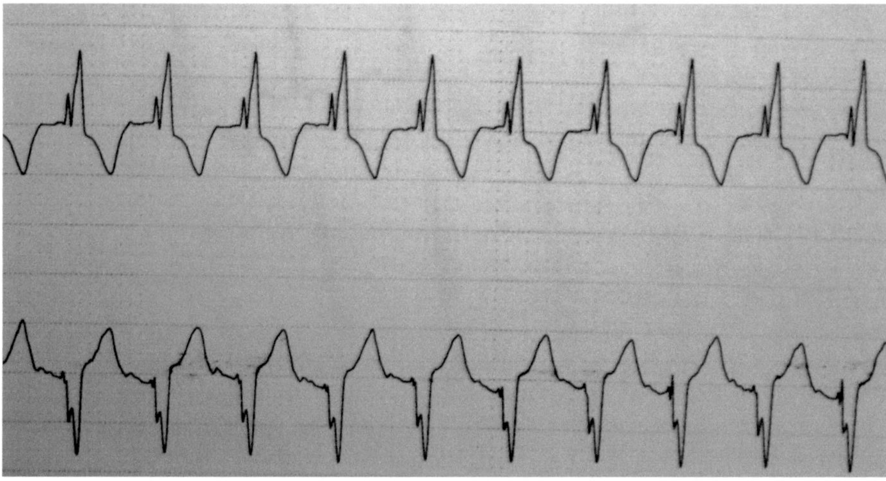

Fig. 8.19 Top, lead V1; bottom, lead II. Many patients with repaired CHD will have a complete right bundle branch QRS pattern, and rapid atrial rates may mimic ventricular tachycardia. Although the rhythm in lead V1 (top) appears to be a wide QRS ventricular tachycardia, a careful search shows normal P waves in lead II (bottom) confirming sinus tachycardia

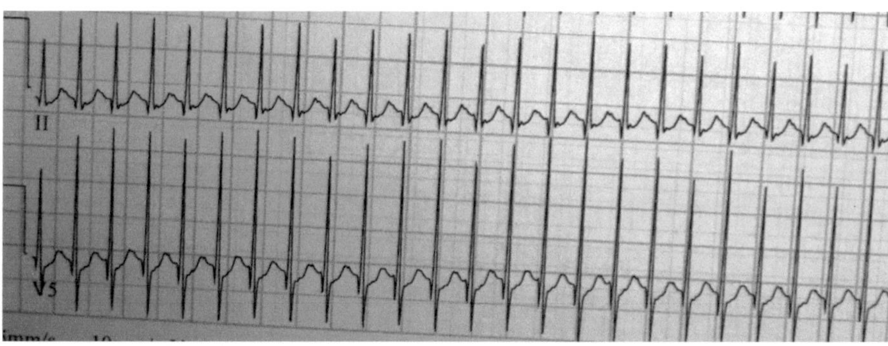

Fig. 8.20 Atrial ectopic tachycardia at 290 bpm. This can easily be confused with sinus tachycardia, but the incessant fixed rate that is much too fast for sinus indicates its origin from an abnormal focus elsewhere in the atria

Atrial ectopic tachycardia or ectopic atrial tachycardia (AET/EAT) is caused by instability of tissue membrane potentials in the atrium and can have heart rates reaching 250–270 bpm. This rhythm is typically faster than can be reached with sinus tachycardia. AET/EAT tachycardia rates are fixed without the usual rate variability seen with sinus rhythms (Fig. 8.20). It results from an automatic focus within the atria. They tend to accelerate (warm up) and get faster after the first few beats or decelerate (cool down) before reverting to sinus rhythm. They tend to have insidious presentation, with a gradual onset of heart failure or even dilated cardiomyopathy. Adenosine and direct current cardioversion are not effective in converting this rhythm. Cardiology consult should be immediately performed for pharmacological control.

Answer: B. In this infant with signs of shock, immediate synchronized cardioversion should be performed. If there was no sign of shock, then a rapid adenosine bolus can be given.

Atrial ectopic tachycardias can have a sudden onset, but it is typically faster than sinus tachycardia, and there is usually an abnormal P wave present (Fig. 8.21).

Primary Atrial Tachycardia (Flutter, IART, Fibrillation)

Case 4

A 45-year-old patient with single ventricle physiology presents with a 24 -h history of sudden-onset palpitations with no other associated symptoms. Physical exam: afebrile, HR100/min, BP 110/70 mmHg, and RR 20/min. Normal S1 and single S2. Lungs: clear to auscultation, no crackles, and no wheezing. Abdomen: soft, no tenderness or hepatomegaly, and well perfused. EKG performed showed the findings in Fig. 8.22.

What would be the most appropriate next step?

(A) Give adenosine.
(B) Admit to cardiology and start IV heparin.
(C) Synchronized cardioversion.
(D) Order an echocardiogram.
(E) External pacing.

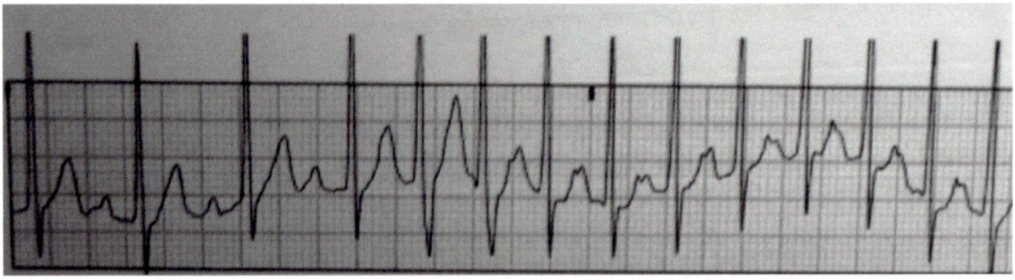

Fig. 8.21 Lead II. In this figure, sinus rhythm at a rate of 100 bpm is evident on the left. There is then a single premature atrial complex with the P wave on top of the T wave causing distortion of the usual rounded T wave appearance. This initiates a rapid atrial tachycardia at 250 bpm

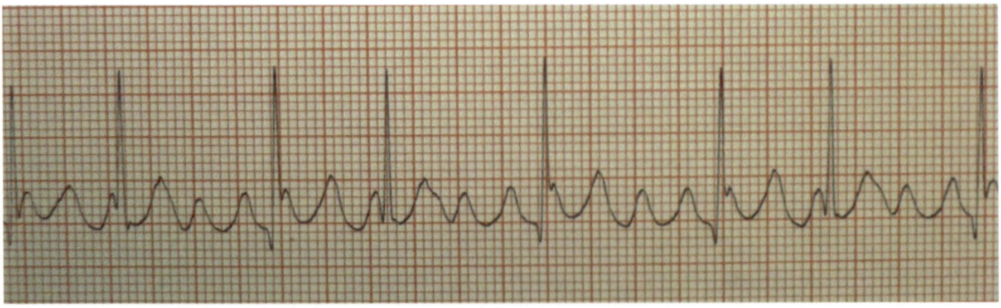

Fig. 8.22 Lead II. Typical "saw tooth" appearance of atrial flutter waves (typically about 300 bpm) with variable AV conduction, in a 3 or 4 to 1 ratio

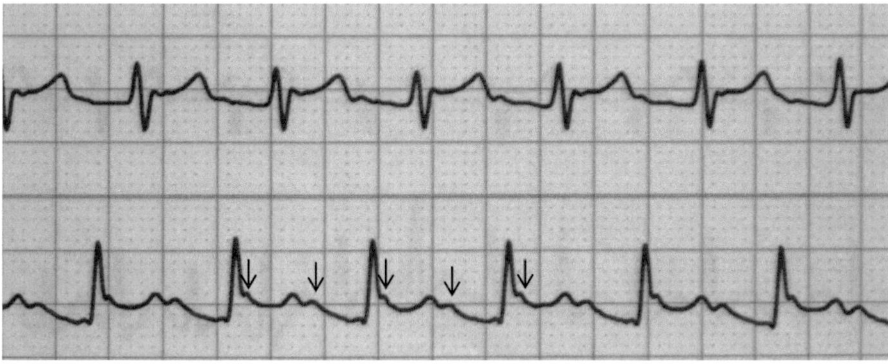

Fig. 8.23 Among patients with repaired CHD with stretched and thickened atria, a slower form of atrial flutter, IART, can occur. As seen, this rhythm can be misinterpreted as sinus tachycardia with 1° AV block. Careful examination of QRS complexes in the bottom lead shows a second atrial wave (black arrow) buried at the end of the QRS complex confirming 2:1 block of this slow atrial flutter

As previously discussed, the atria do not possess special conduction pathways for smooth electrical propagation. Anatomical landmarks such as the tricuspid valve ring, venae cavae, muscle ridges (such as the crista terminalis), and pulmonary vein openings all contribute to interrupt the electrical impulse to create potential re-entrant circuits [12]. In addition, children with repaired CHD have surgical incisions which leave behind scars which can alter electrical conduction. A common result is atrial flutter which can be diagnosed by examining leads II and III for the "saw tooth" pattern of the flutter waves (Fig. 8.22). Any adult with a repaired congenital heart defect presenting with a fast heart rate for no apparent reason should be evaluated for atrial flutter.

Atrial flutter rates range from 240 to 340 bpm and conduct to the ventricles at variable ratios (1:1–4:1) depending on AVN conduction, yielding ventricular rates of 150–200 bpm [9]. Although flutter waves with AVN conduction ratios of 4:1 can readily be appreciated, conduction ratios of 1:1 or 2:1 may be misinterpreted as sinus tachycardia. In such instances, the "T wave" of the QRST may be erroneously identified as a "P wave." Remembering that every QRS has a T wave following it and P waves can be independent will help to make the correct diagnosis.

Among patients with certain repaired CHD, such as single ventricles (Fontan-type surgical repair) a variant of atrial flutter, intra-atrial re-entrant tachycardia (IART), is commonly seen. The atrial rate is typically slower than flutter (150–200 bpm) and, therefore, so is the concomitant ventricular response (75–100 bpm). A misdiagnosis of sinus tachycardia with 1° AV block is often made (Fig. 8.23).

Although less common in children than adults, atrial fibrillation does occur, especially among patients with repaired CHD. The ECG typically shows an irregularly irregular ventricular rate with nonspecific undulating atrial activity (Fig. 8.24).

In instances of primary atrial tachycardias, the administration of adenosine may not terminate the arrhythmia; however, the drug can transiently block AVN conduction and expose the underlying atrial rhythm (Fig. 8.25). This patient can be referred to an electrophysiologist for medical therapy or, if resistant, for an EP study.

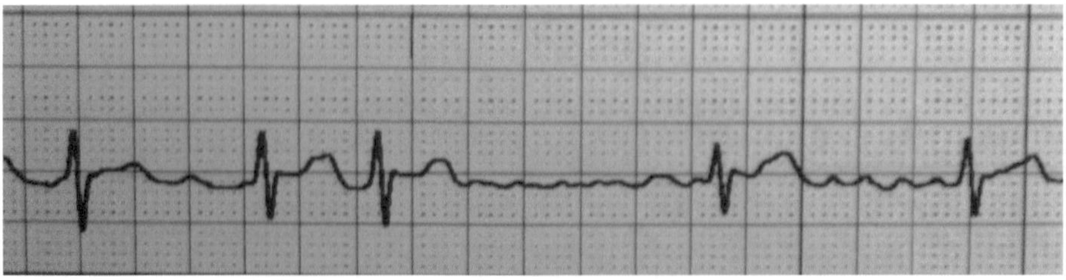

Fig. 8.24 Atrial fibrillation. Coarse wavy baseline is evident with a highly variable rate of QRS complexes

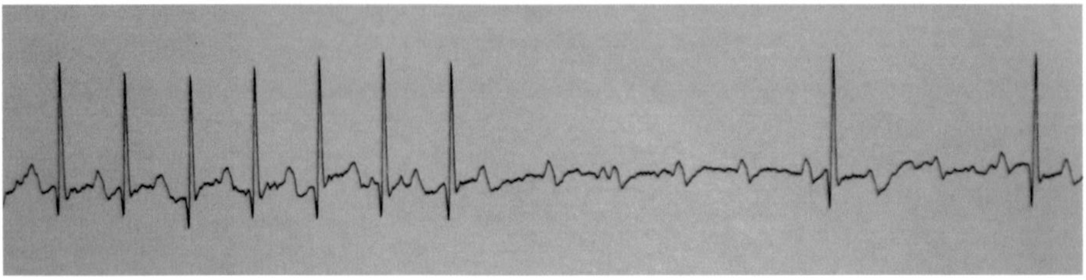

Fig. 8.25 Administration of adenosine during a primary atrial tachycardia typically does not terminate the arrhythmia since the AV node is not part of the circuit. However, it can aid in making the proper diagnosis by transiently delaying AV node conduction where the underlying atrial tachycardia is exposed

AV Node Re-entrant Tachycardia (AVNRT)

AVNRT can be best understood with the concept of "slow" and "fast" conduction as described above. Some children have more than one pathway for electrical impulses to cross the AV node. Atrial tissue connections to the AV node conduct at variable speeds and create a reentry circuit. Typically, the sinus impulse reaches the AV node via the "slow" atrial tissue pathway. It then exits via the "fast" pathway back into the atrium only to reenter the "slow" circuit again. Often, this circuit can be interrupted by vagal maneuvers or medication. The typical ECG shows a rapid narrow QRS (typically >220 bpm) with no visible retrograde P waves (Fig. 8.26). Tachycardia exhibits the qualities of both starting and stopping abruptly. Since the AV node is involved in the arrhythmia circuit, medications such as adenosine can be effective in acutely breaking the re-entrant circuit. The incidence of this type of SVT increases with age and becomes the most common form of SVT by adolescence [13].

Answer: B. Admit to cardiology and start IV heparin. The most likely cause for the sudden onset of a regular tachycardia in an older patient who had a Fontan operation for a "single ventricle" is a slow atrial flutter. This carries a risk for atrial thrombosis, and thus the patient should be admitted for anticoagulation and elective cardioversion once a transesophageal echocardiogram is done to look for a thrombus.

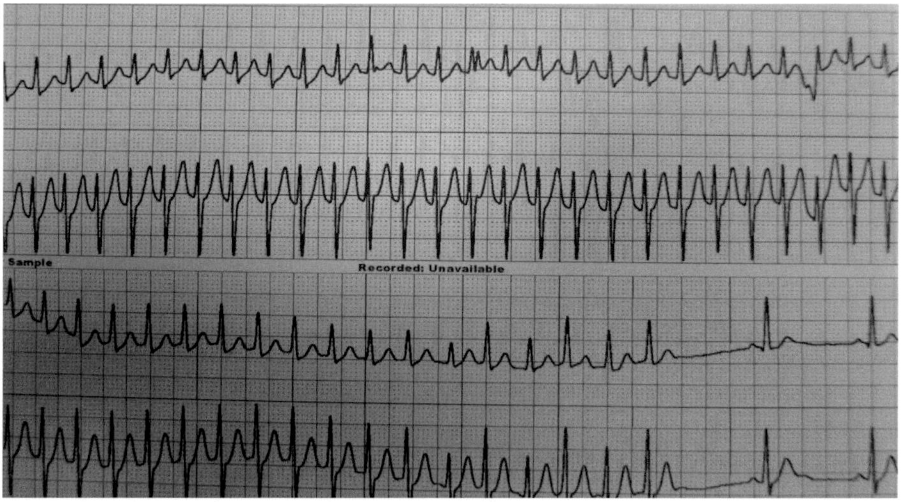

Fig. 8.26 Typical appearance of AVNRT illustrating a narrow QRS tachycardia without evidence of P waves. As shown at the end of the strip, tachycardia terminates abruptly

Atrioventricular Reciprocating Tachycardia (AVRT): Pre-excitation Syndromes

AVRT is the most common form of SVT among infants and represents persistence of embryologic atrioventricular muscle connections. Since any direct tissue-tissue connection may not possess the property of slowing of conduction found in the AV node, the PR interval is typically shorter than normal. Since these direct muscle connections will activate the ventricle earlier than electrical impulses arising via the AV node, the resultant QRS will exhibit varying degrees of pre-excitation or a slur at the onset of the QRS complex referred to as a "delta" (Δ) wave. The QRS may exhibit only a mild slur or a complete bundle branch block pattern, depending on how much of the ventricle is activated via the accessory connection. In addition, the delta wave may be negative, depending on the particular lead. Careful examination of all leads is mandatory to make the correct diagnosis (Fig. 8.27).

In addition, there may be competitive AV conduction between the normal AV node and accessory pathway so that both a normal and a preexcited QRS pattern can occur (Fig. 8.28).

The most common clinical pre-excitation condition is the Wolff-Parkinson-White syndrome (WPW) although there are other types of pre-excitation (Mahaim variants, atrio-nodal and atrio-junctional), which create accessory electrical conduction pathways and predispose to reentry arrhythmias. Among anatomical congenital heart defects, the most common association with WPW is Ebstein anomaly of the tricuspid valve. Other associated congenital cardiac conditions with WPW include Noonan's syndrome and various cardiomyopathies.

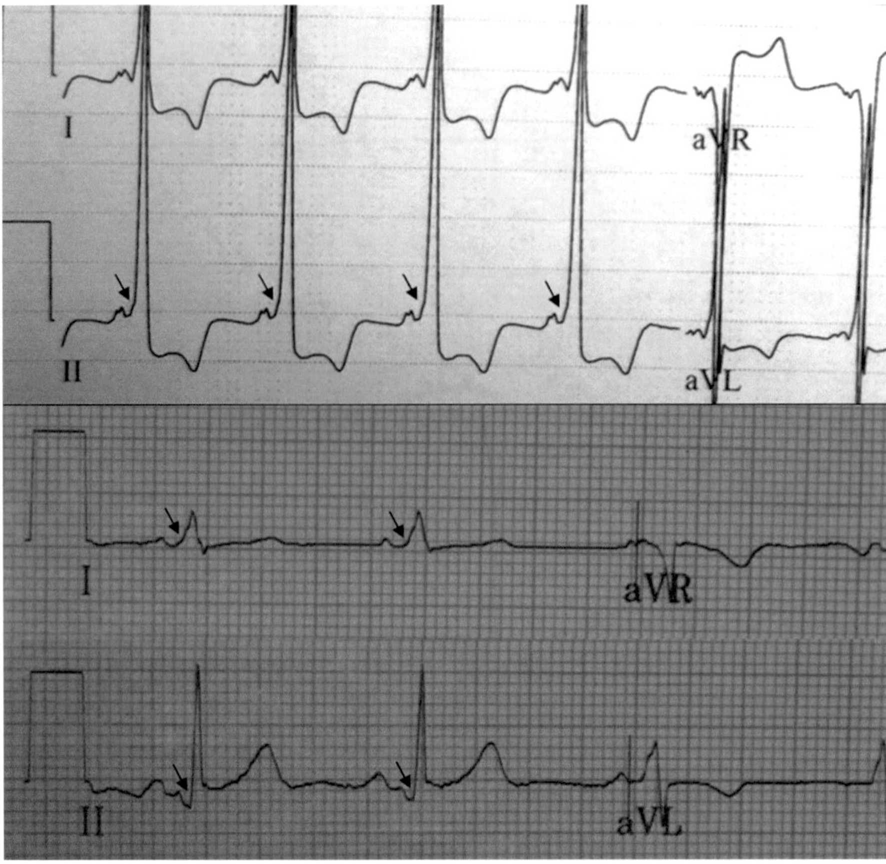

Fig. 8.27 The "delta" wave at the onset of the QRS characteristic of ventricular pre-excitation can be quite obvious or very subtle depending on the particular lead and location of the accessory connection in the heart. The delta wave can be either a positive (top) giving an upward slant to the QRS or a negative deflection as seen in lead II on the bottom tracing

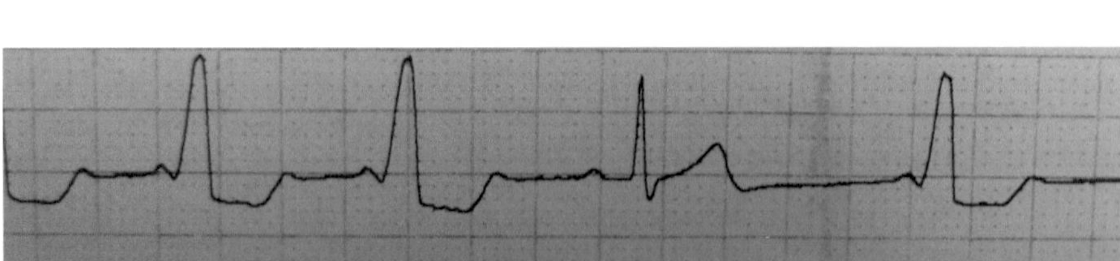

Fig. 8.28 The pre-excitation QRS pattern is not necessarily an "all-or-none" phenomenon. Depending on conduction and refractoriness of tissue, both normal and pre-excitation QRS patterns can occur in the same patient

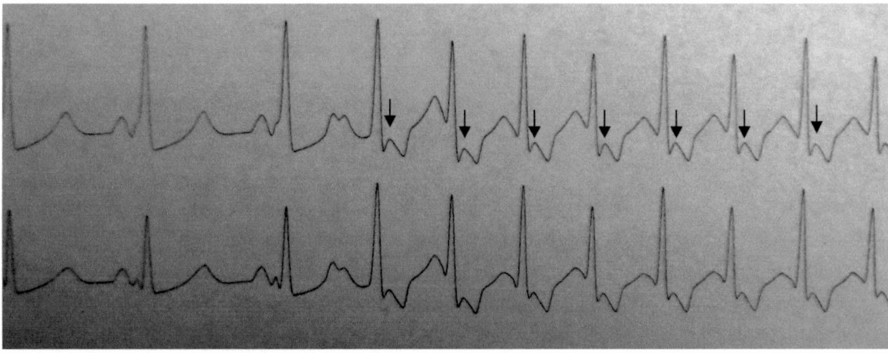

Fig. 8.29 Typical "orthodromic" AVRT (WPW) showing sinus rhythm with preexcited QRS complexes on the left and then a single PAC which is conducted to the ventricle via the AV node with a normal QRS duration. This initiates a narrow QRS tachycardia with retrograde P waves (arrows) evident just following the QRS and distorting the ST segment

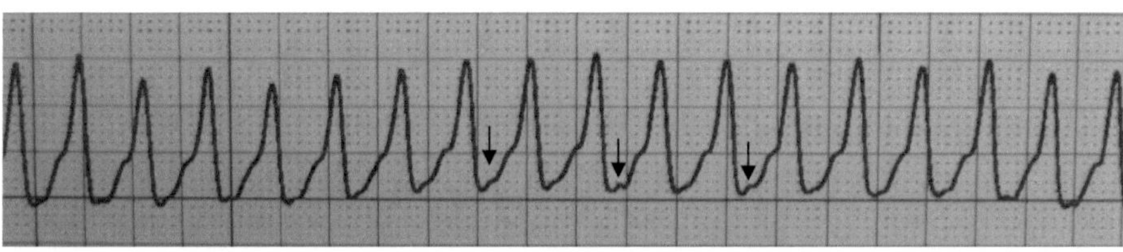

Fig. 8.30 "Antidromic" AVRT can mimic monomorphic ventricular tachycardia. Retrograde P waves are visible following the wide QRS complexes as indicated by the arrows

In the typical form of AVRT, antegrade AV conduction is via the AV node (orthodromic conduction). The accessory pathway then acts to permit retrograde VA conduction, and the circuit is created. The QRS is typically narrow with a heart rate of ≥250 bpm. Due to retrograde atrial activation from the circuit, retrograde P waves are commonly visible immediately after the QRS (Fig. 8.29).

Rarely in children, the antegrade AV conduction utilizes the accessory pathway (antidromic conduction) with the AV node serving to create the retrograde circuit. In these instances, ventricular activation begins where the accessory pathway connects and causes an altered QRS pattern. This may mimic ventricular tachycardia (Fig. 8.30). Since the AV node plays a role in the re-entrant circuit, adenosine can be an effective therapy. Of note, since the accessory tissue connections do not slow the atrial rate, sudden death (about 0.8% of cases) can result if atrial flutter occurs with a very rapid ventricular response (Fig. 8.31) [14].

The flow chart gives a suggested evaluation and therapeutic pathway for patients who present with a wide complex QRS tachycardia. In general, if they are in any distress or show signs of shock, immediate synchronized electrical cardioversion should be performed, with simultaneous emergent cardiology

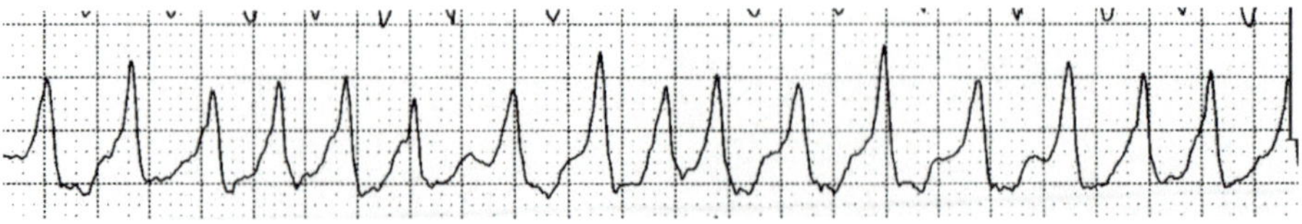

Fig. 8.31 Atrial fibrillation in a patient with WPW and antidromic conduction. Compared with Fig. 8.29, the R-R intervals are variable. The shortest R-R measures about 200 ms (heart rate 300 bpm) which can contribute to sudden death if that conduction rate is persistent

consultation. If they are clinically well, then a more detailed evaluation of the ECG recordings can be done and reviewed with a cardiology consultant (by phone, scanning, or email) to determine if medical therapy may be beneficial in converting the abnormal rhythm.

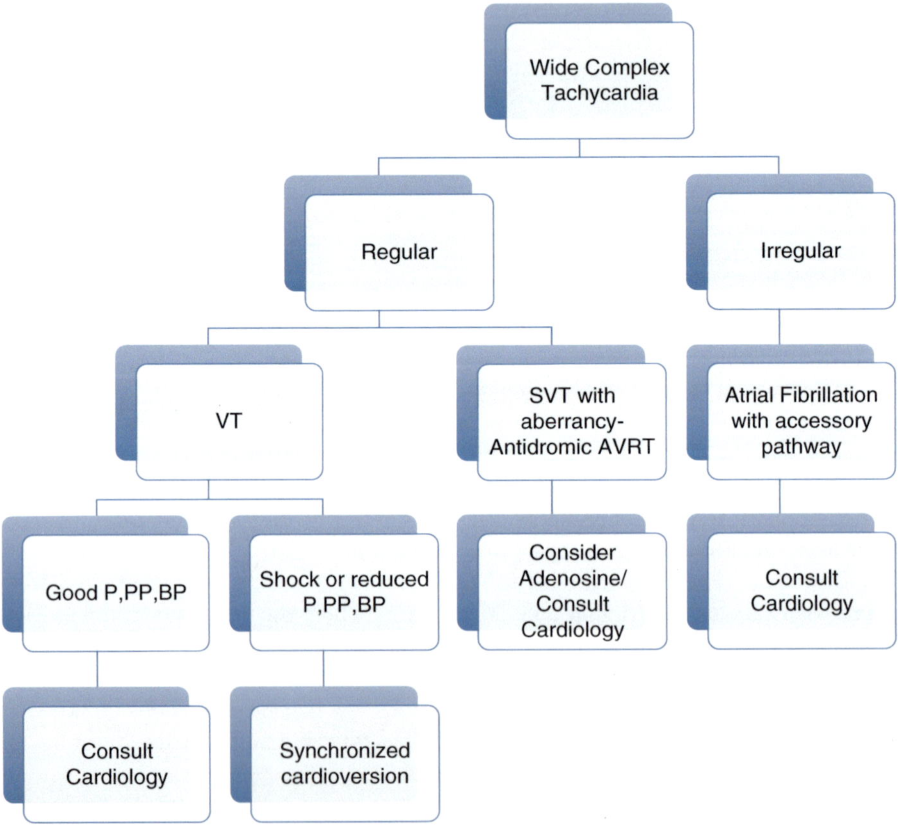

Algorithm for Management of Wide Complex Tachycardia
P/PP/BP = Perfusion/peripheral pulses/blood pressure

AV Node Conduction

First-Degree AV Block

The AV node protects the ventricle from rapid atrial rhythms due to its inherent anatomy and tissue conduction properties which slows the electrical propagation from the atria to the ventricles. This is reflected by the PR interval on the resting ECG. Age-related changes in the PR occur. In addition, changes in the PR interval can be the result of normal vagal tone, medications, myocardial damage, and infections. AVN conduction problems can be associated with certain congenital heart lesions such as septal defects and congenitally corrected transposition of the great arteries as well as with repaired CHD.

First-degree AV block is defined as a PR interval that is prolonged for age (usually >180 ms in young children and >200 ms in older children and adults), and every P wave is followed by a QRS (Fig. 8.32) Typically, no treatment is required although clinical correlation is important if the patient is on any medications that might cause AVN delay (beta- or calcium blockade), has a fever (possible myocarditis or acute rheumatic fever), or has evidence of Lyme disease.

Case 5

A 14-year-old girl sinks to the bottom of the pool while swimming a competitive meet. She is rescued, given CPR, and brought to the ED. She revives but has no memory of what occurred. On examination, her heart rate is 35 and regular, BP is 86/54, and her perfusion is reduced. Her ECG is shown in Fig. 8.35. The first step in her management is:

(A) Emergent temporary pacemaker insertion
(B) IV epinephrine
(C) Oral steroids
(D) Synchronized cardioversion
(E) Chest CT scan

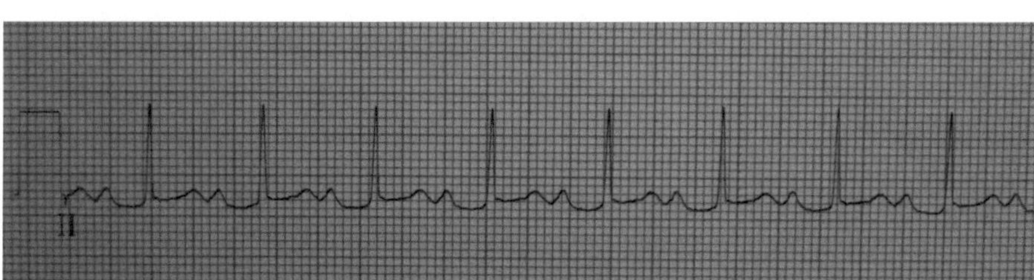

Fig. 8.32 First-degree AV block. P wave axis and morphology are normal. PR interval is prolonged (240 ms); however, every P wave is followed by a QRS complex

Second-Degree AV Block

Progression of the AV node delay which results in intermittently non-conducted P waves is referred to as second-degree AV block (2° AV block). Two distinct patterns are observed: Mobitz type 1 or Wenckebach has progressive PR interval prolongation preceding the non-conducted P wave (Fig. 8.33), while Mobitz type 2 has a fixed PR interval with dropped beats (Fig. 8.34). Most commonly, Wenckebach second-degree block is a benign finding, while Mobitz type 2 is not as this type may progress to third-degree or complete heart block.

Complete or Third-Degree AV Block

Complete independence of the P wave from the QRS is never normal (Fig. 8.35). Complete heart block (3° AV block) may be congenital or the result of inflammation, disease, surgery, CHD, or drug therapy. Complete congenital heart block

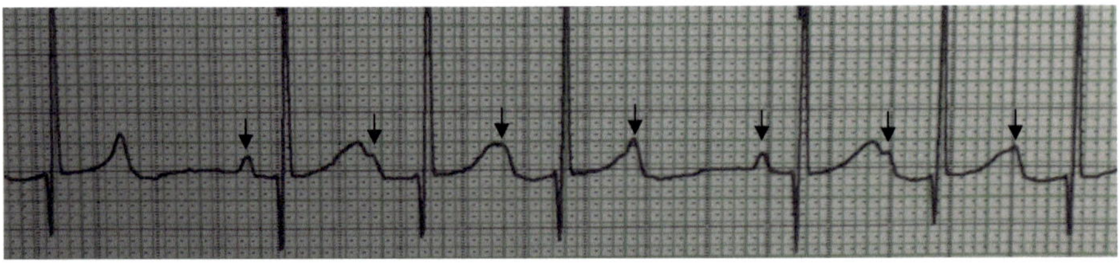

Fig. 8.33 2° AV block Wenckebach (Mobitz type I) is characterized by progressive PR prolongation that precedes the non-conducted P wave (arrows indicate the p waves). It is secondary to increased vagal tone and can occur in normal subjects and athletes without cardiac disease

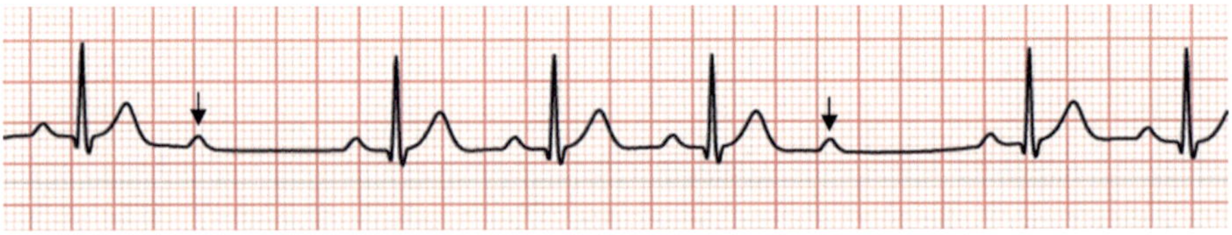

Fig. 8.34 Mobitz type 2 is characterized by a constant PR interval prior to the non-conducted P wave (arrows). It results from conduction system disease below the level of the AV node. This is typically abnormal and rarely seen in children without underlying heart disease

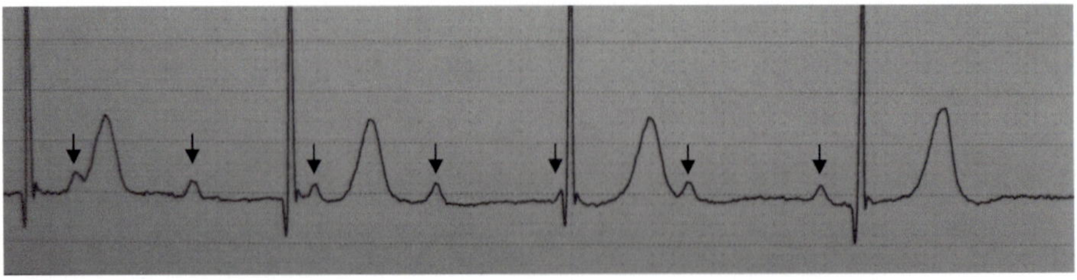

Fig. 8.35 Complete or 3° AV block with independent atrial P waves (arrows) and narrow QRS ventricular complexes

occurs sometimes in babies born to mothers with systemic lupus who have antibodies that affect the developing conduction system in the fetus. If the ventricular rate is too slow, the patient may develop heart failure and require pacemaker therapy.

The flow chart presents a method of quickly evaluating patients with bradycardia. In general, there is urgency in cardiology evaluation and intervention only when shock or near shock accompanies the slow heart rate.

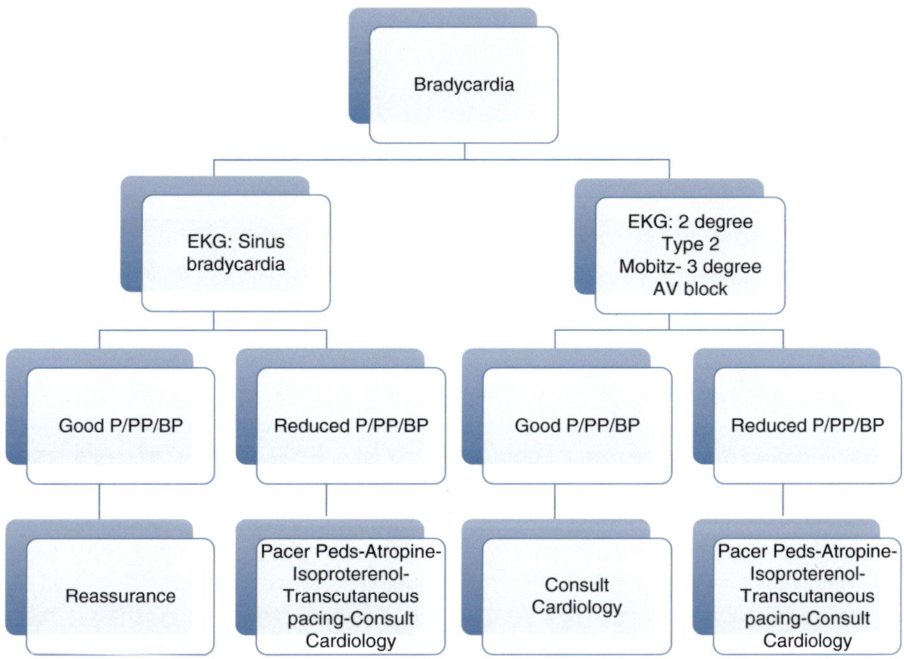

Algorithm for Management of Bradycardia
P/PP/BP = Perfusion/peripheral pulses/blood pressure

Cardiac Devices (Pacemaker/Defibrillator)

Children, even infants, do receive pacemakers and defibrillators (ICD) as a result of AV node issues or ventricular arrhythmias typically resulting from CHD surgery or inherited abnormalities of the conduction system. A full description of device therapy among children and patients with CHD is beyond the scope of this chapter and can be found elsewhere [15]. Basically, a pacemaker emits an electrical pulse which then elicits a cardiac muscle response. Patients who receive a pacemaker are given ID cards to help identify the manufacturer and the device model type. On the ECG, when the device emits an electrical discharge, a spike or sharp signal is seen. Normally, this is followed by either an atrial P or ventricular QRS complex, depending if the device is single (pacing only the ventricle) or dual chamber pacing both the atria and ventricles (Fig. 8.36). ICDs are used for internal defibrillation of potentially life-threatening arrhythmias for those at greatest risk. However, they have risks associated with them. The faster heart rates of children compared with adults may be interpreted as an arrhythmia by the ICD,

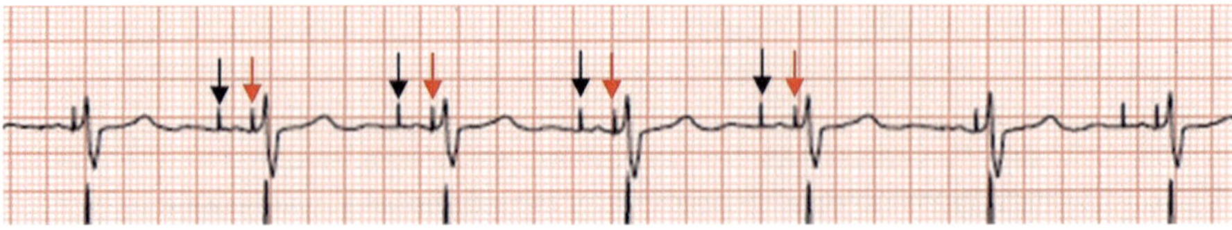

Fig. 8.36 Lead II: normal dual-chamber pacemaker function. Every electrical spike is followed by either an atrial P wave or ventricular QRS complex. Black arrow-atrial spike; Red arrow-ventricular spike

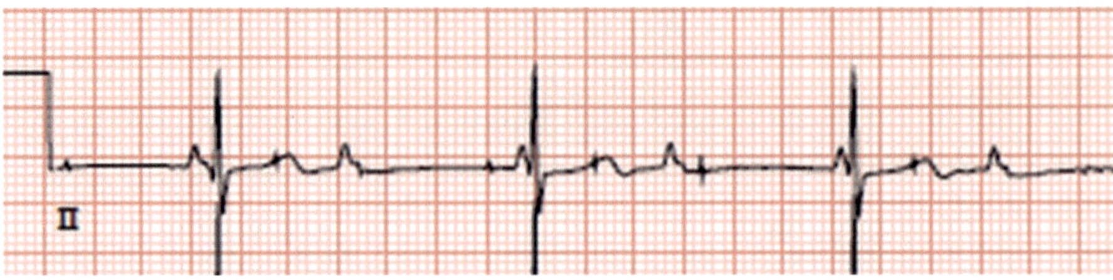

Fig. 8.37 ECG from a 5-year-old with congenital AV block and a fractured pacemaker lead. Note the complete AV block, slow ventricular rate, independent P waves, and intermittent pacemaker spikes that are not followed by any cardiac muscle response

causing an inappropriate ICD discharge. The important concept for the ER physician is to determine if the device is functioning properly (Fig. 8.37). Often a chest radiograph will show a displaced or fractured pacemaker/ICD lead. In instances of suspected device malfunction, or inappropriate ICD discharges, a thorough evaluation of the device is mandatory. Suspected pacemaker malfunction should prompt an urgent cardiology consultation to one familiar with implanted cardiac device technology and has access to the pacemaker interrogating device.

Answer: A. Newly diagnosed complete heart block is a true cardiac emergency requiring cardiac pacing. In the teenager described, this may be due to myocarditis which has affected the conduction system. The cardiology consultant will be able to insert a temporary pacemaker through a femoral vein or jugular approach. If cardiologist is not available, then external pacing may be required until a transvenous pacemaker insertion is available and if the low rate does not maintain adequate cardiac output. Newborns with congenital complete heart block may tolerate ventricular escape rates in the 50s but may require pacemaker insertion for lower rates or if associated decreased ventricular function is present.

Ventricular Arrhythmias

While abnormal and worrisome, ventricular arrhythmias are fortunately less common in children than in adults; it is imperative that the primary care provider is able to identify these findings and provide appropriate initial management [16]. Patients with a history of known and/or repaired CHD represent a high-risk population for serious arrhythmias. However, patients with no prior cardiac history may also sometimes present with serious ventricular rhythm abnormalities.

Repaired Congenital Heart Disease and Bundle Branch Blocks

Following intracardiac repair of CHD or in certain unrepaired defects, the baseline ECG is often abnormal due to surgical incisions and/or altered anatomy. This can cause a bundle branch block or nonspecific intraventricular conduction delay and serve as a diagnostic clue even before a full history is elucidated. In the presence of concerning symptoms (e.g., pre-syncope/syncope and sensed tachycardia), the ER physician should have a high index of suspicion for the presence of serious arrhythmias in such patients even when no arrhythmia has been documented in the ER setting.

Complete right bundle branch block (RBBB) is common in patients with repaired ventricular septal defects and tetralogy of Fallot due to surgical incisions on the right ventricular wall. Complete RBBB (Fig. 8.38) produces a typical "rsR" prime pattern ("rabbit ears") in lead V1 with a wide QRS (>120 ms) with a terminal delay in the left precordial leads representing delayed activation of the right ventricle. A cause of diagnostic error often arises among patients with repaired atrioventricular canal defects in whom the QRS axis is "leftward" or "superior." This finding, combined with a RBBB pattern, often leads to the erroneous diagnosis of bifascicular coronary disease.

A true left bundle branch block (LBBB) is rare and always pathological in the pediatric population and merits full investigation in conjunction with a cardiologist. This is often associated with intrinsic myocardial issues or Kawasaki disease and coronary involvement (Fig. 8.39). The LBBB is characterized by a wide QRS (> 120 ms) with a negative deflection in V1 (QS pattern or sometimes a tiny r wave with rS pattern), late precordial transition (positive R waves beyond lead V3 or V4), and often a notched "M" pattern in the middle of the R wave in lateral precordial leads.

Nonspecific intraventricular conduction delay (IVCD) not meeting the criteria for either a RBBB or a LBBB pattern may be seen in patients with some repaired congenital heart defects, especially patients with a single ventricle (Fontan-type palliation). The QRS duration is typically <120 ms (Fig. 8.40). This finding may not be of concern unless clinical findings suggest an arrhythmia.

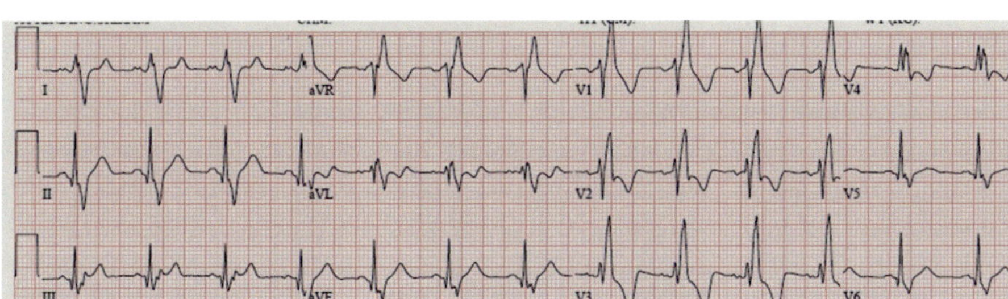

Fig. 8.38 Typical appearance of a RBBB pattern seen among patients with repaired CHD, most commonly tetralogy of Fallot

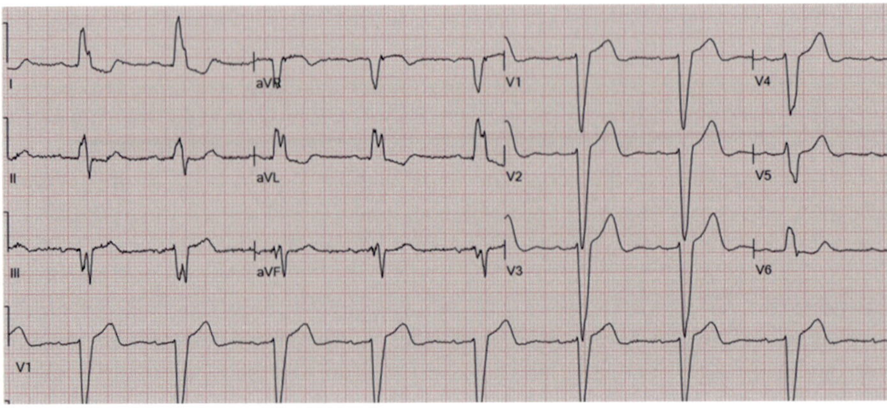

Fig. 8.39 LBBB pattern. In comparison to the more common RBBB pattern, the "rabbit ears" are absent in the right precordial leads

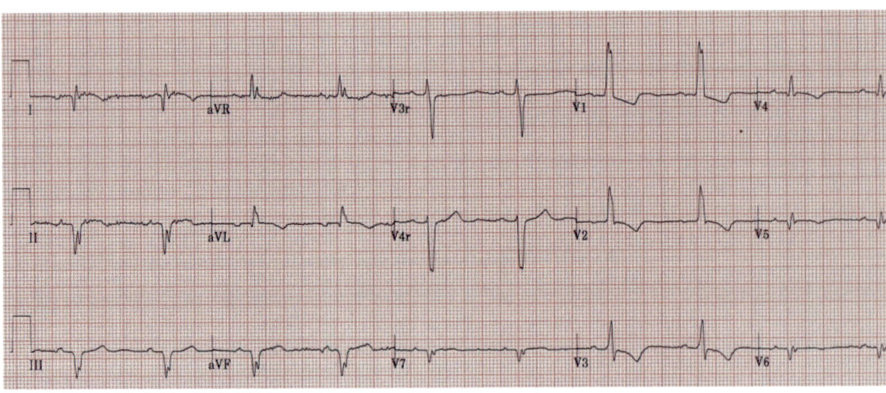

Fig. 8.40 Nonspecific QRS pattern in IVCD showing neither a right nor left bundle branch block pattern. This is common among patients with single ventricle anatomy

Myocardial Injury

Myocardial injury creates a distinct pattern of ST changes, seen at the terminal part of the QRS. Typically, there is diffuse ST segment elevation seen in multiple leads (Fig. 8.41). This is different from the early repolarization pattern described above. Clinical suspicions of inflammatory muscle conditions such as myocarditis or coronary artery problems should be explored. This pattern is always abnormal and requires urgent cardiology consultation and ICU admission. Confirmatory blood tests including cardiac troponins are helpful in this situation.

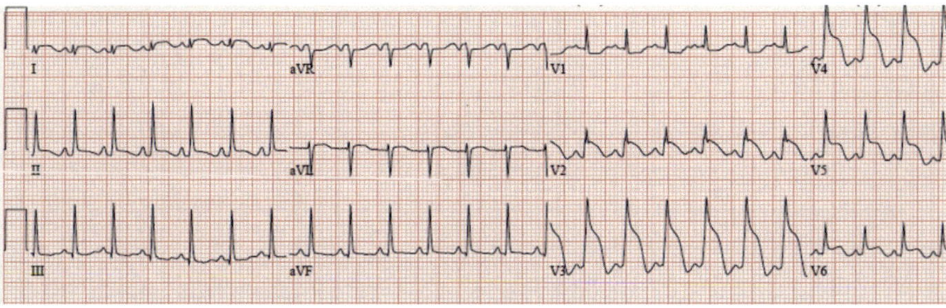

Fig. 8.41 Diffuse ST elevation is seen across the precordial leads in a child presenting with myocarditis

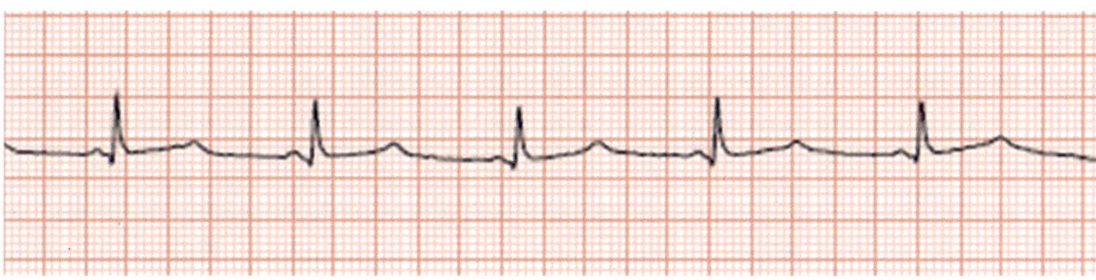

Fig. 8.42 Lead II: QTc >500 ms in a child with familial LQTc syndrome

Genetic Cardiac Channelopathies

A detailed description of the cardiac channelopathies that predispose the patient to serious ventricular arrhythmias and sudden death is beyond the scope of this chapter and can be found elsewhere [17]. A high index of suspicion is needed for the diagnosis in the presence of concerning symptoms and no documented arrhythmia.

A QT interval corrected for heart rate (QTc) ≥ 470 ms in adolescent males or ≥480 ms in adolescent females is considered to be prolonged [18]. A measured prolonged QT interval in the setting of seizures, syncope, or pre-syncope associated with exertional or a sudden startle merits referral to the cardiologist for further evaluation. Discussions should include a family history of long QT syndrome (LQTS) or sudden unexpected death in first-degree relatives. Familial LQTS should be suspected when the QTc interval is ≥500 ms in the absence of any drugs or electrolyte abnormalities which can prolong the QT interval (see above). Other non-cardiac conditions (e.g., trauma, acute intracranial pathology) can also cause QT prolongation (Fig. 8.42).

Another cause of syncope is the Brugada syndrome (BrS) which is rare among children. It is one of the inherited sodium channelopathies and is associated with ventricular arrhythmias. The typical Brugada type I ECG pattern (Fig. 8.43) is denoted by a coved ST segment elevation ≥2 mm in leads V1 and/or V2. Placement of the precordial ECG leads at a higher intercostal space than normal (second intercostal space) improves detection.

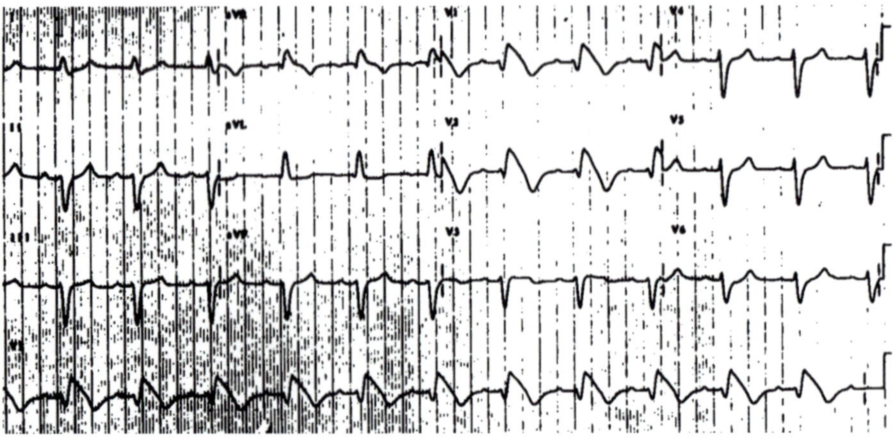

Fig. 8.43 Typical "coved" QRS pattern in lead V1 of Brugada syndrome. Compare this to a RBBB pattern above

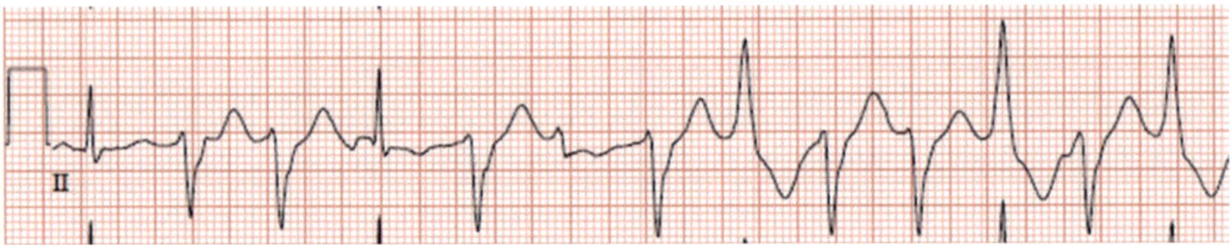

Fig. 8.44 Bidirectional ventricular tachycardia in a patient with CPVT. Note the initial normal QRS pattern (first beat on the left) prior to the arrhythmia onset

Catecholaminergic polymorphic ventricular tachycardia (CPVT) is another inherited myocardial channelopathy associated with sudden death (Fig. 8.44). However, the baseline ECG is normal. Ventricular ectopy and arrhythmias may occur spontaneously but happen more commonly with exercise.

Ventricular Tachycardia

As indicated above, premature ventricular contractions (PVC) are common in children even with structurally normal hearts. However, ventricular tachycardia (VT) is rare. VT can be non-sustained (<30 s and no significant symptoms) or sustained (≥30 s and/or significant symptoms such pre-syncope or syncope). VT can be classified as monomorphic (all QRS complexes with the same morphology), bidirectional (positive and negative QRS), or polymorphic (variable morphologies). The diagnostic criteria for VT include a wide QRS tachycardia without a typical right or left bundle branch block pattern and the presence of AV dissociation. The right ventricular outflow tract (RVOT) is a common site for arrhythmia (Fig. 8.45). Management depends on type of arrhythmia [19, 20].

While polymorphic VT/VF can be the result of channelopathies such as BrS and CPVT, it can also be seen in the setting of ischemia as illustrated in Fig. 8.46 from

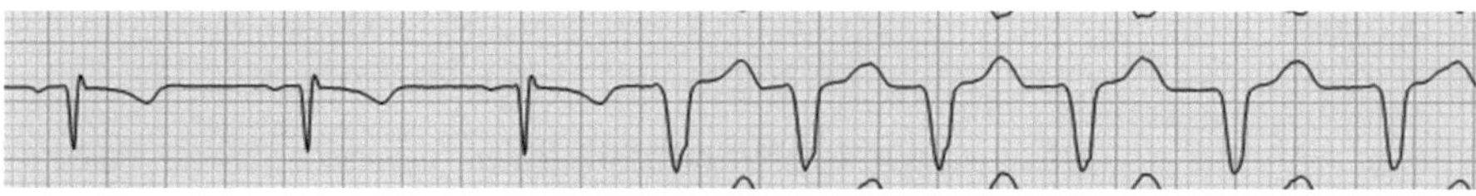

Fig. 8.45 Lead V1: Onset of a wide QRS with LBBB pattern in a teenager arising from the RVOT

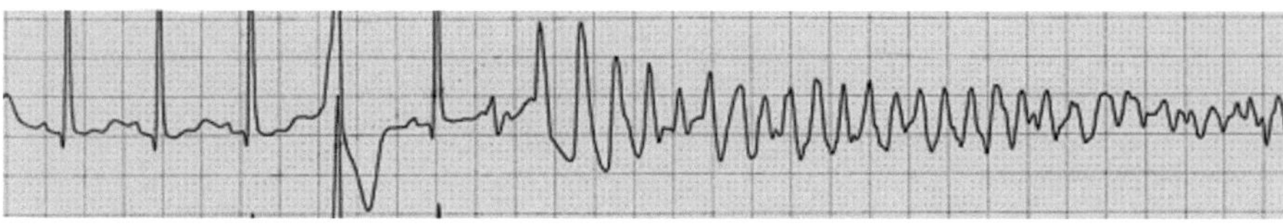

Fig. 8.46 Sinus rhythm followed by a PVC and subsequently the Torsades de pointes variety of VT

a child with coronary artery occlusion following a surgical "unroofing" for anomalous origin of left coronary artery from right aortic sinus. Torsades de pointes is a type of polymorphic VT with gradual variation in the amplitude and "twisting" of QRS axis around the isoelectric line and is the type of VT associated with the long QT syndrome and certain medications. Sustained VT with decreased perfusion always requires immediate action, including electrical cardioversion and emergent cardiology consultation. This most often would be followed by medications in an intensive care setting as recurrence of the arrhythmia is common.

Conclusion

Children at any age can present with arrhythmias. It must be remembered that a repaired congenital heart defect is never normal and even with excellent surgical repair, residual hemodynamic changes and scar tissue can predispose to arrhythmias. In addition, genetically inherited arrhythmogenic conditions can be expressed at any age, and the developing cardiac conduction system predisposes infants and young children to rhythm disturbances. Computer-generated ECG interpretations are frequently erroneous and can cause unnecessary patient anxiety and inappropriate hospital admissions and consultations. Knowledge to interpret real or perceived abnormalities of the ECG is necessary to make appropriate clinical decisions as to management or appropriate cardiology referrals.

References

1. Wier LM, Yu H, Owens P, Washington R. Overview of children in the emergency department 2010. Rockville, MD: Healthcare Cost and Utilization Project, Agency for Healthcare Research and Quality; 2013.
2. Lee YS, Baek JS, Kwon BS, Kim GB, BAe EJ, Noh C, Choi JY, Yun YS. Pediatric emergency room presentation of congenital heart disease. Korean Circ J. 2010;40:36–41.
3. Shah AP, Rubin SA. Errors in the computerized electrocardiogram interpretation of cardiac rhythm. J Electrocardiol. 2007;40(5):385–90.
4. Guglin ME, Datwani N. Electrograms with pacemakers: accuracy of computer reading. J Electrocardiol. 2007;40:144–6.

5. Seppala S, Laitinen T, Tarvainen MP, Tompuri T, Veijalainen SK, Lakka T. Normal values for heart rate variability parameters in children 6-8 years of age: the PANIC study. Clin Physiol Funct Imaging. 2014;34:290–6.
6. Fleming S, Thompson M, Stevens R, Heneghan C, Pluddemann A, Maconochie I, Tarassenko L, Mant D. Normal ranges of heart rate and respiratory rate in children from birth to 18 years: a systematic review of observational studies. Lancet. 2013;19:377–92.
7. Tang CW, Scheinman MM, VanHare GF, Epstein LM, Fitzpatrick AP, Lee RJ, Lesh MD. Use of P wave configuration during atrial tachycardia to predict site of origin. J Am Coll Cardiol. 1995;26:1315–24.
8. Yap Y, Camm J. Drug induced QT prolongation and torsade de pointes. Heart. 2003;89(11):1363–72.
9. Woosley RL, Romero K. Assessing cardiovascular drug safety for clinical decision-making. Nat Rev Cardiol. 2013;10:330–7.
10. Vink AS, Clur SB, Geskus RB, Blank AC, De Kezel CC, Yoshinaga M, Hofman N, Wilde AA, Blom NA. Effect of age and sex on the QTc interval in children and adolescents with type 1 and 2 long-QT syndrome. Circ Arrhythm Electrophysiol. 2017;10(4):pii: e004645.
11. Safa R, Thomas R, Karpawich PP. Electrocardiographic early repolarization characteristics and clinical presentations in the young: a benign finding or worrisome marker for arrhythmias. Congenit Heart Dis. 2017;12(1):99–104.
12. Saoudi N, Cosío F, Waldo A, Chen SA, Iesaka Y, Lesh M, Saksena S, Salerno J, Schoels W, Working Group of Arrhythmias of the European of Cardiology and the North American Society of Pacing and Electrophysiology. A classification of atrial flutter and regular atrial tachycardia according to electrophysiological mechanisms and anatomical bases; a Statement from a Joint Expert Group from The Working Group of Arrhythmias of the European Society of Cardiology and the North American Society of Pacing and Electrophysiology. Eur Heart J. 2001;22(14):1162–82.
13. Blaufox AD, Rhodes JF, Fishberger SB. Age related changes in dual AV nodal physiology. Pacing Clin Electropysiol. 2000;23:477–80.
14. Obeyesekere M, Gula LJ, Skanes AC, Leong-Sit P, Klein GJ. Risk of sudden death in Wolff-Parkinson-white syndrome. How high is the risk? Circulation. 2012;125:659–60.
15. Mond H, Karpawich PP. Pacing options in the adult patient with congenital heart disease. Malden, MA: Blackwell Futura (Pubs); 2007.
16. Khairy P, Van Hare GF, Balaji S, Berul CI, Cecchin F, Cohen MI, Daniels CJ, Deal BJ, Dearani JA, Groot N, Dubin AM, Harris L, Janousek J, Kanter RJ, Karpawich PP, Perry JC, Seslar SP, Shah MJ, Silka MJ, Triedman JK, Walsh EP, Warnes CA. PACES/HRS expert consensus statement on the recognition and management of arrhythmias in adult congenital heart disease. Heart Rhythm. 2014;11:e102–65.
17. Priori SG, Wilde AA, Horie M, Cho Y, Behr ER, Berul C, Blom N, Brugada J, Chiang CE, Huikuri H, Kannankeril P, Krahn A, Leenhardt A, Moss A, Schwartz PJ, Shimizu W, Tomaselli G, Tracy C. HRS/EHRA/APHRS expert consensus statement on the diagnosis and management of patients with inherited primary arrhythmia syndromes:document endorsed by HRS, EHRA, and APHRS in May 2013 and by ACCF, AHA, PACES, and AEPC in June 2013. Heart Rhythm. 2013;10:1932–63.
18. Johnson JN, Ackerman MJ. QTc: how long is too long? Br J Sports Med. 2009;43:657–62.
19. Brugada J, Blom N, Sarquella-Brugada G, Blomstrom-Lundqvist C, Deanfield J, Janousek J, Abrams D, Bauersfeld U, Brugada R, Drago F, de Groot N, Happonen JM, Hebe J, Yen Ho S, Marijon E, Paul T, Pfammatter JP, Rosenthal E, European Heart Rhythm Association; Association for European Paediatric and Congenital Cardiology. Pharmacological and non-pharmacological therapy for arrhythmias in the pediatric population: EHRA and AEPC-Arrhythmia Working Group joint consensus statement. Europace. 2013;15:1337–82.
20. Crosson JE, Callans DJ, Bradley DJ, Dubin A, Epstein M, Etheridge S, Papez A, Phillips JR, Rhodes LA, Saul P, Stephenson E, Stevenson W, Zimmerman F. PACES/HRS expert consensus statement on the evaluation and management of ventricular arrhythmias in the child with a structurally normal heart. Heart Rhythm. 2014;11:e55–78.

9 Hypercyanotic Spells

Tageldin Ahmed, Yamuna Sanil,
and Sabrina M. Heidemann

Case 1

A 6-week-old girl presented to the emergency department with inconsolable crying and bluish discoloration of her lips and mouth. The baby was born full term and prenatally diagnosed with Tetrology of Fallot. She has no previous history of cyanosis and no other symptoms and is not receiving any medication. On examination, the infant is fussy and tachypneic and has central cyanosis. Her heart rate is 180 BPM, respiratory rate of 60 BPM, and blood pressure of 72/48 mmHg, and the oxygen saturation is 50% in room air. Her precordium is quiet with no thrills, S1 is normal, and S2 is single. A faint systolic ejection murmur is heard over the left upper sternal border. Peripheral pulses are palpable. Her lungs are clear and there is no hepatomegaly.

The most likely cause of these symptoms is:

(A) Sepsis
(B) Hypercyanotic spell
(C) Supraventricular tachycardia
(D) Toxic shock syndrome
(E) Severe hypoglycemia

T. Ahmed, M.D. • S. M. Heidemann, M.D. (✉)
Division of Critical Care, Children's Hospital of Michigan, Wayne State University School of Medicine, Detroit, MI, USA
e-mail: tahme@med.wayne.edu; sheidema@med.wayne.edu

Y. Sanil, M.D.
Division of Cardiology, Children's Hospital of Michigan, Wayne State University School of Medicine, Detroit, MI, USA
e-mail: ysanil@dmc.org

© Springer International Publishing AG, part of Springer Nature 2018

A. P. Sarnaik et al. (eds.), *Cardiac Emergencies in Children*,
https://doi.org/10.1007/978-3-319-73754-6_9

Pathophysiology

A hypercyanotic spell is a paroxysmal hypoxic event characterized by severe reduction in pulmonary blood flow that could last minutes to several hours with a multitude of consequences. Several congenital heart lesions are associated with hypercyanotic spells. The common physiology is one of a large unrestricted ventricular septal defect (VSD) resulting in equalization of pressures in both ventricles. The downstream resistance determines the directionality of the shunt across the VSD. Systemic vascular resistance and the pulmonary outflow obstruction determine the amount of net forward flow from the ventricles. An imbalance between pulmonary and systemic vascular resistances favoring systemic blood flow results in shunting of deoxygenated blood from the right ventricle to the systemic circulation through the VSD precipitating the hypercyanotic spell (Fig. 9.1). It is not entirely clear how the hypercyanotic spell starts, yet its progression is fairly predictable from the physiological standpoint. Stimulation of mechanoreceptors in the right ventricle due to an increase in catecholamine-induced cardiac contractility combined with a decrease in right ventricular size may initiate the hypercyanotic spell by increasing right ventricular outflow obstruction. This also triggers a reflex hyperventilation and systemic vasodilation without bradycardia [1]. Woods et al. have postulated that cyanotic spells are a result of right ventricular infundibular spasm leading to right-to-left shunting with progressively worsening hypoxemia and metabolic acidosis [2]. Guntheroth et al. considered the

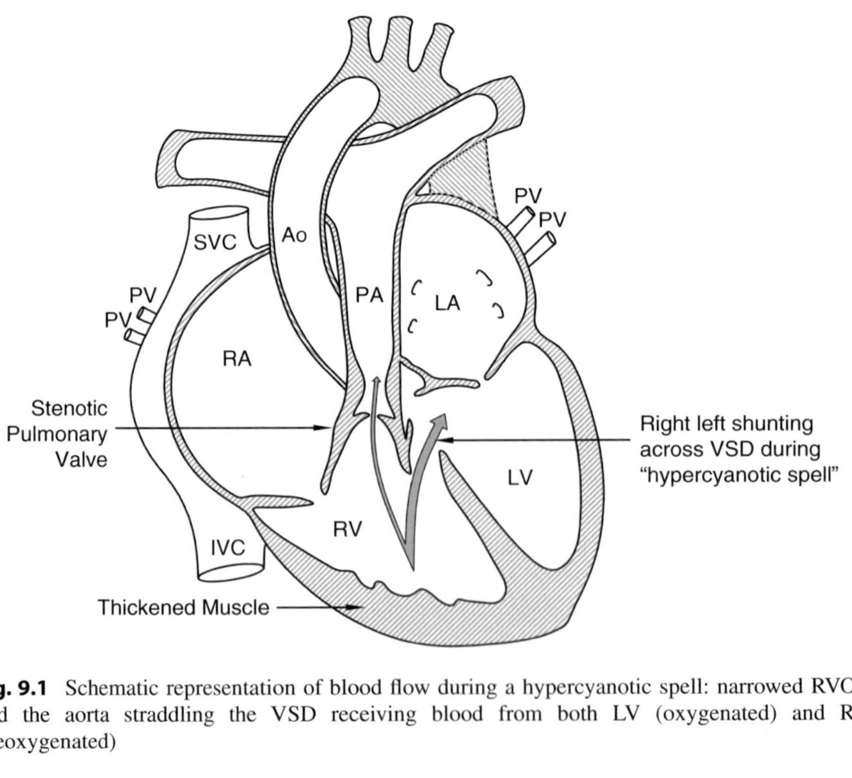

Fig. 9.1 Schematic representation of blood flow during a hypercyanotic spell: narrowed RVOT and the aorta straddling the VSD receiving blood from both LV (oxygenated) and RV (deoxygenated)

paroxysmal hyperpnea a cause rather than a consequence of the cyanotic spell. In this theory, hyperpnea enhances systemic venous return and right ventricular volume load leading to right-to-left shunting, and the vicious cycle continues as the resulting hypoxia stimulates more tachypnea and increased work of breathing [3]. Decreased oxygen delivery to the tissues coupled with increased oxygen demand due to catecholamine surge results in metabolic acidosis that further enhances the hyperpnea creating a vicious cycle. Catecholamine surge also results in tachycardia. This in turn significantly shortens diastolic filling time of the right ventricle with the consequent reduction in the end-diastolic volume—preload—and hence reduced cardiac output [4].

Congenital Heart Lesions Associated with Hypercyanotic Spells

Hypercyanotic spells most commonly occur in Tetrology of Fallot but can also be seen in other congenital heart defects with similar pathophysiology. These include pulmonary atresia with VSD, double outlet right ventricle with pulmonary stenosis (PS), tricuspid atresia with PS, and transposition of great arteries with VSD and PS [5]. With the availability of prenatal diagnosis and early surgical intervention, these "tet spells" are rarely seen in America and Western countries, but they are still commonplace in the rest of the world [6].

Tetralogy of Fallot is the most common cyanotic congenital heart disease comprising about 7% of all congenital heart disease. The four components of this heart defect include large malaligned VSD, overriding aorta, pulmonary stenosis, and right ventricular hypertrophy (Figs. 9.2 and 9.3a, b). Usually the pulmonary stenosis in Tetrology of Fallot is mild early in life, and the net effect is that of a large VSD

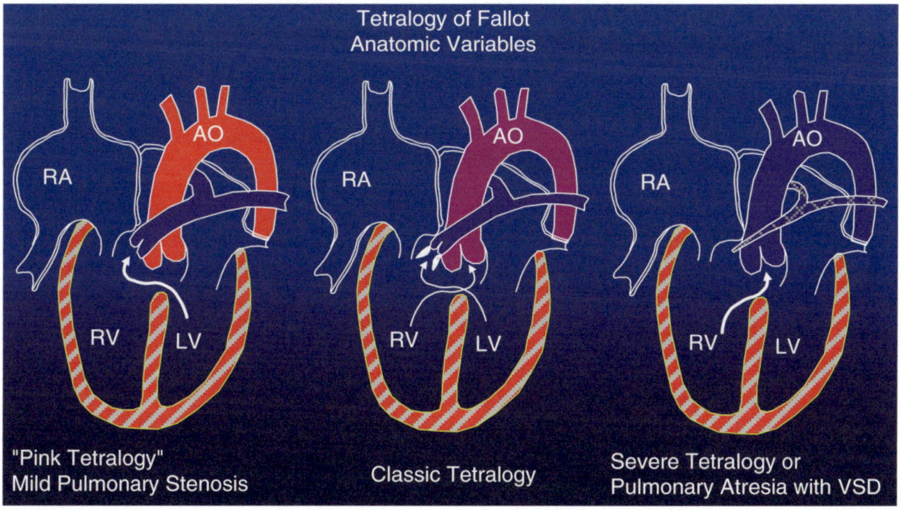

Fig. 9.2 Tetralogy of Fallot: Features include large malaligned VSD, overriding aorta, pulmonary stenosis, and right ventricular hypertrophy

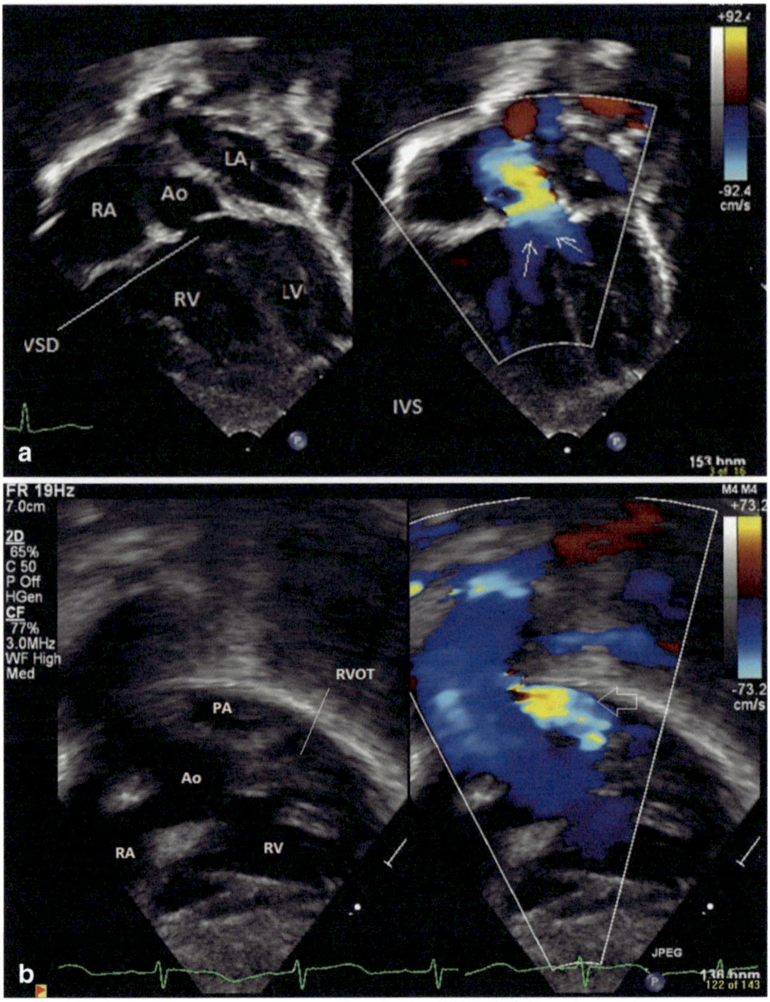

Fig. 9.3 (**a**) The 2D image on the left side demonstrates hypertrophied right ventricle and large VSD with overriding aorta. The image on the right shows the flow from the left as well as right ventricle into the aorta. *RA* right atrium, *LA* left atrium, *AO* aorta, *RV* right ventricle, *LV* left ventricle, *VSD* ventricular septal defect, *IVS* interventricular septum. (**b**) The 2D image on the left side demonstrates hypertrophied right ventricle and large VSD with overriding aorta, severe pulmonary/infundibular stenosis, and hypoplastic main pulmonary artery. The image on the right shows the flow from the right ventricle into the aorta and shows accelerated flow across the narrow right ventricular outflow tract/pulmonary valve (arrow). *RA* right atrium, *AO* aorta, *RV* right ventricle, *PA* pulmonary artery, *RVOT* right ventricular outflow tract

with a large left-to-right shunt, pulmonary overcirculation, and normal oxygen saturation. This is referred to as "pink" tetralogy of Fallot. More often than not, the pulmonary stenosis progressively worsens as the baby grows. As the right ventricular obstruction increases, there is more right-to-left shunting across the VSD resulting in steady decline in resting oxygen saturation. After the newborn period into childhood, these patients can present with hypercyanotic spells.

Clinical Features

Hypercyanotic spells are most often seen in infants who are 2 months to 2 years of age. "Tet spells" commonly happen early in the morning when the intravascular volume is relatively low but can occur anytime of the day. Hypercyanotic spells can be triggered by a variety of different stimuli or can occur spontaneously with no apparent cause. Normal activities such as crying, feeding, or defecation can initiate a cyanotic spell. Anxiety, fever, dehydration, anemia, cardiac catheterization, and supraventricular tachycardia are all known to precipitate these spells. With the onset of hypercyanotic spell, the infant appears fussy and inconsolable with increasing central cyanosis and air hunger. Hyperpnea, defined as rapid and deep breathing, is a hallmark of hypercyanotic spells. During a cyanotic spell, the ejection systolic murmur decreases in intensity and at times becomes inaudible. Cyanotic spells are usually self-limited, lasting about 15–30 min when the infant may be lethargic and somnolent. Prolonged hypercyanotic spells that are not treated can lead to hypoxic neurological injury, seizures, cerebrovascular accidents, and death.

Management of Hypercyanotic Spells

The objectives for treating a hypercyanotic spell include increasing right ventricular filling and pulmonary blood flow while decreasing catecholamine production and increasing systemic vascular resistance. The three initial treatment measures include comforting the infant while holding him in a knee to chest position, giving supplemental oxygen and an intravenous fluid bolus. Calming an agitated and anxious infant is an important initial step in aborting the hypercyanotic spell. Anxiety results in an increase in sympathetic discharge and oxygen consumption. The infant should be picked up by the parent and consoled. Placing the baby supine or on the parent's shoulder with the knee to chest position is beneficial. This kinks the femoral arteries, increases peripheral vascular resistance, and decreases the right-to-left intracardiac shunt [4]. Supplemental oxygen should be administered by nasal cannula or face mask to improve oxygenation. Intravenous access should be obtained and an isotonic fluid bolus of 10 mL/kg given. This improves the intravascular volume and right ventricular preload.

If the hypercyanotic spell persists, sedation with morphine should be given. Morphine blunts the central hyperpneic drive, alleviates pain and discomfort, decreases release of endogenous catecholamines, and reduces the heart rate. Morphine can be given intravenously or intramuscularly at a dose of 0.05–0.1 mg/kg. Mechanical ventilation with paralysis and sedation may be required if morphine is not effective.

If the hypercyanotic spells persist, alpha-adrenergic agonists can be used. Alpha-adrenergic stimulation increases systemic vascular resistance which in turn decreases the right-to-left shunt resulting in improved oxygen saturation [4, 7]. Phenylephrine can be administered as a bolus of 10–20 mcg/kg followed by 2–5 mcg/kg/min. In addition, β-blocker agents are useful in terminating the hypercyanotic spells. Their action is to slow the heart rate, decrease myocardial contractility and oxygen consumption, and reduce the dynamic right ventricular outflow obstruction [5, 8]. Esmolol is given as a loading dose of 500 mcg/kg IV followed by an infusion of 50–300 mcg/kg/min.

If the infant continues to be hypoxic despite all these measures, emergency surgery is indicated. Either palliative modified Blalock-Taussig shunt placement or complete repair with relief of right ventricular outflow obstruction should be performed. However, even if the hypercyanotic spell resolves, surgery should be considered urgent.

Case answer: B.

Clinical Scenario 2

A 2-month-old boy presented to the emergency department because of increased duskiness, lethargy, and diarrhea. A modified Blalock-Taussig (BT) shunt was placed at 5 days of age for pulmonary atresia with ventricular septal defect. Over the last 12 hours, eight episodes of loose stool were noted. His heart rate is 160 BPM, respiratory rate 50 BPM, blood pressure 55/32 mmHg, and oxygen saturation 50% on room air. The anterior fontanelle is sunken. His capillary refill time was 3 seconds and peripheral pulses are barely palpable. The rhythm is regular with a normal S1 and single S2 and no murmur. Lung fields are clear and no hepatomegaly is present.

What is the most likely reason for his current clinical condition?

(A) Septic shock
(B) Acute gastroenteritis
(C) Meningitis
(D) Myocarditis
(E) BT shunt thrombosis

This baby has near-complete occlusion of his modified Blalock-Taussig (BT) shunt. Even though this is not technically a hypercyanotic spell as seen in Tetrology of Fallot, it still is a significant cyanotic episode and a medical emergency. Prompt diagnosis and emergent intervention with immediate cardiology consultation are required in this scenario. Diarrhea led to dehydration that resulted in decreased blood flow in the shunt. With sluggish blood flow, a thrombus formed in the shunt occluding it almost completely. Decreased pulmonary blood flow led to inadequate systemic oxygenation detected by low oxygen saturation. The baby was given oxygen via nasal cannula and isotonic fluids. A bedside echocardiogram was performed which showed no flow in the shunt. The baby had a small aortopulmonary collateral vessel that was supplying a small amount of flow to his lungs. In the cardiac catheterization

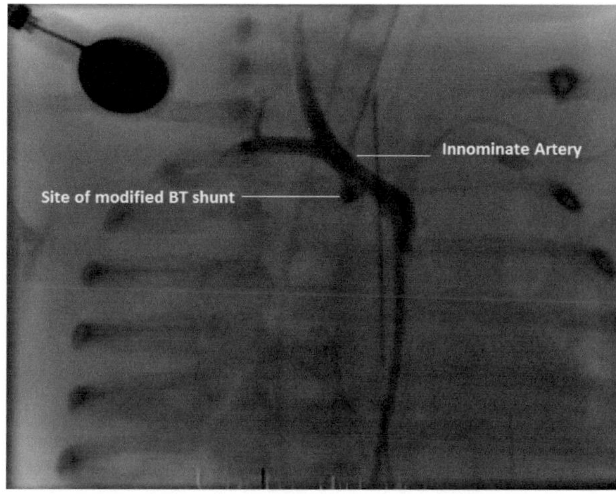

Fig. 9.4 Right innominate artery angiogram showing complete occlusion of the mBT shunt with a small dimple inferiorly at the proximal part of the mBT shunt

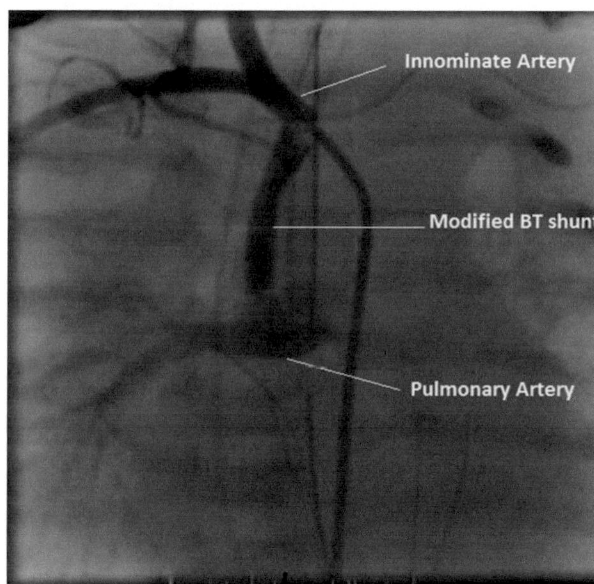

Fig. 9.5 Post-balloon mBT shunt angioplasty and local TPA infiltration: angiogram of the innominate artery and mBT shunt shows normal blood flow in mBT shunt with no evidence of residual thrombus in the shunt or proximal pulmonary arteries. There is no evidence of vessel injury

laboratory, the right innominate artery angiogram showed complete occlusion of the BT shunt with a small dimple inferiorly at the proximal part of the BT shunt (Fig. 9.4). Tissue plasminogen activator was infused locally into the thrombosed shunt after which balloon angioplasty was performed. The BT shunt was successfully re-cannulated establishing adequate pulmonary blood flow (Fig. 9.5). The oxygen saturation improved from 50 to 78% in room air. If cardiac catheterization is unsuccessful in reopening the BT shunt, then emergency cardiac surgery is warranted.

Answer: E.

Conclusion

Hypercyanotic spells continue to be an important clinical presentation to immediately recognize and treat in several cyanotic congenital heart diseases. Accurate diagnosis and appropriate management may prevent the consequences of hypoxia leading to improved outcome and avoiding morbidity or even death.

References

1. Kothari SS. Mechanism of cyanotic spells in tetralogy of Fallot—the missing link? Int J Cardiol. 1992;37(1):1–5.
2. Wood P. Attacks of deeper cyanosis and loss of consciousness (syncope) in Fallot's tetralogy. Br Heart J. 1958;20(2):282–6.
3. Guntheroth WG, Morgan BC, Mullins GL. Physiologic studies of paroxysmal hyperpnea in cyanotic congenital heart disease. Circulation. 1965;31:70–6.
4. Rudolph AM. Wiley Online Library (online service), Congenital diseases of the heart clinical-physiological considerations. 3rd ed. Chichester, Hoboken: Wiley-Blackwell; 2009. http://onlinelibrary.wiley.com/book/10.1002/9781444311822.
5. Moller JH, Hoffman JIE. Pediatric cardiovascular medicine. 1st ed. Philadelphia: Churchill Livingstone; 2000.
6. Allen HD, Driscoll DJ, Shaddy RE, Feltes TF. Moss & Adams' heart disease in infants, children, and adolescents, including the fetus and young adult. Eighth edition. Wolters Kluwer/Lippincott Williams & Wilkins; 2013.
7. Shaddy RE, Viney J, Judd VE, McGough EC. Continuous intravenous phenylephrine infusion for treatment of hypoxemic spells in tetralogy of Fallot. J Pediatr. 1989;114(3):468–70.
8. Garson A Jr, Gillette PC, McNamara DG. Propranolol: the preferred palliation for tetralogy of Fallot. Am J Cardiol. 1981;47(5):1098–104.

Check for updates

Radiographic Evaluation of the Child with Heart Disease

10

Aparna Joshi

Introduction

As technologies such as echocardiography and cross-sectional imaging have advanced, the role of chest radiography in the evaluation of the child with heart disease has evolved. The plain radiograph is now of decreased importance in diagnosis of specific congenital heart lesions, largely supplanted by other modalities. However, in the acute care setting, abnormalities on the chest radiograph may be the first indication of undiagnosed heart disease and can direct further imaging and management in patients with known heart disease. Therefore, it is important to be familiar with the abnormalities in cardiac size and shape, pulmonary vasculature, airway position and morphology, and situs and osseous structures which may be encountered in children with heart disease.

A systematic search pattern should be carried out when evaluating any chest radiograph so as not to miss any findings. The mnemonic "ABCD'S" can be a useful reminder of all the structures to examine when reviewing a chest radiograph:

A: Abdomen
B: Bones
C: Chest (airway, mediastinum/heart, lungs, diaphragm)
D: Devices (catheters, tubes, implants)
S: Soft tissues

(Modified from Haller et al. 2005).

A. Joshi, M.D.
Pediatric Imaging, Children's Hospital of Michigan, Detroit, MI, USA

Wayne State University School of Medicine, Detroit, MI, USA
e-mail: AJoshi@dmc.org

© Springer International Publishing AG, part of Springer Nature 2018

A. P. Sarnaik et al. (eds.), *Cardiac Emergencies in Children*,
https://doi.org/10.1007/978-3-319-73754-6_10

Heart Size and Shape

Evaluation of heart size and shape on the chest radiograph has probably been overemphasized in the past. Over time, it has become clear that many children with mild or even complex heart disease may have normal chest radiographs and that evaluation of cardiac silhouette size and shape on chest radiographs is complicated by multiple factors. Nevertheless, in some cases, abnormalities in the size/shape of the heart on the chest radiograph are the first signs of undiagnosed heart disease or of change in the status of a patient with known heart disease, so it is important to make a reasonable attempt to evaluate the heart size and shape.

Cardiothoracic ratio has been used in adults as a fast and simple way to gauge heart size, but it is of limited use in infants and young children. The ratio is the diameter of the cardiac silhouette on the frontal chest radiograph compared to the inner diameter of the thoracic cage, with a cardiothoracic ratio of greater than 0.55 considered enlarged in adults. Limitations with its use in children include physiologic age-related differences in the heart size and thymus, difficulty obtaining consistently deep inspiration on younger patients during x-ray exposure, rotation of the heart due to cardiac chamber enlargement, and individual variability in thoracic cage shape. Recent attempts at correlating cardiothoracic ratio with actual cardiac volumes calculated by MRI in children with congenital heart disease showed wide variations in ventricular and total heart volumes for any given frontal cardiothoracic ratio, due to the aforementioned factors. However, gross enlargement in any individual child's cardiothoracic ratio compared to previous chest radiographs implies cardiac chamber enlargement, pericardial effusion, or other abnormalities.

The thymus is considered a great mimic because it can have a variable appearance and blend with the cardiac silhouette on the chest radiograph. The thymus may be normally quite prominent in patients up to about 6 years of age. Because the thymus is located anteriorly, evaluation of the cardiac size on the lateral view is often useful in conjunction with the frontal view in younger children.

The anterior tracheal line can be a useful tool: a line drawn along the anterior margin of the trachea on the lateral view when extended inferiorly normally intersects the spine below the diaphragm, but with cardiac enlargement, the line intersects the spine above the diaphragm (Figs. 10.1, 10.2, and 10.3).

Specific chamber enlargement is also more difficult to assess on younger children's chest radiographs due to obscuration of the heart by the relatively large thymus. In older children, it is easier to evaluate and useful to know which chambers form the cardiac borders. (Fig. 10.4). Left atrial enlargement causes widening of the subcarinal angle, whereas right atrial enlargement manifests as a bulge along the right heart border. Right ventricular enlargement may cause obliteration of the retrosternal clear space on the lateral view in an older child (it is filled with thymus in a younger child) and posterior displacement of the trachea. Left ventricular enlargement causes the cardiac apex to turn inferiorly.

Massive enlargement of the cardiomediastinal silhouette in the neonate has a limited differential diagnosis (Table 10.1). Most cases are due to massive right

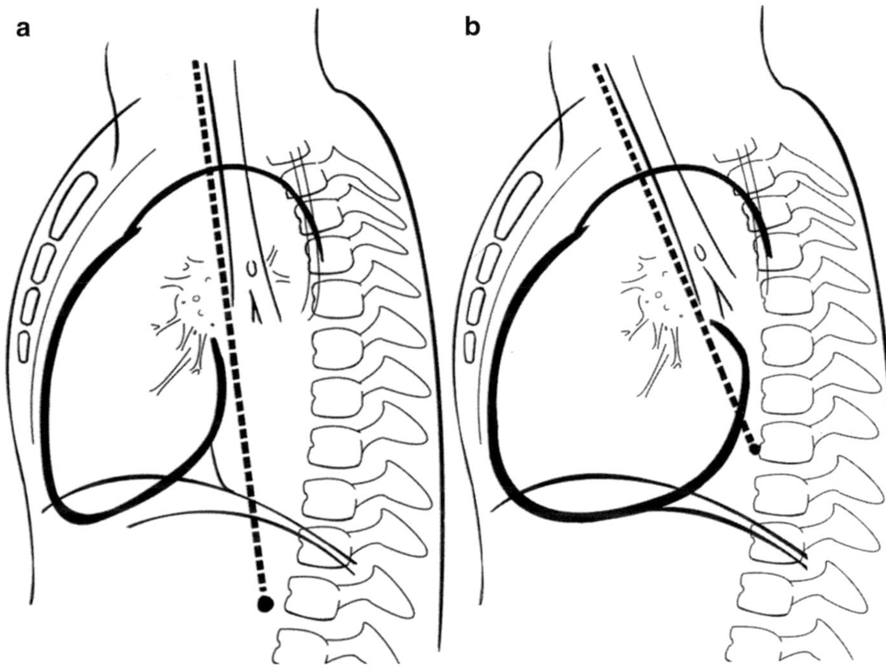

Fig. 10.1 (**a**) In a patient with a normal size heart, when a straight line is drawn along the anterior tracheal wall and extended inferiorly, it intersects the spine below the diaphragm, but in the case of cardiac enlargement (**b**), the large heart alters the tracheal angle, so the anterior tracheal line intersects the spine above the diaphragm (Reproduced with permission from Haller et al. (2005))

atrial enlargement as seen in Ebstein's anomaly of the tricuspid valve (Fig. 10.5) or in pulmonary atresia with intact ventricular septum. "Wall-to-wall" cardiac enlargement may also be caused by hypertrophic cardiomyopathy in infants of diabetic mothers or large arteriovenous shunts (either intracardiac, as in coronary artery-right heart fistula, or extracardiac, as in vein of Galen malformation or hepatic hemangioendothelioma). Large pericardial effusion or cardiac/mediastinal mass (Fig. 10.6) can also mimic massive cardiomegaly on the chest radiograph.

Some characteristic heart shapes have been described. It is useful to be familiar with these, keeping in mind that these shapes are not necessarily specific for the entities with which they are classically associated. The "egg-on-string" appearance of transposition of the great arteries on anteroposterior view is caused by the narrowing of the mediastinal vascular pedicle since the aorta is directly anterior to the pulmonary artery. The "boot-shaped heart" of tetralogy of Fallot (Fig. 10.7) reflects right ventricular hypertrophy and concavity in the main pulmonary artery region due to right ventricular outflow tract obstruction. The "snowman" of supracardiac total anomalous pulmonary venous return (caused by the large ascending vertical vein) was described in older children and is quite specific but is no longer often seen because of earlier diagnosis of this entity.

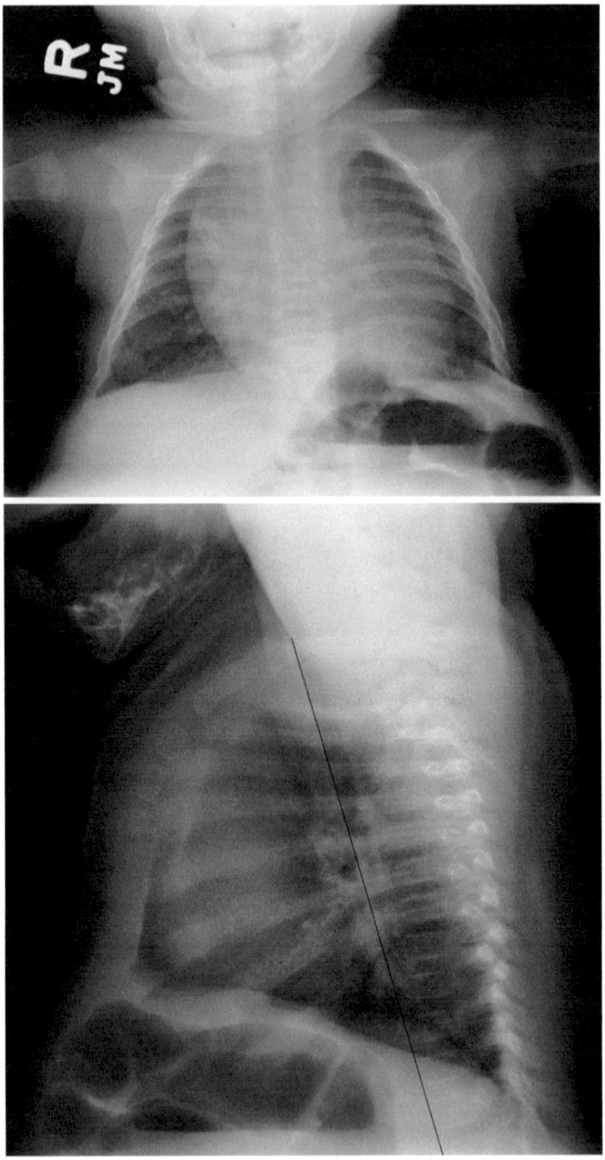

Fig. 10.2 A 2-month-old male presenting with difficulty breathing. Although the cardiomediastinal silhouette appears large on the frontal view, it is not large on the lateral view. The anterior tracheal line (drawn on the lateral view) does not intersect the spine above the diaphragm. The appearance of large cardiothymic silhouette is caused by the normally large thymus in a child this age

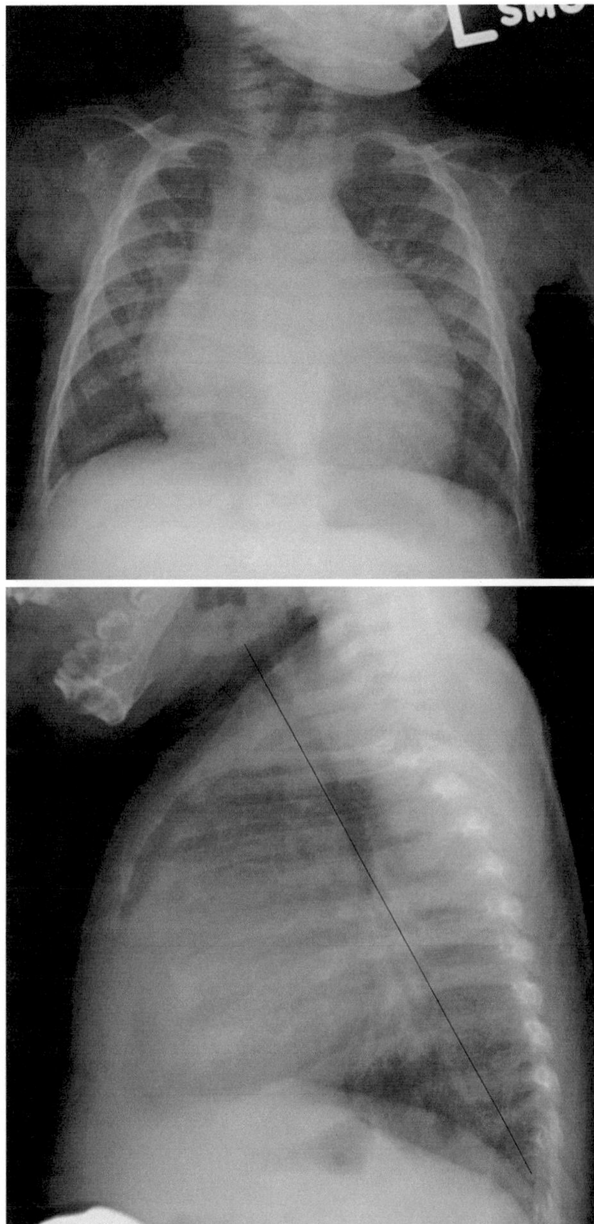

Fig. 10.3 A 3-month-old female who presented with tachypnea. Chest radiograph shows a large cardiac silhouette on the frontal and lateral views and pulmonary venous congestion. The anterior tracheal line (drawn on the lateral view) intersects the spine above the diaphragm on the lateral view. Genetics evaluation yielded a diagnosis of Pompe disease

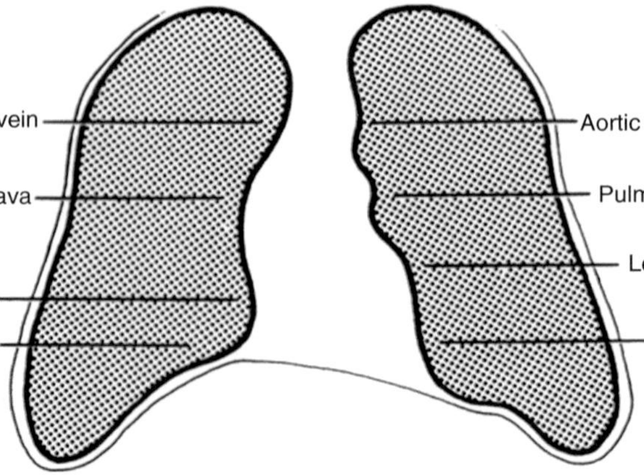

Fig. 10.4 Diagram showing the structures forming the cardiomediastinal borders on a normal chest radiograph. The outlines of the individual structures are difficult to see in young children because the thymus silhouettes the heart, but knowledge of these structures can be useful in determining specific chamber enlargement in older children (Reproduced with permission from Haller et al. (2005))

Table 10.1 Differential diagnosis of "wall-to-wall" cardiothymic silhouette in the newborn

• Massive right atrial enlargement
– Ebstein's anomaly of the tricuspid valve
– Pulmonary atresia with intact ventricular septum
• Hypertrophic cardiomyopathy in infant of diabetic mother
• Large arteriovenous shunt
– Intracardiac: Coronary artery fistula
– Extracardiac: Vein of Galen malformation
• Large pericardial effusion
• Large cardiac/mediastinal mass

Pulmonary Vasculature

Assessment of the pulmonary vasculature on chest radiographs is challenging but provides some of the most useful information from the chest radiograph in patients with heart disease. The pulmonary arterial vascularity may be considered normal, increased, or decreased (Table 10.2). Depending on the degree of pulmonary venous hypertension, one may see cephalization of pulmonary vascular flow, Kerley B lines, or alveolar edema. Vascularity may be more centralized or asymmetric.

Increased pulmonary arterial blood flow is seen in cases where there is a left-to-right shunt, such as ASD, VSD, and PDA. In order to be detectable by chest radiography, the amount of pulmonary blood flow (Qp) must double compared to systemic blood flow (Qs), i.e., Qp/Qs of at least 2:1, and smaller shunts may not be radiographically evident. The vessels seen with increased pulmonary arterial flow are sharply defined and extend into the periphery of the lung (Fig. 10.8).

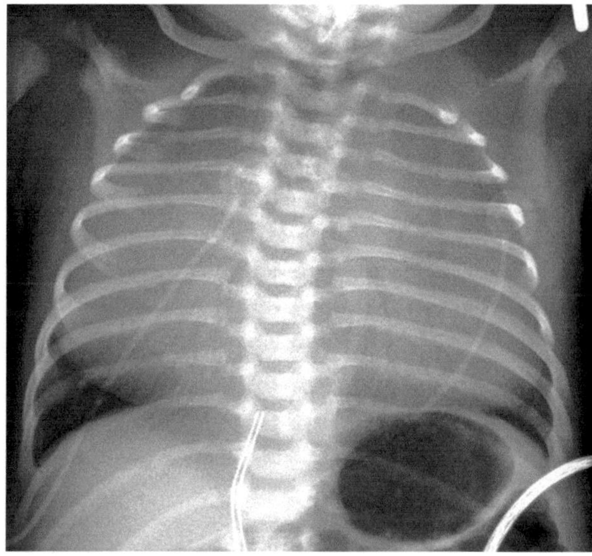

Fig. 10.5 A newborn male on the first day of life with a markedly enlarged cardiac silhouette extending from the right to the left chest wall ("wall-to-wall"). Echocardiogram showed Ebstein's anomaly of the tricuspid valve

Decreased pulmonary arterial flow is reflected by "blacker"-appearing lungs with a paucity of vascular markings. Decreased flow is seen in cyanotic lesions with right heart obstruction and right-to-left shunting. These include tetralogy of Fallot, Ebstein's anomaly, tricuspid atresia, and pulmonary atresia with intact ventricular septum (Fig. 10.9).

Pulmonary venous hypertension secondary to left-heart obstructive lesions (critical aortic stenosis or mitral stenosis, for example) or left ventricular failure results in a series of changes depending on the degree of severity of the venous hypertension. The mildest change is redistribution of the blood flow to the upper lobes of the lungs with increased number and diameter of the upper lung vessels, called "cephalization." This change has been described in adults when the mean pulmonary wedge pressure exceeds 15 mmHg. With further increases in mean pulmonary wedge pressure to greater than 25 mmHg, the plasma oncotic pressure is exceeded, and fluid leaks from capillaries to the adjacent interstitial tissues, leading to indistinct pulmonary vascular margins and septal thickening (Figs. 10.10 and 10.11). Continued leakage will result in fluid in the airspaces or alveolar edema.

Central prominence of the pulmonary vascularity with pruning of peripheral arteries rarely results from pulmonary arterial hypertension in the pediatric age group; this is more typically seen in adult patients with long-standing left-to-right shunts. A small subset of tetralogy of Fallot patients with absent pulmonary valve can have enlargement of the central pulmonary arteries which causes mass effect on the airways and results in respiratory distress.

Asymmetric pulmonary flow may reflect peripheral pulmonary arterial stenosis or hypoplasia or pulmonary venous obstruction. Left pulmonary artery stenosis or isolation may be seen in patients with tetralogy of Fallot.

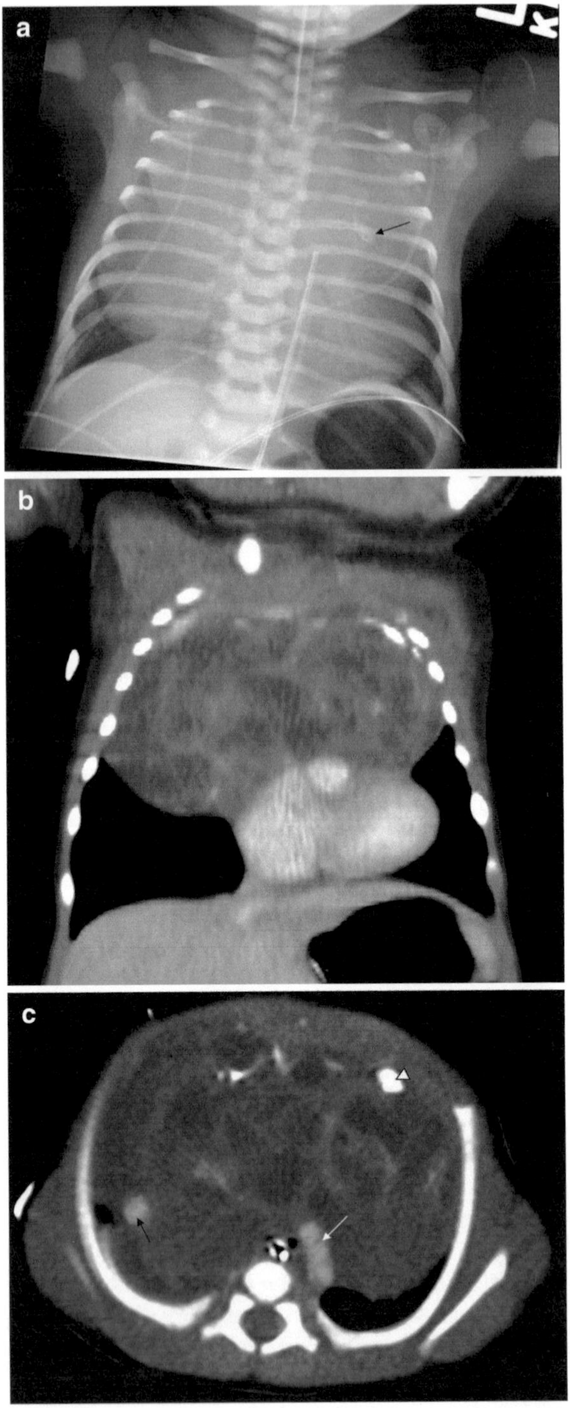

Fig. 10.6 (**a**) Frontal chest radiograph of a newborn male on the first day of life showing marked enlargement of the cardiomediastinal silhouette. Some calcification is seen in the left superior mediastinum (black arrow). (**b**) Coronal CT image shows a large heterogeneous mediastinal mass superior to a normal size heart. (**c**) Axial CT image shows the mixed attenuation mass displacing the aortic arch (white arrow) posteriorly and the superior vena cava laterally. A calcification (white arrowhead) is seen in the mass anteriorly. The mass was resected and confirmed by pathology to be a mediastinal teratoma

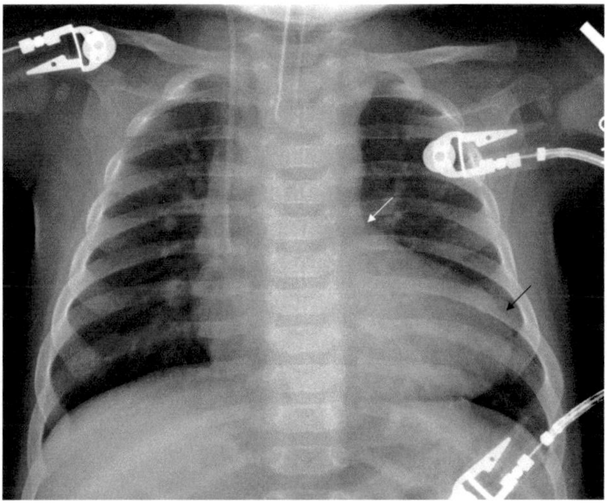

Fig. 10.7 Frontal chest radiograph of a 5-month-old male with tetralogy of Fallot demonstrates concavity of the main pulmonary artery segment (white arrow) due to right ventricular outflow tract obstruction and upturned cardiac apex (black arrow) caused by right ventricular hypertrophy

Table 10.2 Differential diagnosis of congenital heart diseases based on the presence of cyanosis and assessment of pulmonary vascularity

Cyanotic patient with increased pulmonary vascularity	Acyanotic patient with increased pulmonary vascularity
• Truncus arteriosus • Total anomalous pulmonary venous return • Transposition of the great arteries	• Ventricular septal defect • Atrial septal defect • Patent ductus arteriosus
Cyanotic patient with decreased pulmonary vascularity	**Acyanotic patient with normal pulmonary vascularity**
• Tetralogy of Fallot • Ebstein's anomaly • Tricuspid atresia	• Aortic coarctation • Aortic stenosis • Pulmonary stenosis

Airway and Mediastinum

Assessment of the mediastinum and airway proves useful in determining the side of the aortic arch, detecting bronchial abnormalities related to abnormal situs, determining presence of thymus, and evaluating for mediastinal masses.

Inspection of the size and position of the trachea is integral in the detection of vascular rings (typically double aortic arch or right aortic arch with retroesophageal left subclavian artery). Normally, the carina is positioned slightly eccentrically to the right of the midline, displaced by the normal left-sided aortic arch. However, in patients with a right aortic arch or double arch, the carina is often in the midline, and the lateral view shows mild anterior tracheal bowing (Fig. 10.12).

Pulmonary sling, or anomalous origin of the left pulmonary artery from the right, is frequently associated with an abnormal appearance of the airway (Figs. 10.13 and 10.14). The left pulmonary artery frequently compresses the right mainstem or right upper lobe bronchus as it courses to the right, resulting in air-trapping in the right

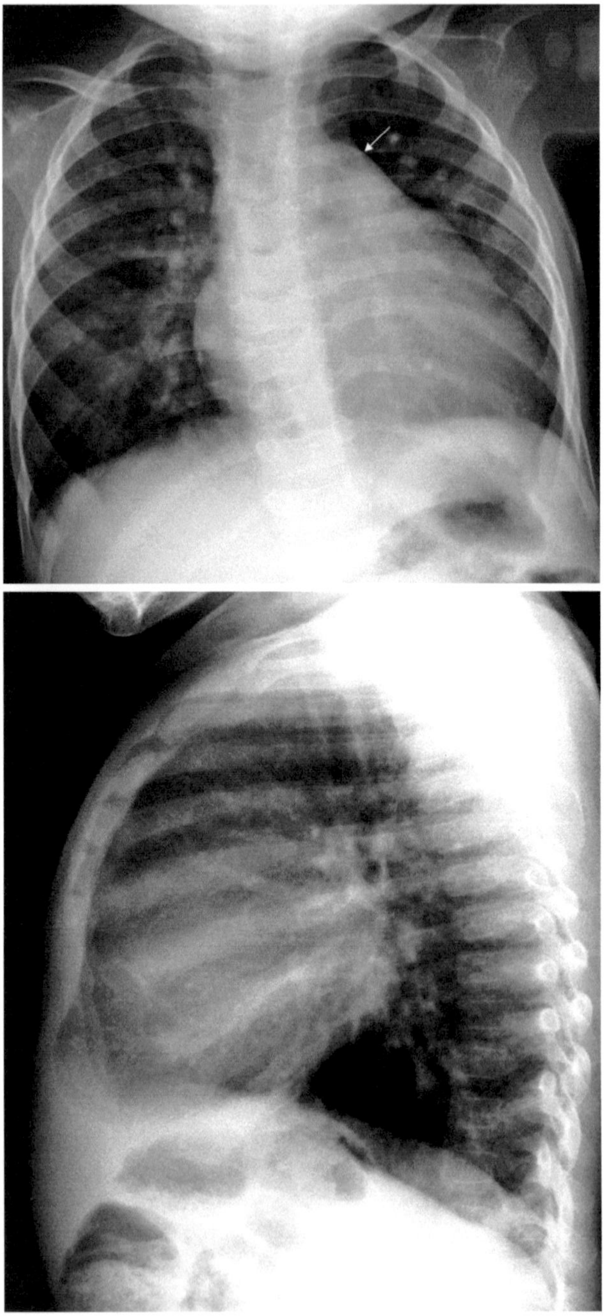

Fig. 10.8 A 7-month-old female with previously diagnosed perimembranous VSD presented to the emergency department with fever. Chest radiograph shows enlargement of the cardiac silhouette, large convex main pulmonary artery segment (white arrow), and large but distinct pulmonary vessels consistent with known left-to-right shunt

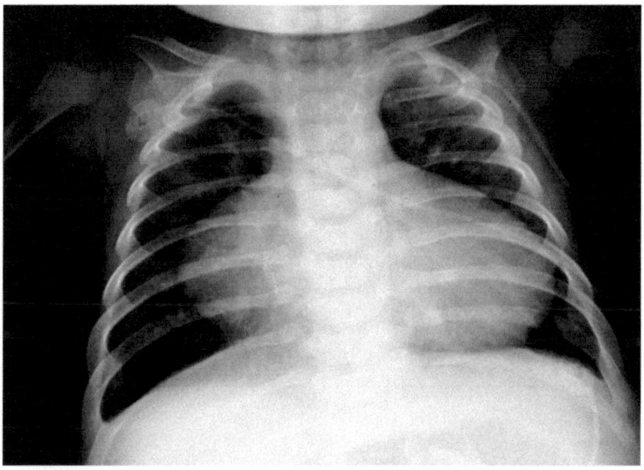

Fig. 10.9 Frontal chest radiograph of a 6-month-old male with Ebstein's anomaly shows cardiomegaly and decreased pulmonary vascularity

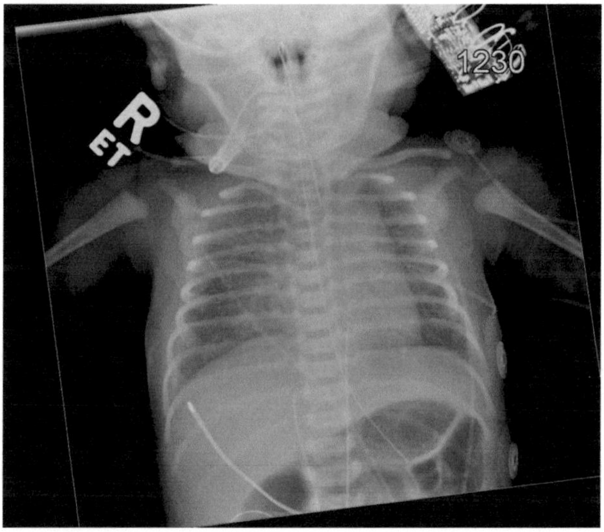

Fig. 10.10 A 3-day-old infant with respiratory distress and cyanosis. Note the lack of cardiomegaly with diffuse pulmonary edema without prominent central pulmonary arterial enlargement. This is representative of pulmonary venous edema. The infant had total anomalous pulmonary venous return with obstruction. Pulmonary venous drainage was entering the portal vein

lung. Approximately 50% of patients with pulmonary sling have intrinsic abnormalities of the airway, including tracheal stenosis from complete tracheal cartilage rings, low carina, and anomalous bronchial branching.

The presence of a mediastinal mass can sometimes mimic cardiomegaly. Conversely, large cardiac masses may cause overall mediastinal enlargement. In these instances, advanced imaging will help to determine the origin of the mass (Fig. 10.6).

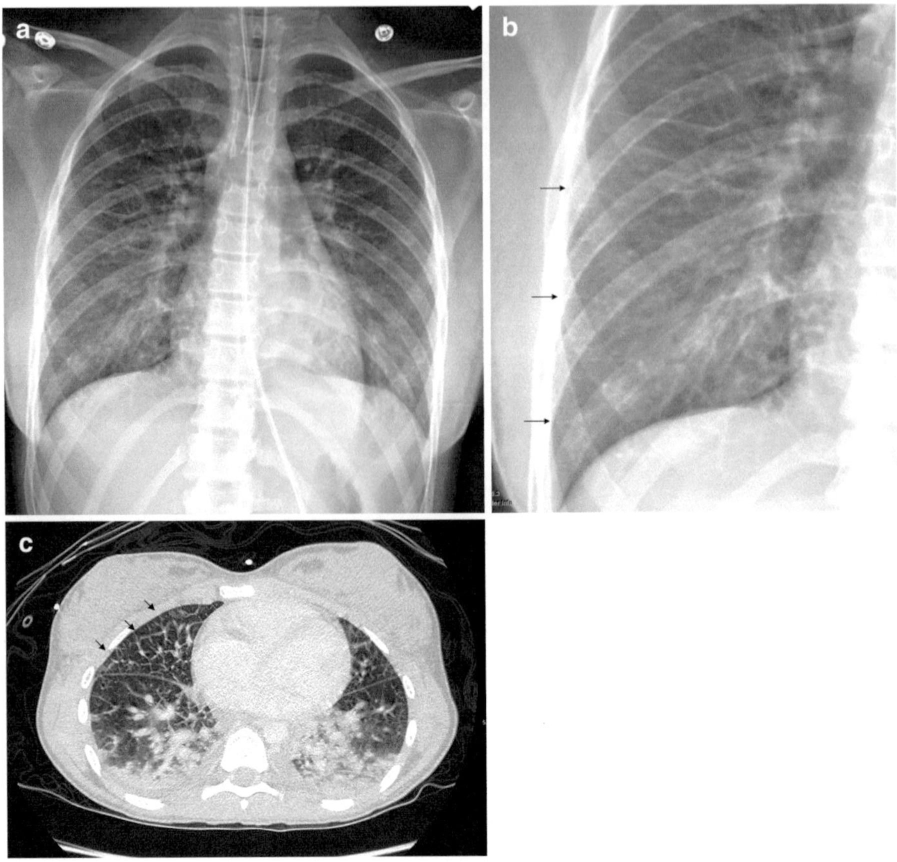

Fig. 10.11 A 13-year-old female hospitalized in pediatric ICU with noncardiogenic (septic) shock. Frontal chest radiograph (**a**) and magnified view of the right lung base (**b**) demonstrate pulmonary interstitial edema with Kerley B lines (black arrows). Lung window image from chest CT (**c**) confirms interlobular septal thickening (black arrows); dependent atelectasis and small pleural effusions were also shown on soft tissue windows

Situs

Noting the location of organs that are normally asymmetrically positioned in the body, or abdominal and thoracic situs, and determining the relationship of the heart to the visceral situs are important steps in the systematic evaluation of the chest radiograph. The position of the liver, stomach, spleen, and heart as well as the anatomy of the tracheobronchial tree should be assessed on the plain radiograph. Other more detailed anatomies indicative of situs abnormalities, such as the atrial appendages and the relationship of the pulmonary arteries to their respective bronchi, cannot be evaluated on plain radiographs but are better demonstrated on cross-sectional

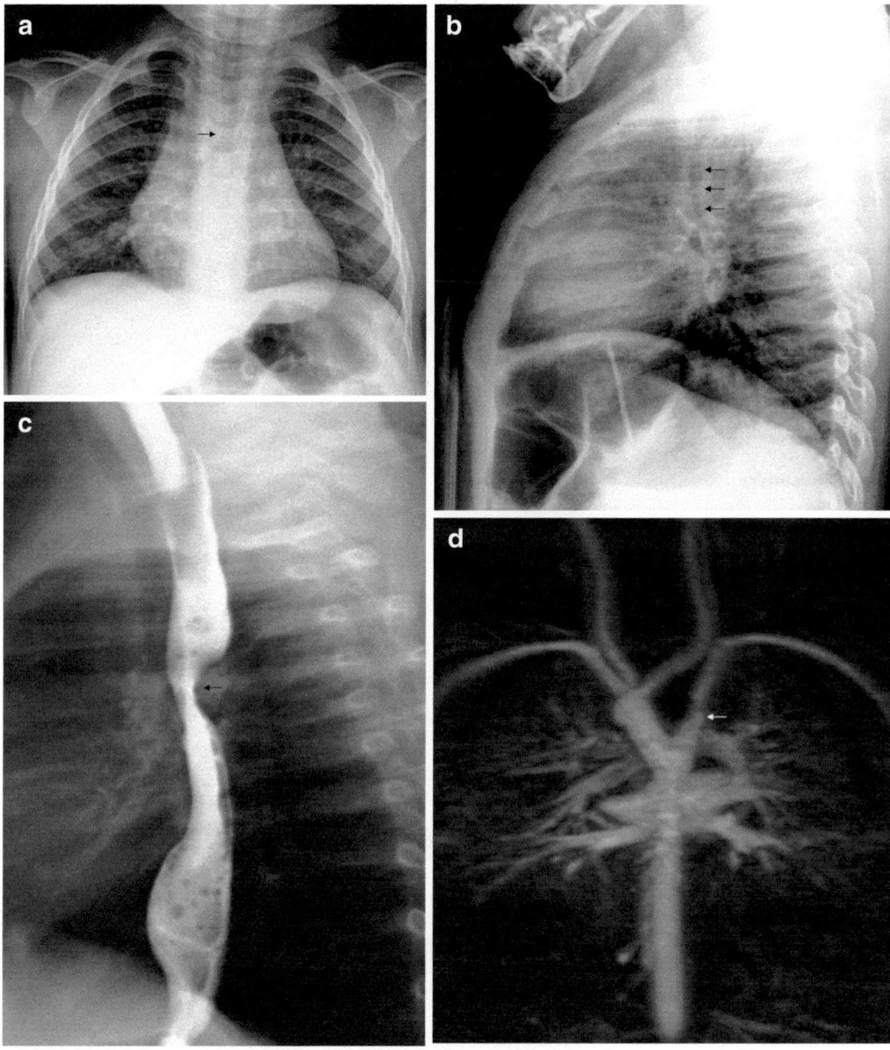

Fig. 10.12 An 8-month-old male with cough. (**a**) Frontal view of the chest shows mass effect on the right side of the distal trachea (black arrow). (**b**) Lateral view shows anterior bowing of the tracheal air column (black arrows). (**c**) Esophagram demonstrates a posterior impression on the esophagus (black arrow). (**d**) MRA confirms a vascular ring with right aortic arch and retroesophageal left subclavian artery (white arrow)

imaging examinations. Ultrasound of the abdomen is typically performed in patients with abnormal situs to delineate infradiaphragmatic venous anatomy (e.g., azygous continuation of the inferior vena cava), to locate the gallbladder and liver, and to determine the location, presence, and number of spleens.

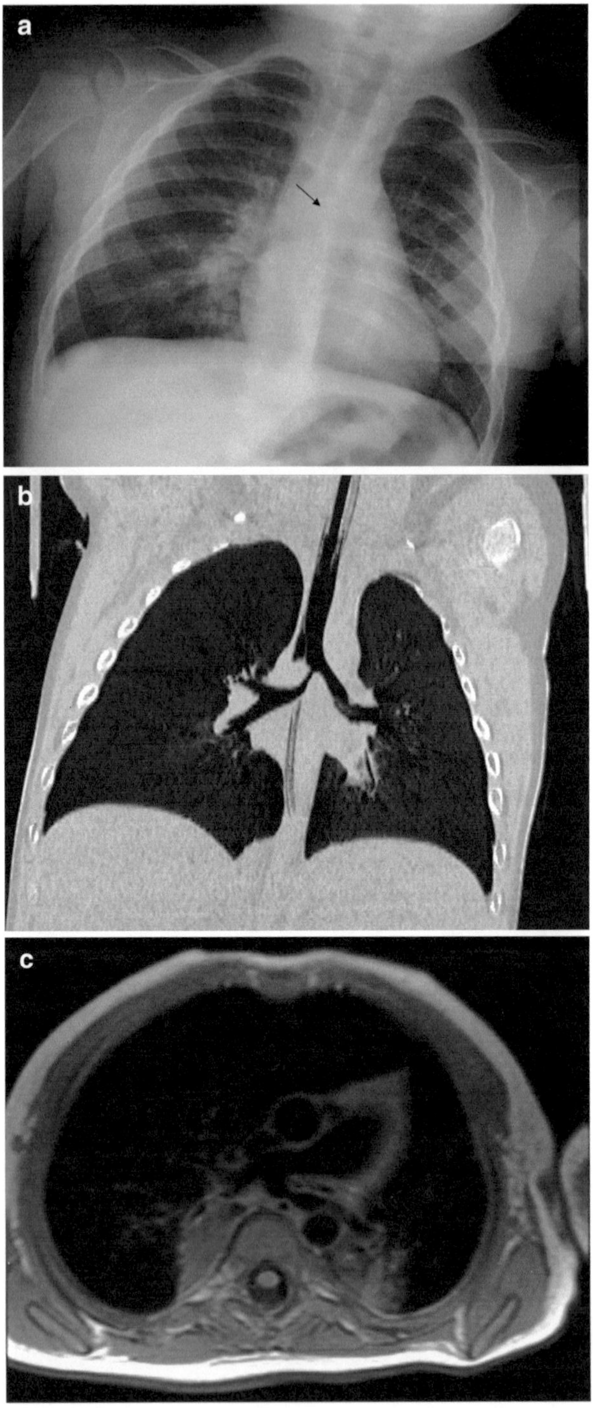

Fig. 10.13 An 11-month-old male with difficulty breathing. (**a**) Chest radiograph shows mass effect on the right side of the tracheal air column (black arrow) and leftward displacement of the carina. (**b**) CT confirms the abnormal course of the airway and also shows marked narrowing of the right main bronchus with air-trapping in the right lung. (**c**) MRI shows a pulmonary artery sling

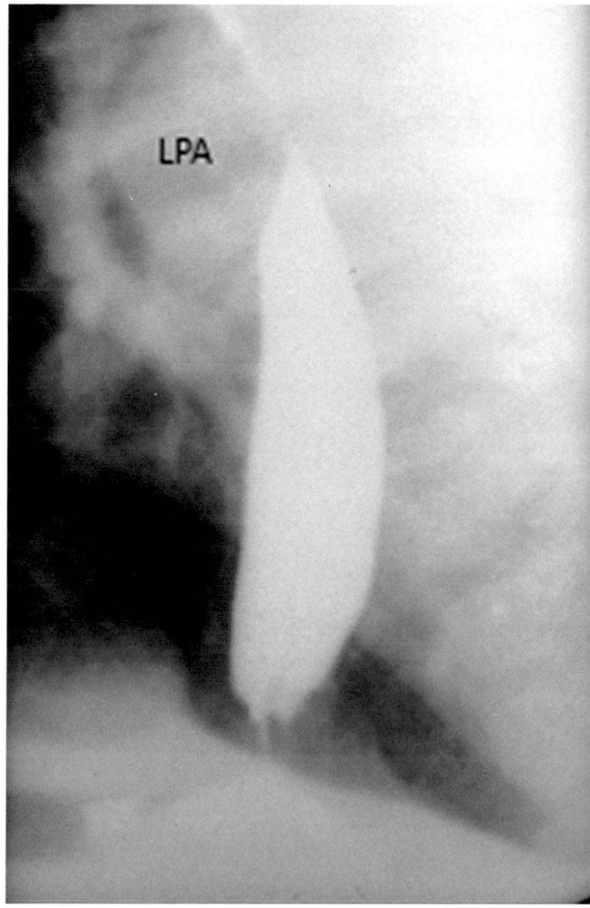

Fig. 10.14 Barium esophagogram lateral projection showing left pulmonary artery (LPA) going behind the trachea and in front of the esophagus resulting in mass effect causing posterior compression of the trachea and anterior compression of the esophagus (pulmonary sling)

The terms levocardia, mesocardia, and dextrocardia are often used to describe the direction of the cardiac apex. However, these terms do not indicate the position or morphology of the atria, which are the true indicators of visceral situs.

Normal position of the above-listed structures is termed “situs solitus.” In this case, the systemic atrium, the trilobed lung, and the liver are on the right, and the pulmonary atrium, the bilobed lung, the spleen, and the stomach are on the left. In children with levocardia and situs solitus, the incidence of congenital heart disease is 0.6–0.8%.

When structures are reversed to the complete mirror image of normal, it is called “situs inversus.” In this case, the pulmonary atrium, the bilobed lung, the spleen, and the stomach are on the right, and the systemic atrium, the trilobed lung, and the liver are on the left. In patients with situs inversus, the incidence of congenital heart disease is slightly increased, 3–5%.

Abnormal position of some structures but not others is called “situs ambiguous” and indicates heterotaxy syndrome (polysplenia or asplenia) (Fig. 10.15). In situs

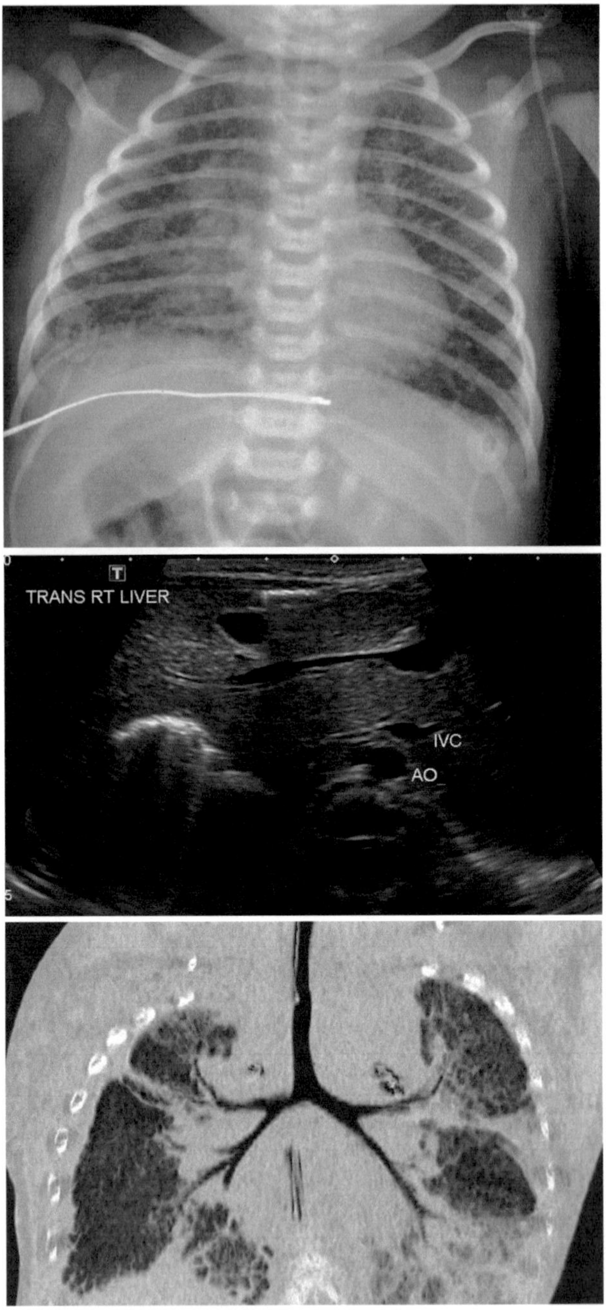

Fig. 10.15 A 1-day-old female with heterotaxy. The cardiac apex is on the left, but the stomach is seen in the right upper abdomen, and there is pulmonary venous congestion and interstitial edema. Abdominal ultrasound showed a transverse liver, midline gallbladder, and no spleen. Coronal minimum intensity projection from CT thorax at 9 months of age shows symmetric bronchial branching pattern. Cardiac lesions included pulmonary atresia, right ventricle-dominant unbalanced common AV canal with aorta arising from the right ventricle, and supracardiac total anomalous pulmonary venous connection. Autopsy after the patient expired at 15 months of age confirmed asplenia

ambiguous, the incidence of congenital heart disease is very high, between 50 and 100%, with cardiac anomalies generally less frequent and less complex in polysplenic than in asplenic patients. Additionally, these patients, particularly those with right-sided isomerism or asplenia, can suffer from life-threatening immune defects and midgut malrotation, which can lead to volvulus.

Bony Abnormalities

Osseous abnormalities may be seen in association with or as a result of congenital heart disease or cardiothoracic surgeries. Abnormalities of the ribs (abnormal number or fusion), spine (vertebral segmentation anomalies and scoliosis), and sternum (decreased number of ossification centers) are sometimes seen in patients with congenital heart disease. Rib notching can be seen in older patients with aortic coarctation, usually over age 8, since time is required for the development of intercostal collateral arteries which are responsible for the effects on the ribs (Fig. 10.16).

One interesting finding seen in the skeleton of infants with cyanotic ductal-dependent congenital heart disease who are being treated with prostaglandin E1 to maintain patency of the ductus arteriosus is prostaglandin-induced periostitis (Fig. 10.17). This symmetric finding is associated more with duration of treatment than with dose and improves with cessation of the drug.

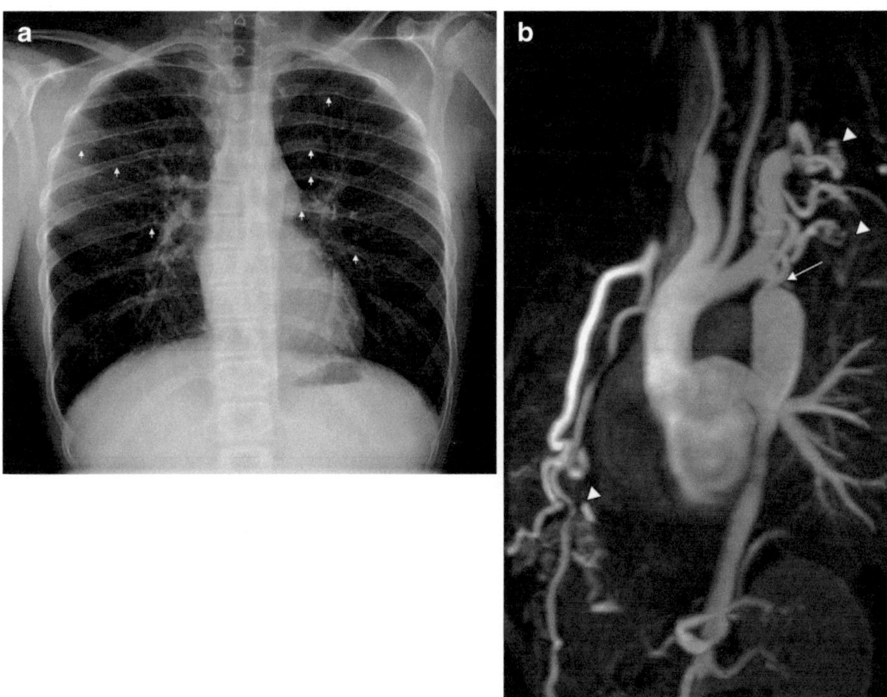

Fig. 10.16 A 15-year-old male with hypertension and 20 mmHg gradient between the upper and lower extremity blood pressures. (**a**) Frontal radiograph shows notching of multiple ribs bilaterally (white arrows). (**b**) Oblique maximum intensity projection from 3D gadolinium MRA demonstrates aortic coarctation (white arrow) with multiple large collateral vessels (white arrowheads)

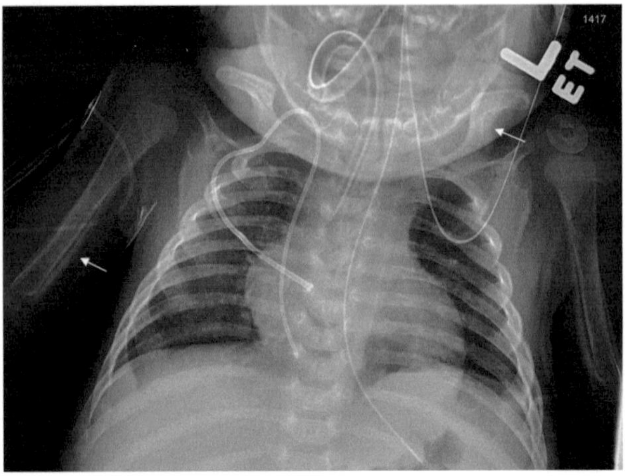

Fig. 10.17 A 9-week-old female with pulmonary atresia/VSD receiving prostaglandin E1 to maintain ductal patency. Radiograph shows periosteal reaction (white arrows) along both humeral diaphyses and clavicles

Careful evaluation of the sternum and ribs in a patient with known heart disease can provide clues to the patient's prior surgical history and sometimes resultant complications.

Intravascular and Surgical Devices

Many children with heart disease have on their radiographs surgically or endovascularly placed devices/material related to cardiovascular repair or vascular access. On any radiograph, it is not only important to identify the device but also its morphology compared to the expected appearance which includes changes in position (Fig. 10.18). Cardiac emergencies can present on radiographs simply with a change in position of a device. It is thus important to include evaluation of catheters/devices as part of the systematic approach to reviewing a chest radiograph.

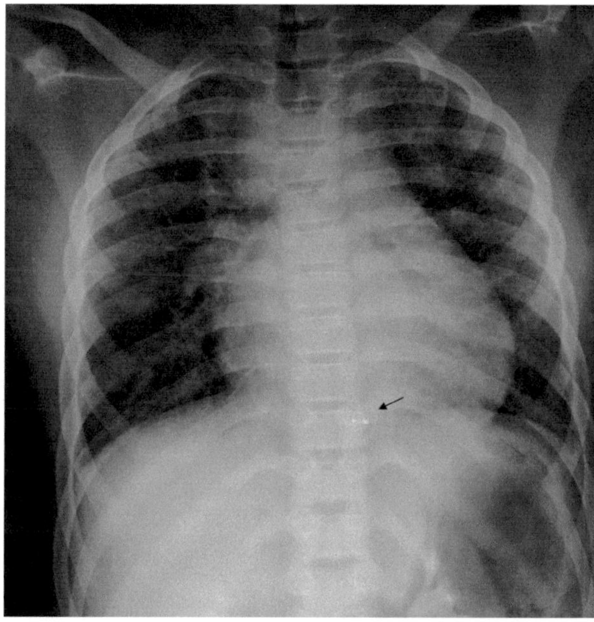

Fig. 10.18 An 11-year-old female with atrial septal defect and patent ductus arteriosus, post occlusion of patent ductus arteriosus. The patient became hypotensive in the post-anesthesia care unit. In addition to increased pulmonary vascularity and pulmonary venous congestion, the chest radiograph shows migration of the occlusion device (black arrow) to the descending aorta. Note contrast from the catheterization procedure being excreted by the kidneys. The patient was immediately taken back to the cardiac catheterization lab for percutaneous retrieval of the migrated device

Bibliography

1. Applegate KE, Goske MJ, Pierce G, Murphy D. Situs revisited: imaging of the heterotaxy syndrome. Radiographics. 1999;19:837–52.
2. Culham JA, Mawson JB. Chest radiography in pediatric cardiovascular disease. In: Coley BD, editor. Caffey's pediatric diagnostic imaging. 12th ed. Philadelphia: Elsevier; 2013. p. 684–8.
3. Donnelly LF, Gelfand KJ, Schwartz DC, Strife JL. The wall to wall heart: differential diagnosis for massively large cardiothymic silhouette in newborns. Appl Radiol. 1997;26:23–8.
4. Grotenhuis HB, Zhou C, Tomlinson G, et al. Cardiothoracic ratio on chest radiograph in pediatric heart disease: how does it correlate with heart volumes at magnetic resonance imaging? Pediatr Radiol. 2015;45:1616–23.
5. Haller JO, Slovis TL, Joshi A. Pediatric radiology. 3rd ed. Heidelberg: Springer; 2005.
6. Laya BF, Goske MJ, Morrison S, et al. The accuracy of chest radiographs in the detection of congenital heart disease and the diagnosis of specific congenital cardiac lesions. Pediatr Radiol. 2006;36:677–81.
7. Ravin CE. Radiographic analysis of pulmonary vascular distribution: a review. Bull NY Acad Med. 1983;59:728–43.
8. Strife JL, Sze RW. Radiographic evaluation of the neonate with congenital heart disease. Radiol Clin N Am. 1999;37:1093–107.

Child with Heart Transplant: Unique Immunologic and Hemodynamic Issues and Their Management

11

Neha Bansal, Swati Sehgal, and Celeste T. Williams

Introduction

The first pediatric heart transplant was performed by Adrian Kantrowitz in the United States in 1967 just 3 days after the first human to human adult heart transplant was performed by Christian Barnard in South Africa. The patient was a neonate with tricuspid atresia. In 1984, Leonard Bailey performed a xenotransplant, with a baboon heart, in a neonate with a 20-day survival. That same year, the first successful infant heart transplant was performed by Denton Cooley, the child lived 13 years after the transplant [1]. Since the first pediatric heart transplant, more than 12,500 heart transplants in children have been reported to the International Society for Heart and Lung Transplantation (ISHLT) registry [2]. Since the 1990s, on an average, approximately 500 pediatric heart transplants are performed worldwide annually.

Heart transplantation is indicated in children with heart failure secondary to various forms of cardiomyopathy refractory to standard medical therapy, in children with congenital heart disease that is not amenable to surgical repair, and in children with failed palliation of congenital heart disease. A small percentage of children will require re-transplantation. The median survival after transplant ranges from 13 to 21 years, with a longer survival seen in infant recipients [3]. Heart transplant recipients can pose unique challenges to emergency room (ER) physicians and primary care providers, including their clinical presentation, the diagnostic testing, and

N. Bansal, M.D. • S. Sehgal, M.D. (✉)
Division of Pediatric Cardiology, Carmen and Ann Adams Department of Pediatrics, Wayne State University School of Medicine, Children's Hospital of Michigan, Detroit, MI, USA
e-mail: NBansal@dmc.org; ssehgal@dmc.org

C. T. Williams, M.D.
Division of Cardiovascular Medicine, Henry Ford Hospital, Heart and Vascular Institute, Detroit, MI, USA
e-mail: CWILLIA6@hfhs.org

© Springer International Publishing AG, part of Springer Nature 2018

A. P. Sarnaik et al. (eds.), *Cardiac Emergencies in Children*,
https://doi.org/10.1007/978-3-319-73754-6_11

the therapeutic interventions that are required. The ER physician is the first to identify and possibly treat the common complications seen after heart transplantation.

The most common post-transplant management issues include allograft rejection, complications and drug interactions of immunosuppressive therapy, life-threatening infections, and malignancies such as post-transplant lymphoproliferative disease (PTLD). These patients are extremely fragile, especially in the first few months post-transplant with the highest risk of rejection and infection being in the first 6 months. To achieve the most favorable outcomes, it is important to work in close collaboration with the patients' transplant team.

Emergency Department (ED) Presentation: Rejection

Clinical Vignette

A 7-year-old female presents to the ED with vomiting, poor appetite, and decreased energy levels for the past 24 h. Her medical history is significant for a heart transplant at 2 years of age for refractory myocardial dysfunction secondary to myocarditis. On physical examination, she is afebrile, the heart rate is 140 beats per minute, the respiratory rate is 20 breaths per minute, and the blood pressure is 112/68 mmHg. The cardiac examination reveals an S3 gallop, a holosystolic murmur at the apex and hepatomegaly. Laboratory testing is significant for an elevated NT-proBNP value at 4200 pg/mL. The AST is 525 U/L, the ALT is 354 U/L, the blood urea nitrogen is 32 mg/dL, and the creatinine is 1.3 mg/dL. The complete blood count is within normal limits.

Signs and Symptoms

Acute allograft rejection is common in the first year post-transplant with 15–20% of the patients requiring treatment [3]. The incidence decreases significantly after the first year of transplant. Rejection is the most common cause of death in the first 5 years after heart transplantation [4]. Rejection can be asymptomatic and detected only on a surveillance endomyocardial biopsy, but when symptomatic, the patient presents with symptoms of low cardiac output, such as poor feeding, vomiting, abdominal pain, and fatigue. Infants and young children may demonstrate lethargy or irritability and feeding intolerance. Older patients may present with dyspnea, abdominal pain, vomiting, palpitations, and near-syncope or syncope. Chest pain is rarely present due to the denervation of the heart during transplant surgery. Arrhythmias are also a common presenting symptom for rejection. Physical examination findings in these patients include tachycardia, an S3 gallop, a new murmur from mitral or tricuspid valve regurgitation, and hepatomegaly, and in severe cases, signs of pulmonary edema and low cardiac output may be present.

Laboratory Studies

Endomyocardial biopsy is the gold standard for the diagnosis of rejection in heart transplant recipients [5]. However, an acutely ill patient may need initiation of treatment prior to obtaining biopsy specimens. Another noninvasive test that can help with the diagnosis is echocardiography. Abnormalities in left ventricular (LV) fractional shortening, LV mass, and mitral E wave amplitude and the presence of a new pericardial effusion support the diagnosis of rejection; however, the absence of these abnormalities does not rule out rejection [6]. An ECG may show sinus tachycardia or new-onset atrial or ventricular arrhythmias. An elevated BNP or NT-proBNP measurement in the blood may aid in diagnosis of rejection [7, 8]. It is important to note that a change in the BNP value from the patient's baseline value is more important than the absolute value in heart transplant recipients. Plasma BNP levels remain elevated for a relatively long period of time after cardiac allograft transplantation, even in the absence of acute rejection [9, 10]. Patients are often taking two–three immunosuppressive agents during the maintenance phase after cardiac transplantation. Obtaining medication levels may be crucial in further management and in distinguishing rejection from medication adverse effect. The adverse effects of major medications used in pediatric cardiac transplants are summarized in Table 11.1.

Table 11.1 Adverse effects of common immunosuppressive medications

Medication	Mechanism	Adverse effect
Cyclosporine (Sandimmune, generic)	– Calcineurin inhibitor, decreasing T-lymphocyte activity and IL-2 function	– Acute or chronic nephrotoxicity, electrolyte derangements (hyperkalemia, hypomagnesemia), gout, hemolytic-uremic syndrome, hirsutism, gingival hyperplasia, hypertension, hyperlipidemia
Tacrolimus (Prograf)	– Calcineurin inhibitor, inhibiting T-lymphocyte activity and IL-2 function	– Similar to cyclosporine above
		– Neurotoxicity (headache, tremor, paresthesias, seizures), hair loss instead of hirsutism, less hypertension/hyperlipidemia, no gingival hyperplasia
Azathioprine (Imuran)	– Block nucleotide production for immune cell replication	– Bone marrow suppression, macrocytosis, anemia, hepatotoxicity, pancreatitis
Mycophenolate mofetil (CellCept)	– Cytostatic effect on B and T cells, decreasing proliferation through inhibiting nucleotide synthesis	– Abdominal pain, decreased oral intake, nausea/vomiting, diarrhea, anemia, leukopenia, thrombocytopenia

(continued)

Table 11.1 (continued)

Medication	Mechanism	Adverse effect
Corticosteroids	– Impairs phagocyte function	– Weight gain, cataracts, acne, skin thinning, bruising, osteoporosis, GI bleeding, hyperglycemia, hyperlipidemia, psychologic effects, Cushingoid appearance
	– Attenuates production of proinflammatory mediator	
	– Decreases T-cell activity	
	– Decreases cell signal transduction	
Sirolimus (Rapamune)	– Blocks mTOR receptor and immune cell signal transduction, reducing B- and T-cell activity	– Thrombocytopenia, leukopenia/ anemia (less common), hyperlipidemia, mucosal irritation, buccal ulceration, diarrhea, interstitial pneumonitis
Polyclonal antibodies (antithymocyte gamma-globulin)	– Antilymphocyte antibody	– Fever, serum sickness, anaphylaxis, anemia, thrombocytopenia
	– Used for immunosuppression when nephrotoxic agent is held	
	– Used for treatment of corticosteroid-resistant rejection	
Monoclonal antibodies (OKT3, IL-2 receptor antibody)	– Antilymphocyte antibody	– OKT3: During first 3 days of therapy, may have headache, aseptic meningitis, encephalopathy, seizures, nausea, vomiting, diarrhea, pulmonary edema, nephrotoxicity: After 3 days, low risk of adverse effects
	– Used for prophylaxis against rejection in early period	
	– Used for immunosuppression when nephrotoxic agent is held	
		– IL-2 receptor antibodies have rare adverse effects such as anaphylaxis
	– Used for treatment of corticosteroid resistant rejection	

Reproduced with permission from Elsevier [16]

Management

Heart transplant recipients are on lifelong maintenance immunosuppressive therapy to prevent allograft rejection. These agents are used typically in combination, composed of a calcineurin inhibitor (cyclosporine or tacrolimus) and an antiproliferative agent (azathioprine or mycophenolate mofetil). Oral steroids are often used in addition. Other agents, like sirolimus and everolimus, are used if there is intolerance to standard therapy or when there is evidence of transplant coronary artery disease, as there is data that these agents may halt or slow the progression of transplant coronary artery disease [11]. Allograft rejection can be cellular or antibody-mediated (previously known as humoral rejection) with the latter being more commonly associated with hemodynamic compromise and accelerated coronary allograft vasculopathy [12, 13].

Acute cellular rejection (ACR) is predominantly mediated by T cells. The hallmark of ACR is the presence of lymphocytes in the myocardium (diagnosis made by biopsy), with more severe rejection being associated with greater myocardial injury [14]. The International Society for Heart and Lung Transplantation (ISHLT) grading system (revised in 2004) is used to stratify acute cellular rejection in order of severity. Grading is as follows:

Grade 0: No rejection
Grade 1R: Mild, interstitial, and/or perivascular infiltrates with up to one focus of myocyte damage
Grade 2R: Moderate, two or more foci of infiltrates with associated myocyte damage
Grade 3R: Severe, diffuse infiltrate with multifocal myocyte damage, with or without edema, hemorrhage, or vasculitis

Antibody-mediated rejection (AMR) is defined by the presence of clinical evidence of allograft dysfunction, histological evidence of acute capillary injury, and immunopathological evidence for antibody-mediated injury, such as C4d capillary positivity on endomyocardial biopsy sample [5]. As per the 2013 ISHLT working formulation for pathological diagnosis of antibody-mediated rejection, the grading is as follows:

pAMR0: Negative for pathologic AMR; histologic and immunopathologic studies are both negative
pAMR1 (H+): Histologic findings positive, immunopathologic findings negative
pAMR1 (I+): Histologic findings negative, immunopathologic findings positive (C4d+ and/or CD68+)
pAMR2: Positive pathologic AMR, histologic and immunopathologic findings both present
pAMR3: Severe pathologic AMR; interstitial hemorrhage, capillary fragmentation, mixed inflammatory infiltrates, endothelial cell pyknosis, and/or karyorrhexis and marked edema

The transplant center/transplant team should be notified if there is suspicion for rejection as prompt treatment can improve the outcomes. Patients with suspected rejection undergo cardiac catheterization and endomyocardial biopsy for confirmation and grading of the rejection, if present. If an endomyocardial biopsy is not readily available and suspicion for rejection is high, consider initiation of empirical treatment for rejection. Rejection is typically treated with high-dose intravenous methylprednisolone with the use of anti-thymocyte globulin reserved for severe cases. Intravenous immunoglobulin and plasmapheresis are used to treat antibody-mediated rejection. In severe cases of antibody-mediated rejection, aggressive therapies involving monoclonal antibodies like rituximab, proteasome inhibitors like bortezomib, and anticomplement antibodies like eculizumab have been used. Patients with hemodynamically significant rejection may present with cardiogenic shock. The initial management of these patients is similar to the treatment of other causes of cardiogenic shock and includes diuretics, intravenous inotropes, and mechanical ventilation in addition to aggressive immune modulating therapy.

Mechanical Circulatory Support

The preemptive use of extracorporeal membrane oxygenation (ECMO) or a short-term ventricular assist device in the setting of hemodynamic compromise from AMR has been shown to have survival benefit over patients who received salvage therapy. Kittleson and colleagues described the use of ECMO in 32 patients with heart transplant rejection. Twenty-five of these patients had presumed rejection, and 15 had biopsy-proven rejection. Of these, nine had grade 2R or 3R cellular rejection, and six had AMR. After support with ECMO, five of the six with AMR improved. At 1 year, 26% of the preemptively treated patients were alive compared with only 7% of the salvage patients. Thus, ECMO or other temporary mechanical supports can be considered as salvage therapy in those with AMR and hemodynamic compromise refractory to medical therapy [15].

Complications

Antibody-mediated rejection frequently leads to decreased graft and patient survival. Allograft function may not fully recover, especially if there is a dramatic decrease in the ventricular function [16]. It is also associated with the development and rapid progression of transplant coronary allograft disease, an aggressive form of coronary artery disease, which is the most common cause of graft loss in heart transplant recipients. Recurrent episodes of acute cellular rejection, similarly, can also lead to poor long-term outcomes [17].

Emergency Department Presentation: Infection

Clinical Vignette

A 10-year-old female presents to the emergency room with a 3-day history of cough, runny nose, and fever. She underwent heart transplant in infancy for medically refractory myocardial dysfunction secondary to dilated cardiomyopathy. In the ER, her vital signs are: HR 120, RR 32, T 38.5C, BP 100/70, room air oxygen saturation 92%. On examination, she is in mild distress. She has crackles in the left lower lobe but good air entry bilaterally. Cardiac examination is normal with no gallop rhythm. Her chest x-ray is unremarkable. Her medications include tacrolimus, mycophenolate mofetil, and prednisone, as well as trimethoprim sulfamethoxazole for pneumocystis prophylaxis. Echocardiography shows normal biventricular function.

Signs and Symptoms

Infections continue to remain a major complication after heart transplantation [18]. Potent immunosuppressive agents have dramatically reduced the incidence of rejection of transplanted organs. This is a double-edged sword as this immunosuppressed state increases the susceptibility to opportunistic infections. Pre-transplant factors such as malnutrition from chronic myocardial dysfunction, mechanical ventilation with colonization of pathogens in the respiratory tract, and previous surgical palliation in children with congenital heart defects can increase the risk of infections post-transplant even further. The signs and symptoms of infections in immunocompromised patients are like any other patient presenting with similar infections. The patients may or may not present with fever with or without an apparent source, upper respiratory symptoms like cough and nasal congestion, lower respiratory symptoms which may include tachypnea and respiratory distress, and urinary tract infections with increased frequency of urination and dysuria. Disseminated disease may present with fever, malaise, and end-organ dysfunction in the form of acute kidney injury or elevated transaminases from liver involvement. Gastrointestinal symptoms like abdominal pain, nausea, vomiting, and diarrhea may be seen with gastroenteritis from local infection or disseminated disease from *Cytomegalovirus* (CMV). However, signs and symptoms of infection may be diminished (e.g., fever may be absent in patients with florid infections) making it more difficult to recognize infection in a transplant patient [19]. The risk of infection after transplantation changes over time, especially if immunosuppressive therapy can be weaned over time. In addition, noninfectious causes of fever, such as allograft rejection, may complicate the clinical picture in transplant recipients.

Differential Diagnosis

Infections in heart transplant recipients may be caused by a wide variety of organisms including bacteria, fungi, viruses, and protozoa. Nonetheless, bacterial and viral infections account for 80–90% of all infections in these patients. According to a large single-center study of heart transplant recipients, 44% of infections were bacterial, 42% were viral, 10% were fungal, and 4% due to *pneumocystis jiroveci*. Parasitic infections were rare, accounting for 0.6% of the infections. In their experience, the most common bacterial infection sites were the pulmonary and urinary tracts. *Escherichia coli* and *Pseudomonas aeruginosa* were the most common

Gram-negative infectious bacterial agents, whereas *Staphylococcus aureus* was the most common Gram-positive bacterial agent. The most common viral infections were herpes simplex (stomatitis) and cytomegalovirus infection. *Aspergillus* and *Candida* species accounted for the majority of the fungal infections (83%) with the most common site being the pulmonary followed by disseminated infection. *Pneumocystis jiroveci* pneumonia was diagnosed in almost two-thirds of the patients in the first 6 months post-transplant, and another 10% developed within the first year. The parasitic infections were *Toxoplasma gondii* and intestinal giardiasis. Toxoplasma infection was more common in serologically negative recipients who had donors with positive toxoplasma serology. None of the patients on trimethoprim-sulfamethoxazole prophylaxis developed toxoplasmosis. The authors also note that the rate of infections with *Cytomegalovirus* (CMV), herpes simplex virus (HSV), varicella-zoster (VZV), *Aspergillus* species, bacteria, *Nocardia* species, *Listeria* species, and *P. jiroveci* has significantly reduced since 1990, primarily due to the introduction of effective antimicrobial prophylaxis in addition to targeting lower levels of immunosuppressant medications [19]. Infants and younger children however suffer more commonly from community-acquired viruses like respiratory syncytial virus, parainfluenza, and adenovirus. They are also at risk for primary infection from CMV and Epstein-Barr virus (EBV) as opposed to older children and adults in whom reactivation of the disease is seen. Additionally, infants who undergo heart transplant prior to completing a primary vaccination series are at risk for contracting vaccine-preventable diseases. Vaccination after transplantation is not as effective as completing it before transplantation. A detailed history, including all possible exposures, is essential for creating a differential diagnosis. Postoperative infections, acquisition of nosocomial or community pathogens, and reactivation of latent infections and opportunistic infections are all possible etiologies in patients with a heart transplant.

Time after transplantation is an important determinant of the nature of infection and causative organism (Table 11.2). Opportunistic infections are not common in the first month after transplantation as the full effect of immunosuppression is not yet established. Viral and candida infections in this period are mainly donor-derived. However, occasionally they may be recipient-derived or even related to the surgery itself. Beyond the first month, viral pathogens are responsible for most of the infections seen in transplant recipients. *Pneumocystis jiroveci* pneumonia is another important pathogen causing infection in the first 6 months. Other infections in the interval between 1–6 months postoperatively include endemic fungi, *Aspergillus*, *Cryptococcus*, *Trypanosoma cruzi*, or *Strongyloides* [18]. Newer immunosuppressive approaches, including the use of tacrolimus, sirolimus, and mycophenolate mofetil, have largely replaced high-dose corticosteroids and azathioprine. Sirolimus-based regimens can sometimes lead to idiosyncratic noninfectious pneumonitis, which can be easily confused with pneumocystis pneumonia or viral pneumonia [18]. Reactivation of latent viral infections like *Cytomegalovirus* (CMV), Epstein-Barr virus (EBV), or human immunodeficiency virus (HIV) can be seen early after cardiac transplant. The risk of these infections is higher if there is donor-recipient mismatch with regard to these infections. One example is a donor who is CMV

Table 11.2 Common infections based on transplant period

Transplant period	Infection
Early: First month after transplantation	– Donor-derived: Donor-derived bacteria (MRSA, VRE, tuberculosis), fungi (*Candida*), and parasite (toxoplasmosis, Chagas disease)
	– Nosocomial/surgery-related: Aspiration pneumonia, surgical site infection, urinary tract infection, superinfection of graft tissue, vascular access infection, *Clostridium difficile* colitis
Intermediate: 1–6 months after transplantation	– Most at risk for opportunistic infection: *Pneumocystis jirovecii, Histoplasma, Coccidioides, Cryptococcus*, hepatitis B/C, BK polyomavirus, Kaposi sarcoma, cytomegalovirus, tuberculosis, Epstein-Barr virus (EBV)
	– Surgical site infections may arise in this period.
	– Reactivation of dormant host infection (CMV, HZV, HSV, EBV)
Late: >6 months after transplantation	– Community-acquired infection: Respiratory viruses, *Pneumococcus, Legionella, Listeria, Influenza*, EBV

MRSA methicillin-resistant *Staphylococcus aureus*, *VRE* Vancomycin-resistant enterococci
Reproduced with permission from Elsevier [16]

positive and a recipient who is CMV negative. CMV infection may be asymptomatic, but CMV disease can present as fever and neutropenia, lymphadenopathy, pneumonitis, gastrointestinal symptoms (bleeding, gastritis, colitis, ulcers, and pancreatitis), chorioretinitis, meningoencephalitis, or disseminated disease [18]. There is a potential for acquiring donor-derived infections that are not known at the time of organ procurement, for example, *Mycobacterium tuberculosis*, West Nile virus, hepatitis B and C, and HIV. Although very rare, it is important to have a high index of suspicion for these agents, especially in the early post-transplant phase [19]. The risk of infection diminishes 6 months after transplantation, due to the ability to wean immunosuppression in patients with a favorable post-transplant course who do not have recurrent rejection episodes. However, transplant recipients maintain a persistently increased risk of infection from community-acquired pathogens due to their chronic immunosuppressed state compared to the normal population.

Management

Antimicrobial prophylaxis has significantly reduced the incidence and severity of post-transplantation infections [18]. Preventive strategies, in addition to antimicrobial prophylaxis, include accelerated vaccination of transplant recipients prior to transplant and continuing the vaccination series with the exception of live vaccines, post-transplant, as well as preemptive therapy. Ganciclovir, valganciclovir, and acyclovir are commonly used for antiviral prophylaxis. Trimethoprim-sulfamethoxazole is used for prophylaxis primarily against *Pneumocystis jiroveci* pneumonia and toxoplasmosis. However, it also provides protection against other infectious agents like *Isospora belli*, *Cyclospora cayetanensis*, many *Nocardia* and *Listeria* species, and common urinary, respiratory, and gastrointestinal pathogens [17]. Alternatives in this class are dapsone, atovaquone, and inhaled pentamidine if the transplant recipient is allergic to trimethoprim-sulfamethoxazole. Nystatin is used for prophylaxis against oral candidiasis. This is most commonly used as swish-and-swallow or swish-and-spit formulation. Some centers also use amphotericin B for antifungal prophylaxis. These antimicrobials are frequently prescribed for the first 6 months post-transplant. Priority should be given to the prevention and preemptive treatment of these infections to effectively reduce the mortality. Preemptive treatment is made possible by antigen detection assays like sensitive polymerase chain reaction tests that allow identification of infection prior to symptoms and disease manifestation. Reduction in immunosuppressant dosages, institution of antimicrobial therapy, and intensive monitoring at this stage decrease morbidity associated with post-transplant infections. Due to the patient's immunocompromised status, it is imperative to have an aggressive approach with empirical management, as the spectrum of potential pathogens is broad and infection can progress rapidly. Early and specific microbiological diagnosis is essential for guiding treatment and minimizing nonessential and toxic antimicrobial drug therapy.

When faced with a transplant recipient with a fever and no obvious source, it is reasonable to start empiric antibiotic therapy while awaiting microbiology results. Initial microbiological testing should include blood and urine cultures along with sensitivity testing and quantitative viral assays for CMV and EBV, and in patients with diarrhea, stool should be analyzed for not only stool culture but also for presence of *C. difficile*, ova, parasites, and norovirus. Central nervous system (CNS) infections, although uncommon, should be treated as a medical emergency. Causative organisms include *Listeria*, herpes simplex virus, JC virus, and *Cryptococcus neoformans*. Empirical treatment should be initiated while awaiting results of CSF fluid analysis and imaging studies. The differential diagnosis of CNS infections should include calcineurin inhibitor toxicity. Techniques currently under development, such as more sensitive microbiologic assays and immunoassays, may provide the potential for individualized immunosuppression and prophylactic strategies. In adults, an infectious disease consult, to help with the diagnosis of infections in solid organ transplant patients, has shown improved outcomes [16]. Confirmatory diagnosis may require advanced testing, like biopsy, which may not be obtainable in the ED, and often the results of advanced testing may not return during the ED stay. It is important to note that antimicrobial therapy frequently has interactions with immunosuppressive agents requiring close monitoring of immunosuppression medication levels during the antimicrobial treatment period. Certain antibiotics may increase or decrease the level of tacrolimus in the blood due to altered drug metabolism, thus requiring frequent dose adjustments. Infections in transplant recipients can have lasting effects over and beyond the acute stage. Chronic viral infections can lead to allograft injury, for example, CMV infection is implicated in the early development and progression of transplant coronary artery disease [17]. EBV infection is associated with the development of post-transplant lymphoproliferative disease (PTLD). Recurrent infection may develop in some patients despite minimization of their immunosuppression. These patients may benefit from lifelong prophylactic medications.

Clinical Pearls [5–7]

- It is important to have a high index of suspicion for rejection. Timely initiation of treatment with high-dose intravenous methylprednisolone may prevent damage to the allograft and decrease morbidity and mortality.
- Endomyocardial biopsy is the gold standard for the definitive diagnosis of cellular and antibody-mediated rejection. In collaboration with the transplant team, empiric treatment can be initiated prior to the confirmation of rejection.
- There is a diverse group of organisms causing infections in the immunocompromised transplant patient. The inflammatory responses are often impaired, resulting in decreased symptoms and atypical clinical presentations and radiological findings.
- Empiric treatment with broad-spectrum antimicrobials must be initiated in a sick transplant recipient with suspected infection.
- Antimicrobial treatment is more complex in heart transplant recipients due to medication interactions with immunosuppressant drugs.
- To achieve favorable outcomes, close consultation with the primary heart transplant team is essential for management of these complex and fragile patients.

References

1. Bailey LL. The evolution of infant heart transplantation. J Heart Lung Transplant. 2009;28(12):1241–5. PubMed PMID: 19818649. Epub 2009/10/13. eng.
2. Rossano JW, Dipchand AI, Edwards LB, Goldfarb S, Kucheryavaya AY, Levvey Rn BJ, Lund LH, et al. The registry of the International Society for Heart and Lung Transplantation: nineteenth Pediatric heart transplantation report-2016; focus theme: primary diagnostic indications for transplant. J Heart Lung Transplant. 2016;35(10):1185–95. PubMed PMID: 27772670. Epub 2016/10/25. eng.
3. Dipchand AI, Rossano JW, Edwards LB, Kucheryavaya AY, Benden C, Goldfarb S, Levvey BJ, et al. The registry of the International Society for Heart and Lung transplantation: eighteenth official pediatric heart transplantation report—2015; focus theme: early graft failure. J Heart Lung Transplant. 2015;34(10):1233–43. PubMed PMID: 26454737. Epub 2015/10/12. eng.
4. Waltz DA, Boucek MM, Edwards LB, Keck BM, Trulock EP, Taylor DO, Hertz MI. Registry of the International Society for Heart and Lung Transplantation: ninth official pediatric lung and heart-lung transplantation report—2006. J Heart Lung Transplant. 2006;25(8):904–11. PubMed PMID: 16890110. Epub 2006/08/08. eng.
5. Stewart S, Winters GL, Fishbein MC, Tazelaar HD, Kobashigawa J, Abrams J, Andersen CB, et al. Revision of the 1990 working formulation for the standardization of nomenclature in the diagnosis of heart rejection. J Heart Lung Transplant. 2005;24(11):1710–20. PubMed PMID: 16297770. Epub 2005/11/22. eng.
6. Moran AM, Lipshultz SE, Rifai N, O'Brien P, Mooney H, Perry S, Perez-Atayde A, et al. Non-invasive assessment of rejection in pediatric transplant patients: serologic and echocardiographic prediction of biopsy-proven myocardial rejection. J Heart Lung Transplant. 2000;19(8):756–64. PubMed PMID: 10967269. Epub 2000/09/01. eng.

7. Rossano JW, Denfield SW, Kim JJ, Price JF, Jefferies JL, Decker JA, Smith EO, et al. B-type natriuretic peptide is a sensitive screening test for acute rejection in pediatric heart transplant patients. J Heart Lung Transplant. 2008;27(6):649–54. PubMed PMID: 18503965. Epub 2008/05/28. eng.
8. Lindblade CL, Chun DS, Darragh RK, Caldwell RL, Murphy DJ, Schamberger MS. Value of plasma B-type natriuretic peptide as a marker for rejection in pediatric heart transplant recipients. Am J Cardiol. 2005;95(7):909–11. PubMed PMID: 15781032. Epub 2005/03/23. eng.
9. Kittleson MM, Skojec DV, Wittstein IS, Champion HC, Judge DP, Barouch LA, Halushka M, et al. The change in B-type natriuretic peptide levels over time predicts significant rejection in cardiac transplant recipients. J Heart Lung Transplant. 2009;28(7):704–9. PubMed PMID: 19560699. Epub 2009/06/30. eng.
10. Ogawa T, Veinot JP, Davies RA, Haddad H, Smith SJ, Masters RG, Hendry PJ, et al. Neuroendocrine profiling of humans receiving cardiac allografts. J Heart Lung Transplant. 2005;24(8):1046–54. PubMed PMID: 16102440. Epub 2005/08/17. eng.
11. Kindel SJ, Pahl E. Current therapies for cardiac allograft vasculopathy in children. Congenit Heart Dis. 2012;7(4):324–35. PubMed PMID: 22613206. Epub 2012/05/23. eng.
12. Hathout E, Beeson WL, Kuhn M, Johnston J, Fitts J, Razzouk A, Bailey L, et al. Cardiac allograft vasculopathy in pediatric heart transplant recipients. Transpl Int. 2006;19(3):184–9. PubMed PMID: 16441766. Epub 2006/01/31. eng.
13. Pahl E, Naftel DC, Kuhn MA, Shaddy RE, Morrow WR, Canter CE, Kirklin J. The impact and outcome of transplant coronary artery disease in a pediatric population: a 9-year multi-institutional study. J Heart Lung Transplant. 2005;24(6):645–51. PubMed PMID: 15949722. Epub 2005/06/14. eng.
14. Kirk R, Edwards LB, Kucheryavaya AY, Aurora P, Christie JD, Dobbels F, Rahmel AO, et al. The registry of the International Society for Heart and Lung Transplantation: thirteenth official pediatric heart transplantation report—2010. J Heart Lung Transplant. 2010;29(10):1119–28. PubMed PMID: 20870166. Epub 2010/09/28. eng.
15. Kittleson MM, Patel JK, Moriguchi JD, Kawano M, Davis S, Hage A, Hamilton MA, et al. Heart transplant recipients supported with extracorporeal membrane oxygenation: outcomes from a single-center experience. J Heart Lung Transplant. 2011;30(11):1250–6. PubMed PMID: 21676629. Epub 2011/06/17. eng.
16. Long B, Koyfman A. The emergency medicine approach to transplant complications. Am J Emerg Med. 2016;34(11):2200–8. PubMed PMID: 27645810. Epub 2016/09/21. eng.
17. Kfoury AG, Renlund DG, Snow GL, Stehlik J, Folsom JW, Fisher PW, Reid BB, et al. A clinical correlation study of severity of antibody-mediated rejection and cardiovascular mortality in heart transplantation. J Heart Lung Transplant. 2009;28(1):51–7. PubMed PMID: 19134531. Epub 2009/01/13. eng.
18. Fishman JA. Infection in solid-organ transplant recipients. N Engl J Med. 2007;357(25):2601–14. PubMed PMID: 18094380. Epub 2007/12/21. eng.
19. Green M. Introduction: infections in solid organ transplantation. Am J Transplant. 2013; 13(Suppl 4):3–8. PubMed PMID: 23464993. Epub 2013/03/08. eng.

Pediatric Mechanical Circulatory Support

12

Katherine Cashen, Swati Sehgal, and Henry L. Walters III

Introduction

Pediatric mechanical circulatory support has continued to evolve as a therapeutic treatment option for children with severe ventricular dysfunction, refractory to medical and/or surgical therapy. Since the first pediatric heart transplant in 1967, advancements in surgical technique, organ preservation, and immune modulation have improved survival in children after heart transplantation. Despite these successes, limitations remain. Wait-list mortality and morbidity remain high in some cases necessitating a "bridge" to transplant via mechanical circulatory support. Technological advances have improved and expanded applications of mechanical circulatory support devices for children. The two major forms of mechanical support for pediatric patients include extracorporeal membrane oxygenation (ECMO) and ventricular assist devices (VADs.) These modalities have different indications, advantages, and disadvantages.

Mechanical circulatory support is used as a bridge to heart transplant, a bridge to recovery, a bridge to decision, or, if circulatory support is needed in a patient who may

K. Cashen, D.O. (✉)
Department of Pediatrics, Division of Critical Care Medicine, Children's Hospital of Michigan, Wayne State University School of Medicine, Detroit, MI, USA
e-mail: kcashen@med.wayne.edu

S. Sehgal, M.D.
Department of Pediatrics, Division of Cardiology, Children's Hospital of Michigan, Wayne State University School of Medicine, Detroit, MI, USA
e-mail: ssehgal@dmc.org

H. L. Walters III, M.D.
Department of Cardiovascular Surgery, Children's Hospital of Michigan, FTA, Wayne State University School of Medicine, Detroit, MI, USA
e-mail: hwalters@dmc.org

© Springer International Publishing AG, part of Springer Nature 2018
A. P. Sarnaik et al. (eds.), *Cardiac Emergencies in Children*,
https://doi.org/10.1007/978-3-319-73754-6_12

not be a candidate for heart transplantation, destination therapy. The indications and decision to use a specific device depend on the clinical scenario, stability of the patient, and whether short-term or long-term support is needed. In general, short-term mechanical circulatory support via ECMO is used in the acute treatment of cardiogenic shock or ventricular dysfunction after cardiac surgery with the expectation of patient recovery or as a bridge to a more long-term device, whereas mechanical circulatory support with a VAD is typically employed for long-term support in a child who is unlikely to recover from the cardiac dysfunction and may require support for longer than 14 days.

In this chapter, through clinical vignettes, we describe specific scenarios and applications of different mechanical circulatory support devices. In addition, we discuss the indications, management strategies, short- and long-term outcomes, complications, limitations of the available pediatric support devices, and the role of the emergency department physician in their application.

Emergency Department (ED) Presentation: ECMO

Clinical Vignette

An 8-year-old girl presents to the emergency department with complaints of shortness of breath, fatigue, and decreased exercise tolerance. She felt dizzy at school, and the teacher called her mother to pick her up today during recess. She has no past medical history and was well until she developed nasal congestion, cough, and fever 10 days ago. Her siblings also had a "cold." She seemed to improve but has been more tired the last few days. She does not take any medications. Vital signs show a heart rate of 160 beats per minute, a respiratory rate of 40 breaths per minute, and a temperature of 38.1 °C. On physical examination, she is ill appearing. She has an S3 gallop on cardiac examination and cool extremities with delayed capillary refill. Lung examination reveals crackles in the bases bilaterally. On abdominal examination, she has hepatomegaly with the liver palpable 4 cm below the right costal margin. The chest radiograph shows mild cardiomegaly. The electrocardiogram shows nonspecific ST-segment changes and multiple isolated ectopic ventricular beats. The echocardiogram is in process and shows severely depressed left ventricular function. During this time, the child starts having runs of non-sustained ventricular tachycardia that quickly degenerate into pulseless ventricular tachycardia. The algorithm for pulseless ventricular tachycardia in the pediatric advanced life support (PALS) guidelines is initiated. What is the etiology of this child's cardiac dysfunction? What management strategies should be considered? Is ECMO an option for this child?

Epidemiology

Myocarditis is an inflammatory process involving the myocardium. These disease processes have a wide spectrum of clinical presentations and multiple etiologies. As the inflammatory process progresses, it may lead to myocyte necrosis and development of congestive, dilated cardiomyopathy. The diagnosis may be challenging due to the wide range of presentations and symptoms, and it may be based upon circumstantial evidence, including a recent viral illness. A bimodal pattern is reported with a higher incidence in infants and teenagers, but all ages may be affected. Etiologies include a large spectrum of infectious and noninfectious agents. The majority of cases in North America are of viral etiology with enteroviruses and adenovirus as the most common agents. A combination of direct viral infection and immunologic reaction in the myocardial cells causes inflammatory changes and promotes myocardial apoptosis.

Acute fulminant myocarditis is a distinct entity associated with an aggressive course and increased risk of cardiovascular collapse. These patients typically present with a viral prodrome, distinct onset of symptoms, and rapid hemodynamic deterioration. Although they have a high severity of illness, most will have myocardial recovery if end-organ function is supported. ECMO and other modes of mechanical circulatory support have been successfully utilized as rescue strategies when cardiogenic shock is refractory to maximum medical therapy.

Signs/Symptoms

Children with myocarditis may be asymptomatic, or they may present with obvious signs of congestive heart failure. Older children may have an acute febrile illness, tachycardia, and isolated electrocardiogram changes. The most common cardiovascular complaint in older children is chest pain. Sudden death is a severe presentation after which the myocarditis is diagnosed on autopsy. Signs of myocardial dysfunction including cardiomegaly, hepatomegaly, and third or fourth heart sounds may be present. Symptoms of dyspnea, exercise intolerance, and tiredness may be present. In neonates and infants, irritability and poor feeding followed by signs of shock and pulmonary congestion may be present.

Laboratory and electrocardiographic findings are generally nonspecific. Elevation in creatine phosphokinase, lactate dehydrogenase, and cardiac troponin I may be seen. Half of these patients have leukocytosis on a complete blood count. Elevation of the erythrocyte sedimentation rate has also been reported. Electrocardiographic findings include nonspecific ST changes, ventricular and atrial ectopy, and T wave inversion.

Management

Treatment for myocarditis includes removal of any toxic or infectious agent and supportive care to maintain cardiac output and systemic oxygen delivery. The acute management of the myocardial dysfunction is based upon optimizing preload by avoiding intravascular volume depletion, reducing systemic vascular resistance, reducing myocardial oxygen consumption, maintaining myocardial synchrony, and unloading the heart, if possible, to allow for repair. Intubation and mechanical ventilation to decrease afterload (LV wall stress) and inotropic support may be required. A child who is unresponsive to these therapies and has ongoing cardiac dysfunction may require mechanical support. In addition, a child with shock and increasing arrhythmias may require ECMO or a VAD.

In our clinical vignette, the child had signs and symptoms of acute fulminant myocarditis and developed pulseless ventricular tachycardia in the emergency department. Prompt defibrillation, cardiopulmonary resuscitation (CPR), and antiarrhythmic therapy, if the ventricular tachycardia is refractory to defibrillation, should be employed. In addition, extracorporeal cardiopulmonary resuscitation (ECPR) (ECMO during CPR) should be mobilized, if available. The American Heart Association's pediatric advanced life support guidelines for in-hospital pediatric cardiac arrest recommend consideration of ECPR in children with heart disease if the conditions are likely reversible or amenable to heart transplant. Most centers utilizing ECPR have established rapid deployment teams with pre-primed circuits, and some institutions have protocols in place to cannulate patients in the emergency department.

ECMO

ECMO is the most common mechanical circulatory support option for pediatric patients. Data from the Extracorporeal Life Support Organization (ELSO) Registry indicates that as of 2017, 21,462 children have been supported with ECMO for a cardiac or ECPR indication. This modality provides both cardiac and pulmonary support using a blood pump to augment cardiac output and a membrane oxygenator for oxygen and CO_2 exchange (Fig. 12.1). Venoarterial (VA) ECMO is the mode required in infants and children with myocardial dysfunction. Three modes of ECMO cannulation used in pediatric patients include (1) transthoracic cannulation, with direct cannulation of the right atrium and aorta through a median sternotomy incision; (2) cannulation of the right internal jugular vein and right carotid artery percutaneously or through a cervical incision or, less frequently; and (3) femoral vein and femoral artery cannulation percutaneously or through a femoral incision. The location of cannulation depends on the size of the vessels, presence of occluded vessels, cardiac anatomy, surgeon preference, and circumstances surrounding initiation of extracorporeal support.

Peripheral cannulation via the carotid artery and the internal jugular vein is commonly used in infants and children who do not have contraindications to the use of these vessels. The right internal jugular vein is a large vessel with a straight course to the right atrium and is generally preferred. The right carotid artery is cannulated with advancement of the cannula to the aortic arch. In older children and adolescents, peripheral cannulation via the femoral vessels may be used. Venous cannulation is performed from the femoral vein to the inferior vena cava (IVC) or to the right atrium-IVC junction, and arterial cannulation is performed in the femoral artery. The biggest barrier to femoral cannulation in pediatric patients is the size of the vessels and limitation in venous flow. Limb ischemia is a significant problem in pediatric and adult patients when using femoral cannulation and remains a limiting factor when considering cannulation sites.

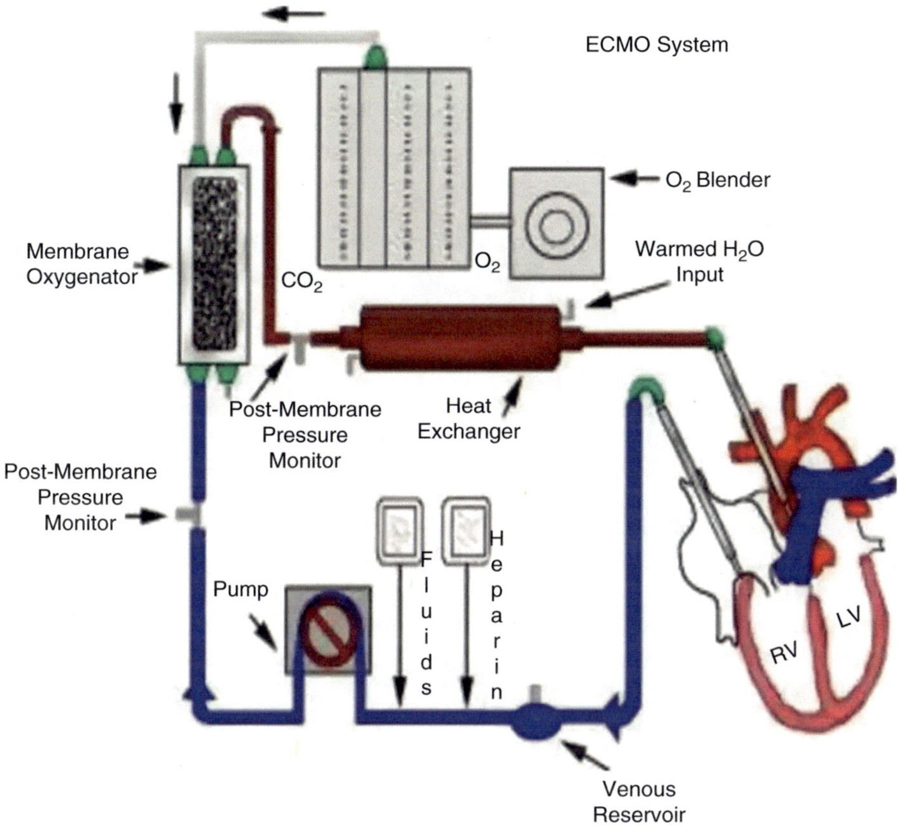

Fig. 12.1 Schematic of a typical ECMO system. O_2 is oxygen, H_2O is water, and CO_2 is carbon dioxide and represents the gas blender with arrows showing the sweep gas flow. Image retrieved 28 April 2017 from https://amprandom.blogspot.com/2016/12/ecmo-extracorporeal-membrane-oxygenation.html. Commons License associated: https://creativecommons.org/licenses/by-nc/4.0/

ECMO may serve as a bridge to recovery, a bridge to transplant, a bridge to more permanent mechanical assist device placement, or an adjunct to cardiopulmonary resuscitation (ECPR). ECMO has been used in postoperative congenital heart patients, children with acquired heart disease, and children with respiratory failure. ECMO should be employed for potentially reversible conditions. Absolute contraindications to ECMO include lethal chromosomal abnormalities, severe irreversible neurological injury, and extreme prematurity. Relative contraindications include intracranial hemorrhage, late pre-term birth, and weight <2 kg.

The main advantage of ECMO is that it can be rapidly deployed, may be performed in a child with a closed chest, provides pulmonary as well as cardiac support, and may be more readily available in different institutions globally. Major liabilities of ECMO are the presence of infection and stroke and that it may cause platelet damage and consumption with resultant hemorrhagic complications. In addition, ECMO is a time-limited therapy used for shorter-term circulatory support.

Complications

Although ECMO may be lifesaving, many complications have been reported. Hemorrhagic complications are most common. Acute kidney injury, infection, and serious neurologic injury are other known complications that contribute to the mortality and morbidity seen in survivors of ECMO. Hemorrhagic complications include cannulation site bleeding, surgical site bleeding, pulmonary hemorrhage, and hemothorax. Infection is a serious complication of ECMO and increases mortality. Bizzarro et al. reviewed the ELSO Registry and reported an 11.7% prevalence of infections with a rate of 15.4 per 1000 ECMO days. Rates for the pediatric and neonatal populations were 20.8 and 10.1 infections per 1000 ECMO days. VA ECMO was associated with the highest infection rate and increased in those patients who required ECMO for more than 14 days. The most common organism identified was coagulase-negative staphylococcus followed by candida species and pseudomonas.

Children undergoing ECMO are at risk for neurological injury for many of the same reasons they are placed on ECMO. Pre-ECMO clinical factors such as hypotension, low cardiac output, hypoxemia, acidosis, and infection all increase the risk of neurological injury. In addition, ECMO factors (anticoagulation, hemolysis, air or clots) increase the risk of hemorrhage, ischemia, seizures, and abnormal cerebral autoregulation. Neurological injuries are recorded in the ELSO Registry under the categories hemorrhage, infarct, seizure, and brain death. Neonates and specifically those placed on ECMO for cardiac indications have the highest risk of injury. In a recent publication, Poliito et al. reported 14% of neonates with congenital heart disease on ECMO had neurological injury and identified the need for CPR prior to ECMO as the strongest risk factor for injury. Intracranial hemorrhage is poorly tolerated due to anticoagulation on ECMO and has the highest incidence in cardiac neonates at 11.1% followed by 4.9% of pediatric cardiac patients. Ischemic injury from embolic clots or air is reported in 3.5% of neonates. Clinical seizures have been reported in 7.2% of neonatal cardiac patients and 6.8% of pediatric cardiac patients. Nonconvulsive electroencephalographical seizures may be even more common than previously recognized with 11–17% reported in neonatal studies. Pineda et al. reported 21% seizures in a cohort of pediatric ECMO patients, and 16% of patients had exclusively nonconvulsive seizures. These reports highlight the difficult neurological complications that must be identified and managed by care providers.

Outcomes

ECMO remains a highly invasive therapy with significant cost, high short-term mortality, and significant long-term dysfunction in survivors. Overall survival to discharge in pediatric cardiac ECMO patients is 50% and 41% for ECPR. This survival varies by age, indication, and cardiac diagnosis. Children with myocarditis have the highest survival to discharge of any cardiac ECMO diagnosis in the ELSO Registry at 72%. Multiple pediatric studies report survival to recovery or bridge to transplant at 63–87%.

The ELSO Registry reports only survival to hospital discharge and not long-term survival. Individual centers have survival to discharge at 88–96% with median follow-up ranging from 1 to 5 years after discharge. Data shows that hospital readmission and late mortality significantly affect ECMO survivors. Late deaths for pediatric ECMO survivors are likely a reflection of the severity of the underlying medical condition and associated comorbidities.

General ED Presentation: VAD

Clinical Vignette

A 15-year-old male presents to the emergency room with shortness of breath, decreased appetite, and fatigue for the past 2 days. He is known to have idiopathic dilated cardiomyopathy and is on oral heart failure therapy that includes lisinopril, carvedilol, spironolactone, and furosemide. Vital signs are notable for a heart rate of 140 beats per minute and a respiratory rate of 30 breaths per minute. On physical examination, he has an S3 gallop and a grade II/VI holosystolic regurgitant murmur at the apex. The lung examination is notable for crackles at the bases bilaterally. On abdominal examination, his liver is palpated 3 cm below the costal margin. He has 2+ pitting edema bilaterally at the level of the ankles. An echocardiogram is obtained in the emergency room, and it demonstrates a severely dilated left ventricle with severely reduced function and mildly reduced function of the right ventricle. There is mild-to-moderate mitral valve regurgitation. How would you manage this patient?

Epidemiology

Dilated cardiomyopathy (DCM) is a heart muscle disorder characterized by systolic dysfunction and dilation of the left or both ventricles. Based upon two large, international registries, the North American Pediatric Cardiomyopathy Registry (PCMR) and the National Australian Childhood Cardiomyopathy Study (NACCS), the incidence of idiopathic dilated cardiomyopathy is 1.1–1.2/100,000 people, and its prevalence in the pediatric age group is 1:170,000 in the United States. DCM accounts for >50% of all cardiomyopathies combined, with the highest proportion made up by infants (children <1 year of age). The various etiologies of dilated cardiomyopathy include infection (myocarditis), mutations in myocardial proteins (familial, >20 genes identified), neuromuscular disorders (Duchenne's and Becker's muscular dystrophy), inborn errors of metabolism (amino acid and organic acid disorders; fatty acid oxidation defects; glycogen, glycoprotein, and lysosomal storage disorders; mitochondrial and oxidative phosphorylation defects), myocardial toxins, and idiopathic. According to PCMR registry, idiopathic cases accounted for 66% of the patients with DCM. According to the same registry, the 1- and 5-year rates of death or transplantation in this population were 31% and 46%, respectively.

Signs and Symptoms

Seventy-one percent of patients with dilated cardiomyopathy have congestive heart failure at presentation according to the PCMR registry data. Some patients may be diagnosed during surveillance on screening echocardiograms that are obtained due to a family history of dilated cardiomyopathy. Neonates and infants present with symptoms of increased work of breathing, poor feeding, decreased urination, lethargy, and failure to thrive. Older children manifest shortness of breath and may complain of orthopnea. Signs of heart failure on physical examination can include tachycardia, gallop rhythm, tachypnea, rales, wheezing, hepatomegaly, and pedal edema. In severe cases, there may be frank pulmonary edema with respiratory distress and respiratory failure.

Management

Acute heart failure management focused on the strategies listed in the previous section should be employed. Treatment goals focus on optimizing preload, reducing systemic vascular resistance, reducing myocardial oxygen consumption, and establishing myocardial synchrony. Despite these medical interventions, a patient with heart failure who cannot be weaned from mechanical ventilation and/or multiple inotropes should be considered for mechanical cardiac support.

Brief Overview of Pediatric-Specific Devices

A left ventricular assist device (LVAD) is a pump connecting the left ventricle to the aorta. It helps to unload the ventricle and provide adequate cardiac output for tissue perfusion by drawing blood from the heart chamber, most commonly the left ventricle, running it through the pump and ejecting it into the aorta.

Since their first use in the 1960s and 1970s, there has been tremendous growth and sophistication in VAD technology. Today, ventricular assist devices are used in different capacities in children with heart failure. They could be used as a bridge to transplant when there is not much hope for cardiac recovery or bridge to recovery in situations where the cardiac function is likely to recover. They can also be used as a bridge to decision when it is unclear if the patient is a suitable candidate for heart transplant or a long-term VAD. Commonly in adults and increasingly in pediatrics, VADs are also being used as destination therapy (DT) with no plans to bridge it to transplant. This option is reserved for patients who are not suitable candidates for heart transplant due to other major comorbidities.

VADs can be classified into different categories based on their mechanism of action or duration of use. Based on the type of flow that they generate, they can be divided into pulsatile and continuous-flow devices. Table 12.1 outlines the different types and characteristics of pediatric VADs. Berlin Heart EXCOR is an example of a pulsatile device (Fig. 12.2a). Continuous-flow pumps generate a flat, non-pulsatile

Table 12.1 Features of commonly used ventricular assist devices in children

Name	Location/route of insertion	Type of flow/ mechanism	FDA approval/size range	Max flow
Berlin heart EXCOR (berlin heart GmbH)	Paracorporeal/ sternotomy	Pulsatile/ pneumatic	Approved for use in pediatrics	10–60 mL stroke volume
HeartMate II (Thoratec Corp)	Intracorporeal/ sternotomy	Continuous flow/axial	Approved for BTT, DT/ BSA > = 1.3, >45 kg	10 L/min
HeartWare (Medtronic)	Intracorporeal/ sternotomy	Continuous flow/ centrifugal	Approved for BTT	10 L/min
PediMag (Thoratec Corp)	Paracorporeal/ sternotomy	Non-pulsatile/ centrifugal	CE mark approved for short-term use	0.4–1.7 L/ min
Rotaflow (MAQUET)	Sternotomy	Pulsatile/ pneumatic	CE certificate	9.9 L/min
Thoratec PVAD (Thoratec Corp.)	Sternotomy/intra- or paracorporeal	Pulsatile/ pneumatic	Approved for BTT and postcardiotomy recovery from open heart surgery and home discharge	6.5 L/min
Impella 2.5, 5.0 (Abiomed)	Intracorporeal/ percutaneous-femoral access	Non-pulsatile/ microaxial	Approved for short-term support up to 6 h Smallest size – 12 F	2.5–5 L/ min
Intra-aortic balloon pump (MAQUET)	Extracorporeal/ percutaneous-femoral access	Pulsatile/ pneumatic	2.5 to 50 mL balloon sizes/4.5 to 7.5 F catheters	+0.5 L/ min
TandemHeart (Kardia)	Extracorporeal/ percutaneous-femoral access *or* transthoracic	Continuous, centrifugal	Few hours up to 14 days of support, 21 F transseptal cannula	8 L/min
Total artificial heart (SynCardia)	Intracorporeal/ sternotomy	Pulsatile/ pneumatic	70 cc – Approved for BTT and humanitarian status for DT Sizes – 50, 70 cc BSA >1.2	9.5 L/min

BTT bridge to transplant, *DT* destination therapy, *BSA* body surface area, *F* French

flow and can be further divided into axial flow or centrifugal flow devices. HeartMate II is an axial flow device (Fig. 12.2b), whereas the HeartWare (Fig. 12.2c) and HeartMate III devices are centrifugal flow pumps.

Temporary VADs: Temporary devices are preferred when the underlying etiology of heart failure is believed to be reversible like viral myocarditis. Additionally, if the patient is too critical to undergo the major surgery that would be required to implant a long-term device or if it is not known whether the patient is a suitable candidate for a long-term device, it may be advisable to implant a temporary device first and then plan for the long-term device or use the temporary device as a bridge to a decision. ECMO is most widely used for temporary mechanical support due to the ease of peripheral cannulation and avoiding the need for a sternotomy. However,

a

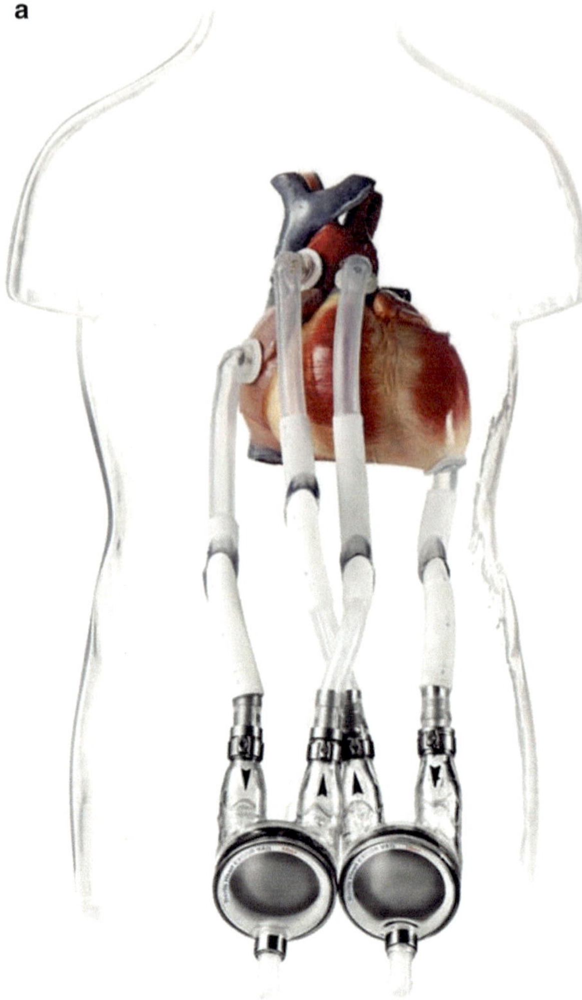

Fig. 12.2 (**a**) Berlin Heart EXCOR. (**b**) HeartMate II https://commons.wikimedia.org/wiki/File%3AVad_heartmateii.jpg public domain. (**c**) HeartWare. Reproduced with permission from Medtronic, Inc

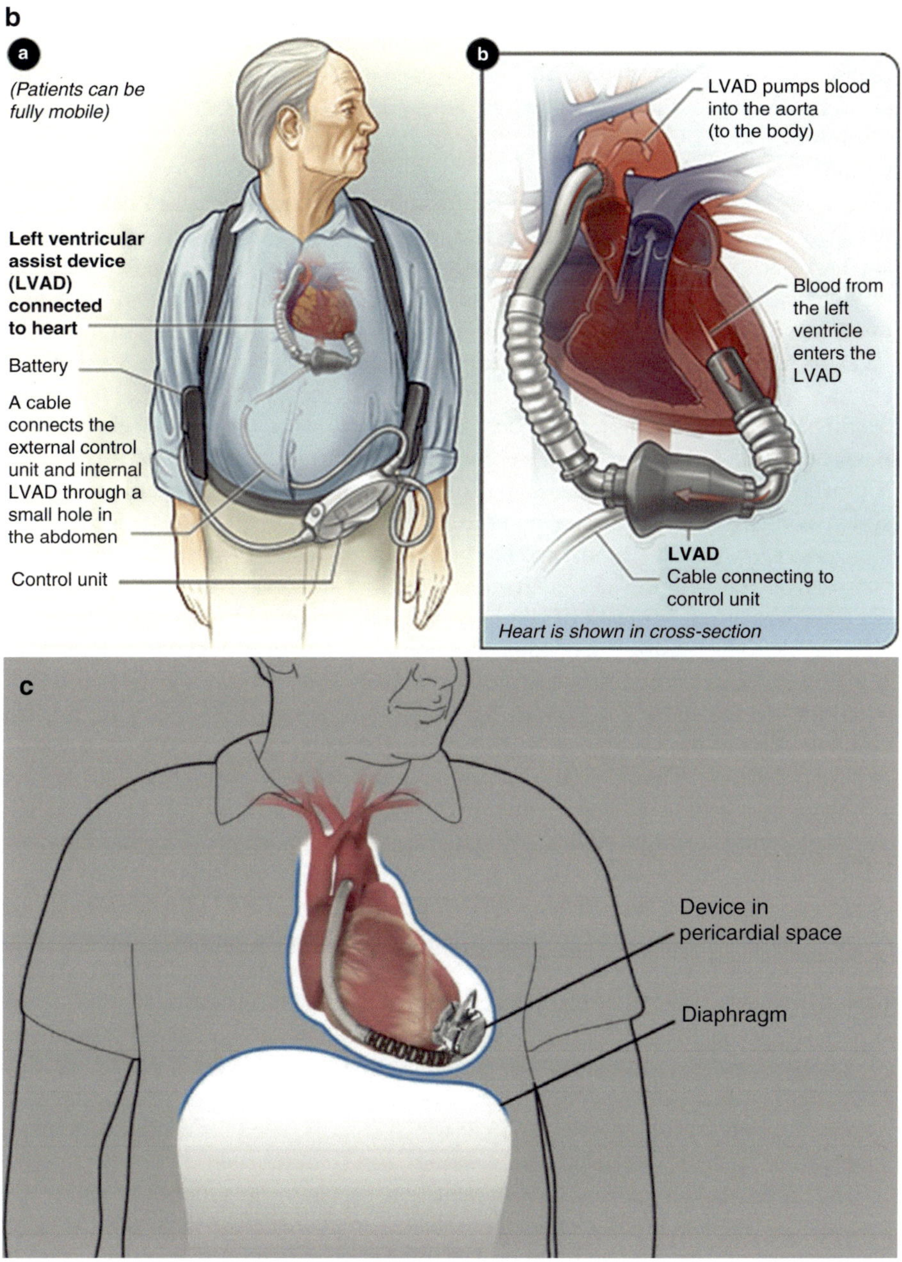

Fig. 12.2 (continued)

a ventricular assist device is better able to decompress a failing ventricle and thereby may facilitate recovery of function in certain reversible causes of dysfunction. Examples of temporary devices that can be used in children are CentriMag/PediMag (Thoratec Corp., Pleasanton, CA) (Fig. 12.3a) and Rotaflow (MAQUET Cardiovascular LLC, Wayne, NJ) that are both centrifugal flow, extracorporeal (pump is outside the body) devices. Percutaneously placed devices, like Impella (Fig. 12.3c), are commonly used in adults with acute decompensated heart failure, but their use in children is limited. The main limitation of this device is that the smallest size available is 12 F which cannot be used in small children. Other temporary devices like intra-aortic balloon pump and TandemHeart are also used mainly in adults and occasionally in older children (Fig. 12.3b, d).

Durable devices: In chronic heart failure, the chances of recovery of LV function are low as in the patient described in the vignette. In these circumstances, the patient would benefit from a long-term device. In smaller children, the VAD of choice is the Berlin Heart EXCOR. At present, Berlin Heart EXCOR is the only device that is FDA approved for use in children. It is a paracorporeal air-driven (pneumatic) pump. This system contains several different pump sizes (10, 15, 25, 30, 50, and 60 mL) and cannula sizes (5, 6, 9, and 12 mm) and has been used in infants as small as 3 kg. A large prospective trial with this device demonstrated that survival at 12 months was 75%, but there was also a 33% risk of neurological complications like stroke and bleeding. This has led to increasing use of adult continuous-flow devices in children. HeartMate II and HeartWare are currently the most commonly used devices. HeartMate II is an axial flow device and a good option for an adolescent with a BSA of $\geq$1.3 m^2. The pump housing of the HeartMate II is placed in the abdomen. HeartWare is a smaller device and therefore has a wider application in the pediatric population, having been implanted in a 4-year-old child with a BSA of 0.65 m^2. HeartWare is a magnetically levitated, centrifugal flow device. Its pump housing is located in the pericardial space adjacent to the cardiac apex. These durable devices allow patients to be discharged home and managed as outpatients, unlike the Berlin Heart EXCOR where the patient needs to stay in the hospital for the duration of pump use. In certain situations where the traditional left ventricular assist devices may not be applicable, the total artificial heart (SynCardia, Fig. 12.4) has been used by select centers. These situations include certain congenital heart defects where the left ventricular configuration is not amenable to traditional devices, restrictive cardiomyopathy, and severe biventricular dysfunction. The total artificial heart can also be used in situations of chronic graft dysfunction after heart transplantation in which case the need for continued immune suppression, with its associated complications, can be eliminated.

The international registry for patients on mechanical support is called the Interagency Registry for Mechanically Assisted Circulatory Support (INTERMACS). This registry was created with the goal of improving patient selection, with the ultimate goal of improving outcomes with the use of mechanical assist devices. Seven INTERMACS profiles are described that help choose the appropriate candidate and optimal timing for VAD implantation as shown in Table 12.2. Patients with profiles

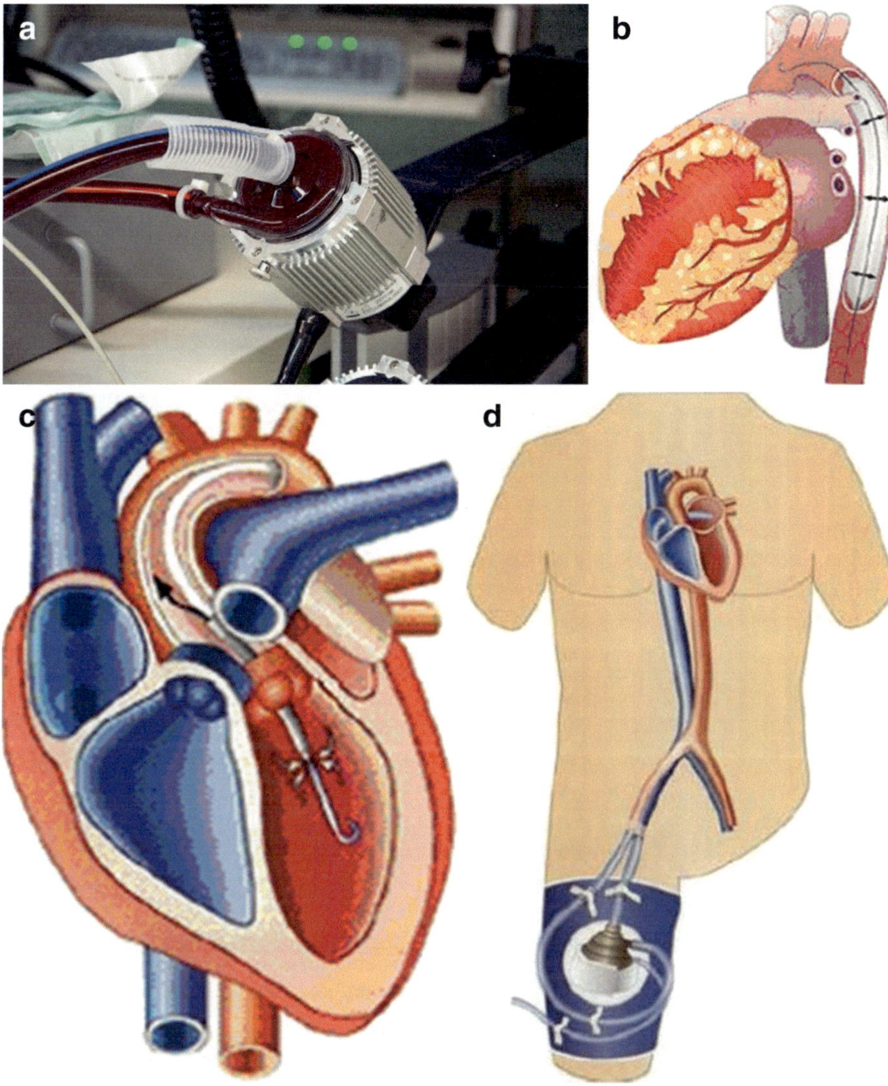

Fig. 12.3 (**a**) PediMag/CentriMag Image retrieved 30 April 2017 from https://www.flickr.com/photos/ec-jpr/9243359624/in/photolist-f5NCMo-f5NDAL Commons License associated: https://creativecommons.org/licenses/by-nc-nd/2. (**b**) Intra-aortic balloon pump. Image retrieved 30 April 2017 from https://www.flickr.com/photos/libertasacademica/16443744239. Commons License associated: https://creativecommons.org/licenses/by-nc-nd/2. (**c**) Impella. Image retrieved 30 April 2017 from https://www.flickr.com/photos/libertasacademica/16443744239. Commons License associated: https://creativecommons.org/licenses/by-nc-nd/2. (**d**) TandemHeart. Image retrieved 30 April 2017 from https://www.flickr.com/photos/libertasacademica/16443744239. Commons License associated: https://creativecommons.org/licenses/by-nc-nd/2

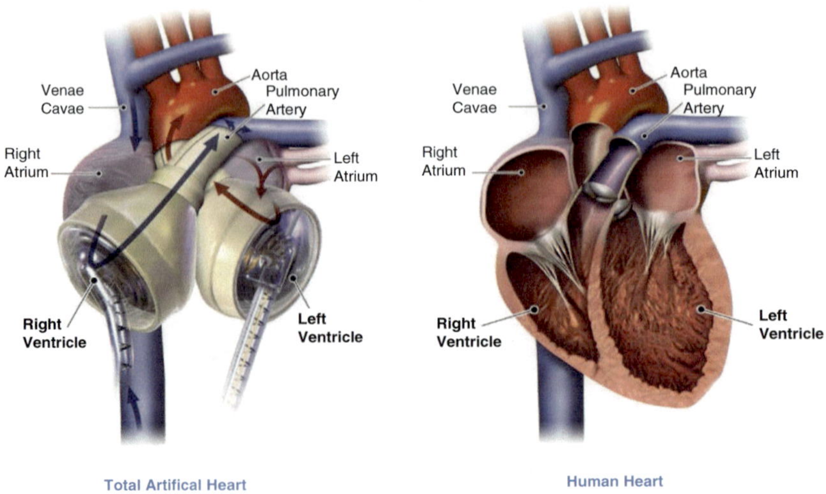

Fig. 12.4 Total artificial heart. Image retrieved 30 April 2017 from https://commons.wikimedia.org/wiki/File:Graphic_of_the_SynCardia_temporary_Total_Artificial_Heart_beside_a_human_heart.jpg. Commons License associated: http://creativecommons.org/licenses/by-sa/3.0)

Table 12.2 INTERMACS profiles

Profiles	Brief Description	Details
INTERMACS 1	Critical cardiogenic shock (crash and burn)	Life-threatening hypotension despite rapidly escalating inotropic support
INTERMACS 2	Progressive decline (sliding fast on inotropes)	Declining function despite intravenous inotropic support
INTERMACS 3	Stable but inotrope dependent (dependent stability)	Stable on continuous intravenous inotropic support
INTERMACS 4	Resting symptoms on oral therapy at home	Patient experience daily symptoms of congestion at rest or during activities of daily living
INTERMACS 5	Exertion intolerant	Patient is comfortable at rest and with activities of daily living but unable to engage in any other activity
INTERMACS 6	Exertion limited (walking wounded)	Patient has fatigue after the first few minutes of meaningful activity
INTERMACS 7	Advanced NYHA class III (placeholder)	Patient living comfortably with meaningful activity limited to mild physical exertion

4–7 are believed to be better surgical candidates than profiles 1 through 3. Patients in INTERMACS profile 1–3 may benefit from a temporary device prior to implanting a long-term durable device.

Select Patient Populations

Ventricular assist device implantation in patients with congenital heart disease is challenging. Anatomic limitations in patients such as missing the left ventricle in patients with hypoplastic left heart syndrome, prior surgeries, and different pathophysiology of heart failure are some of the reasons. Berlin Heart EXCOR has been used in children with single ventricles, but the outcomes are poorer than in children with two ventricles (42% successfully bridged to transplant compared to 73% with two ventricles). Although the success rate of VAD use in single ventricles is lower than in two-ventricle anatomy, it is better than ECMO support in these patients as bridge to transplant.

Complications

The major adverse effects common to all ventricular assist devices are bleeding, stroke, device thrombosis, and infection. Nearly one-third of the patients supported with the Berlin Heart EXCOR suffer neurological complications. Bleeding, device thrombosis, stokes, and driveline infections are complications sometimes seen in HeartMate II and HeartWare. According to data from the PediMACS registry (Pediatric INTERMACS), the most frequent adverse events in children on VADs (both pulsatile and continuous-flow devices) are device malfunction, infection, neurological dysfunction, and bleeding. Most events occur in the first 30 days after implantation.

Outcomes

Since the wait times for pediatric transplants often exceed the time that patients can be supported successfully with ECMO, the use of durable left ventricular assist devices is increasing in pediatric end-stage heart failure prior to transplant. Older children and adolescents with dilated cardiomyopathy are successfully bridged to transplant in 80% of the cases. As compared to patients bridged to transplant by ECMO, there is higher success rate when patients are bridged using a ventricular assist device.

A large prospective trial with Berlin Heart EXCOR demonstrated that survival at 12 months was 75%, including 64% who reached transplantation, 6% who recovered, and 5% who were alive on the device. Thirty percent of the patient cohort in this study had congenital heart disease.

According to the PediMACS report, 99 of the 2375 children undergoing heart transplantation between 1993 and 2003 were bridged with a VAD. The median age at VAD implantation was 13.3 years (range, 2 days to 17.9 years). Most patients in this cohort had DCM (78%); 22% had congenital heart disease. The mean duration of support was 57 days (range, 1 to 465 days). Seventy-seven percent survived the transplantation, 5 patients were successfully weaned from support and recovered, and 17 (17%) died on support. In the recent era (2000–2003), successful bridge to transplantation with a VAD was achieved in 86% of the patients. Another report describing the use of Berlin Heart EXCOR in younger children demonstrated successful bridge to transplant in 70% of the children and bridge to recovery in 7%. The median age of the cohort in this study was 2.1 years.

The use of durable VADs has improved the quality of life of children with end-stage heart failure as they can be discharged and return to school while awaiting heart transplant. However, successful use of these devices in the community requires educating not only the families but also the schools and local medical centers so that they can manage routine care as well as emergencies that can arise.

Clinical Pearls

- Mechanical circulatory support should be considered for children with acute heart failure refractory to medical management.
- The management of acute heart failure should be focused on optimizing preload, reducing systemic vascular resistance, reducing myocardial oxygen consumption, maintaining myocardial synchrony, and unloading the heart.
- ECMO is the preferred modality for inhospital pediatric cardiac arrest (not responsive to CPR) and should be considered for children with heart disease that is likely reversible or amenable to heart transplant.
- The Interagency Registry for Mechanically Assisted Circulatory Support (INTERMACS) helps aid clinicians in choosing appropriate candidates and optimal timing for VAD implantation.
- Complications of mechanical circulatory support devices include bleeding, infection, device thrombosis, and neurologic injury.

Board Exam Questions

1. A 15-year-old boy presents with shortness of breath, fatigue, and decreased exercise tolerance. He has no past medical history but did have a cold 1 week ago. Vital signs show a heart rate of 130 beats per minute, a respiratory rate of 40 breaths per minute, and a temperature of 38.1 °C. On physical examination, he has an S3 gallop and cool extremities with delayed capillary refill. Lung examination reveals crackles in the bases bilaterally. On abdominal examination, he has hepatomegaly with the liver palpable 4 cm below the costal margin. Which of the following is this child's chest radiograph most likely to show?
   (A) Massive cardiomegaly with pneumothorax
   (B) **Mild cardiomegaly with pulmonary edema**
   (C) Moderate cardiomegaly with right middle lobe pneumonia and parapneumonic effusion
   (D) Narrow cardiac silhouette with hyperinflated lungs

2. The same boy, as described in Question 1, develops ventricular ectopic beats. This child has an electrocardiogram showing nonspecific ST-segment changes. These findings are most likely due to:
   (A) Direct antibodies affecting the cardiac conduction system
   (B) Tumor infiltration in the myocardium
   (C) Pericardial inflammation
   (D) **Myocyte inflammation**
3. Initial management of this same child, described in Question 1, should focus on:
   (A) **Removing the offending agent, supportive care with attempts to improve preload, contractility, and decrease afterload**
   (B) Antibiotic therapy and mechanical ventilatory support
   (C) Initiation of ECMO
   (D) Implantation of a VAD
4. An 8-year-old girl with dilated cardiomyopathy presents to the ED after failing outpatient therapy for congestive heart failure. She is intubated and started on inotropic support in the intensive care unit. Although she remains normotensive, she still shows signs of poor perfusion despite mechanical ventilation and three inotropes. The next step in her management should include?
   (A) Initiation of ECPR
   (B) Treatment with intravenous immunoglobulin
   (C) Treatment for Pompe disease
   (D) **Consideration of VAD implantation**

Conflicts of Interest *Disclosures*: The authors have not disclosed any potential conflicts of interest.

Selected Reading

1. de Caen AR, Maconochie IK, Aickin R, et al. Part 6: pediatric basic life support and pediatric advanced life support: 2015 international consensus on cardiopulmonary resuscitation and emergency cardiovascular care science with treatment recommendations. Circulation. 2015;132(16 Suppl 1):S177–203.
2. Bergmann KR, Kharbanda A, Haveman L. Myocarditis and pericarditis in the pediatric patient: validated management strategies. Pediatr Emerg Med Pract. 2015;12(7):1–22.
3. Bizzarro MJ, Conrad SA, Kaufman DA, Rycus P. Infections acquired during extracorporeal membrane oxygenation in neonates, children, and adults. Pediatr Crit Care Med. 2011;12(3):277–81.
4. Polito A, Barrett CS, Wypij D, et al. Neurologic complications in neonates supported with extracorporeal membrane oxygenation. An analysis of ELSO registry data. Intensive Care Med. 2013;39(9):1594–601.
5. ELSO. Registry of the extracorporeal life support organization. Ann Arbor, MI: ELSO; 2017. http://www.elsonet.org. Accessed 25 Apr 2017.
6. Towbin JA, Lowe AM, Colan SD, Sleeper LA, Orav EJ, Clunie S, Messere J, Cox GF, Lurie PR, Hsu D, Canter C, Wilkinson JD, Lipshultz SE. Incidence, causes, and outcomes of dilated cardiomyopathy in children. JAMA. 2006;296(15):1867–76.

7. Adachi I, Burki S, Zafar F, Morales DL. Pediatric ventricular assist devices. J Thorac Dis. 2015;7(12):2194–202.
8. Fuchs A, Netz H. Ventricular assist devices in pediatrics. Images Pediatr Cardiol. 2001;3(4):24–54.
9. Almond CS, Morales DL, Blackstone EH, et al. Berlin Heart EXCOR pediatric ventricular assist device for bridge to heart transplantation in US children. Circulation. 2013;127(16):1702–11.
10. Stevenson LW, Pagani FD, Young JB, Jessup M, Miller L, Kormos RL, et al. INTERMACS profiles of advanced heart failure: the current picture. J Heart Lung Transplant. 2009;28:535–41.
11. Rosenthal DN, Almond CS, Jaquiss RD, et al. Adverse events in children implanted with ventricular assist devices in the United States: data from the Pediatric Interagency Registry for Mechanical Circulatory Support (PediMACS). J Heart Lung Transplant. 2016;35(5):569–77.

13 Recognition, Stabilization, and Management of Children with Pulmonary Hypertension in the Emergency Department

Robert D. Ross and Patrick Hines

Introduction

Pulmonary hypertension (PH) is an uncommon but potentially life-threatening condition in children, and improved survival makes it more likely that acute care practitioners will encounter children with PH. This is due in part to better outcomes of extremely preterm infants who develop PH from chronic lung disease and children with congenital heart and lung defects who survive surgery but have residual PH, increased diagnosis of PH due to expanded screening indications, and better diagnostic modalities. The goal of this chapter is to provide an overview of the types of pediatric PH likely to be encountered in the acute care setting and discuss the recognition and initial management of this disease. Specific clinical cases will be presented to illustrate various pulmonary hypertensive emergencies in the five categories of PH as classified by the World Health Organization. These consist of (1) pulmonary arterial hypertension, (2) PH with left heart disease, (3) PH associated with lung diseases and/or hypoxemia, (4) PH due to chronic thrombotic and/or embolic disease, (5) and miscellaneous.

R. D. Ross, M.D. (✉)
Pediatrics, Division of Cardiology, Children's Hospital of Michigan and Wayne State University School of Medicine, Detroit, MI, USA
e-mail: rross@dmc.org

P. Hines, M.D., Ph.D.
Division of Critical Care Medicine, Children's Hospital of Michigan, Wayne State University School of Medicine, Detroit, MI, USA
e-mail: phines@med.wayne.edu

© Springer International Publishing AG, part of Springer Nature 2018

A. P. Sarnaik et al. (eds.), *Cardiac Emergencies in Children*,
https://doi.org/10.1007/978-3-319-73754-6_13

Case 1

A 3-month-old infant presents with tachypnea and poor feeding for the last week. The mother states that the baby has decreased her formula intake to 2 ounces per feed, which takes 40 min to get in. On examination, she is noted to have a respiratory rate of 65, a heart rate of 170, a grade 3/6 harsh holosystolic murmur at the lower left sternal border, and a grade 2 diastolic rumble at the apex. She has tachypnea and retractions with mildly reduced perfusion, and the liver edge is palpated 4 cm below the right costal margin.

What is the most likely etiology of this collection of signs and symptoms?

(a) RSV bronchiolitis
(b) Large ventricular septal defect
(c) *Staphylococcus aureus* sepsis
(d) Tetralogy of Fallot
(e) Aortic insufficiency

Pulmonary artery hypertension from congenital heart disease may present several weeks to months after birth since the pulmonary vascular resistance (PVR) is high at the time of delivery due to the lungs being filled with amniotic fluid in utero. Normally, this PVR decreases dramatically after birth as the lung fluid decreases and oxygen is introduced with the first breaths. PVR then decreases to normal adult levels usually by 6 months of age as the smooth muscle in the pulmonary arterioles resorbs. When there is a large intracardiac communication present such as a ventricular septal defect (VSD), this fall in pulmonary pressure and PVR does not occur as rapidly. Thus, early in life, the infants are typically asymptomatic, and no murmur or only a very soft systolic murmur is present as not much shunting occurs through the defect. Over the next few weeks, the PVR gradually decreases, and the left to right shunting through the VSD increases. This leads to progressive pulmonary overcirculation and fluid retention, which produces the symptoms described above. The infants breathe fast to compensate for reduced lung compliance, which leads to poor feeding and post-feeding emesis. With increased flow across the VSD, the systolic murmur becomes louder, and a diastolic murmur may appear from the excess flow across the mitral valve. Fluid backs up into the liver accounting for the hepatomegaly, and there is activation of the sympathetic nervous system causing the tachycardia [1]. If the pulmonary overcirculation is severe, there is a decrease in systemic output producing the reduced peripheral perfusion, which on occasion can present as a shock-like state.

Diagnostic Clues

A chest x-ray will reveal significant cardiomegaly and diffuse pulmonary congestion. The ECG typically shows left ventricular or biventricular hypertrophy. Echocardiography is diagnostic and will show the dilated left atrium and ventricle and the large VSD (Fig. 13.1). A large PDA can present the same way; however, the murmur would be continuous and is described as “machinery” in quality.

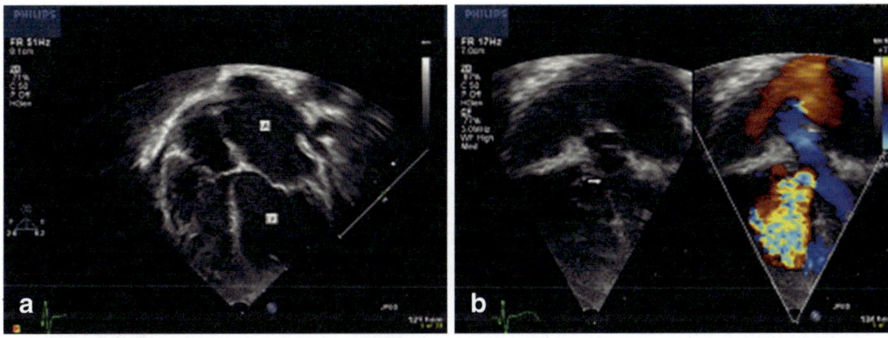

Fig. 13.1 (**a**) Apical four chamber view showing the dilated left atrium (LA) and left ventricle (LV). (**b**) Color comparison of apical five-chamber view showing a large ventricular septal defect (arrow) and the color flow from the LV to the right ventricle

Emergency Management Principles

Unlike other causes of near shock or shock in infants, large fluid boluses may be detrimental in those with large left to right shunts who are already fluid overloaded. They require a delicate balance of cautious intravenous fluid administration to maintain intravascular volume and aggressive diuresis to remove the extracellular fluid. If the echocardiogram shows any decrease in cardiac function, then low doses of intravenous inotrope administration are helpful acutely. These infants typically respond quickly to diuretics, most commonly intravenous furosemide (1 mg/kg/dose) which can be given two to three times a day and then changed to the oral form. Spironolactone is recommended to maintain electrolyte balance at a dose of 1 mg/kg/dose twice daily. Once the infant is stabilized, oral feeding can be resumed, and concentration of the formula is recommended to maximize the calories and minimize the water intake. Standard 20 cal/oz formulas can be concentrated gradually up to 24, 27, and even 30 cal/oz as long as no osmotic diarrhea occurs. In the most severe cases, the formula needs to be given through a nasal gavage tube, and if bolus feedings are not tolerated, then continuous low volumes can be delivered. As the metabolic demands are greater in pulmonary overcirculation, 140–150 kcals/kg/day may need to be given to achieve steady growth. If the infant continues to struggle despite these maneuvers, then surgical repair is indicated.

Correct answer: b-Large ventricular septal defect

Case 2

A 6-month-old is brought to the ED with 2 weeks of decreased feeding, increased post-feeding emesis, and increased work of breathing. The mother states that he had heart surgery just after birth for abnormally connected veins from the lungs. On examination, there is a well-healed median sternotomy scar with an active precordium and a right ventricular lift. The baby is afebrile but tachypneic, and there is a loud second heart sound with no murmur. The liver edge is palpated 6 cm below the right costal margin. Oxygen saturation is 96%.

What is the most likely etiology of this collection of signs and symptoms?

(a) Pyloric stenosis
(b) Pneumonia
(c) Post-pericardiotomy syndrome
(d) Idiopathic pulmonary arterial hypertension
(e) Obstructed pulmonary venous return

A loud pulmonic component of the second heart sound is an important diagnostic clue to the presence of pulmonary hypertension, as a high diastolic pulmonary pressure will force the pulmonary valve shut with greater intensity. Pulmonary vein stenosis is an example of obstruction to blood flow returning to the left atrium and acts like obstruction in the left heart at other levels including cor triatriatum, mitral stenosis, and aortic stenosis. Isolated pulmonary vein stenosis is a rare cause of such obstruction but can occur in up to 11% of children who have undergone repair of total anomalous pulmonary venous return [2]. This leads to transmission of back pressure into the pulmonary arteries and progressive lung and hepatic congestion, poor feeding and growth, and heart failure.

It is important to auscultate the second heart sound and become familiar with the normal sound intensity so that when the sound is increased, it will be recognized and the patient evaluated for PH. The other forms of left heart obstruction should be accompanied by a heart murmur, systolic ejection in the case of aortic outflow obstruction, and a diastolic inflow murmur for cor triatriatum or mitral stenosis. Many of these lesions are amenable to surgery or catheter-based intervention; however, pulmonary vein stenosis may be due to a progressive, fibrosing, endothelial proliferation that can be resistant to such treatments.

Diagnostic Clues

A chest x-ray will reveal diffuse pulmonary venous congestion. The ECG will have large R waves in lead V1 and/or large S waves in leads V5-6 indicating right ventricular hypertrophy (Fig. 13.2). Echocardiography is important to evaluate the surgical repair, quantify the right ventricular size and function, and estimate the pulmonary pressures. Often a cardiac catheterization is required to evaluate the extent of stenosis in the pulmonary veins, and if two or more are affected, there is a poor prognosis [3].

Emergency Management Principles

Young children with left heart obstruction often present with respiratory or gastrointestinal (GI) symptoms that can mimic pneumonia, bronchiolitis, asthma, or GI

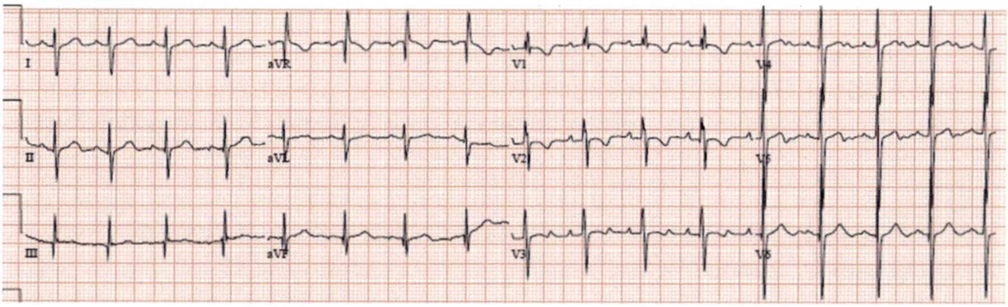

Fig. 13.2 ECG showing right axis deviation and right ventricular hypertrophy with an "rSR" in lead V1 and deep S waves in V5.6

obstruction. If they are critically ill, basic resuscitative efforts should be performed for stabilization and restoration of circulation. Those who are less sick on presentation should be given intravenous diuretics and oxygen while cardiology consultation is obtained. Fluid overload should be avoided, and evaluation for infection should be undertaken. Frank heart failure is often brought on by an acute infection in the face of previous cardiac compensation for the obstruction with myocardial hypertrophy to maintain cardiac output.

Correct answer: e-Obstructed pulmonary venous return

Case 3

A 9-month-old is brought in by ambulance after being found by her mother in bed unresponsive and blue in appearance. She performed CPR and called 911. History reveals a preterm birth at 24 weeks' gestation with a prolonged NICU stay and severe bronchopulmonary dysplasia (BPD) requiring tracheotomy and home ventilation. Home medications include diuretics, sildenafil, albuterol, and Pulmicort inhalers. Examination shows a heart rate of 135, respiratory rate of 45 (above the set ventilator rate), blood pressure of 70/30, oxygen saturation of 75%, harsh and course breath sounds throughout, and a loud second heart sound with a capillary refill of 3–4 s. An NT-proBNP is 4400 pg/mL.

What is the most likely etiology of this collection of signs and symptoms?

(a) TET (hypercyanotic) spell
(b) Ventricular tachycardia
(c) Pulmonary hypertensive crisis
(d) Tracheal tube obstruction
(e) Aspiration pneumonia

A common complication of severe BPD is pulmonary hypertension, which in the revised WHO classification of PH is class 3, "associated with lung diseases and/or hypoxemia" [4]. The presence of PH in children with BPD puts them at risk for significant morbidity and a mortality with independent risk factors for death being severe PH at systemic or suprasystemic levels and small for gestational age status with a birth weight less than the third percentile for gestational age [5]. The presence of a patent foramen ovale or patent ductus arteriosus provides a communication for mixing of saturated and unsaturated blood, and any stimulus which acutely increases the pulmonary vascular resistance will cause more right to left shunting and desaturation. This may herald a pulmonary hypertensive crisis with progressive hypoxemia, which may escalate to decreased cardiac output, bradycardia, hypotension, and cardiac arrest.

Diagnostic Clues

An arterial blood gas will show a low-oxygen level and CO2 retention, some of which may be chronic. In a crisis, metabolic acidosis may be present as well. The chest x-ray will show the chronic lung disease of BPD (Fig. 13.3) but may also show a new pneumonia, atelectasis, or pleural effusion that has tipped the patient into a PH crisis. Other studies (ECG, echo, MRI, cardiac catheterization) may be useful after the patient has been stabilized in the ICU setting.

Emergency Management Principles

Emergency interventions include 100% oxygen delivery, sedation, suctioning to clear the airways of any mucous plugging, and transient hyperventilation. The addition of inhaled nitric oxide at a dose of 20 ppm can produce effective pulmonary vasodilation and reverse such a crisis allowing for transfer to an intensive care setting for further management [6].

Correct answer: c-Pulmonary hypertensive crisis

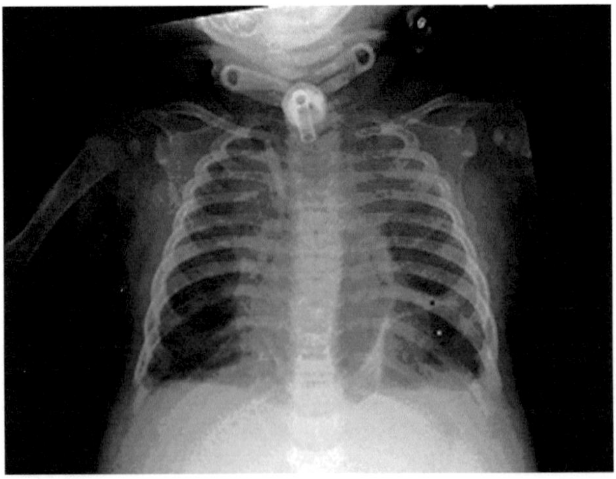

Fig. 13.3 CXR showing the tracheostomy tube, chronic lung changes of BPD, with atelectasis and hyperinflation

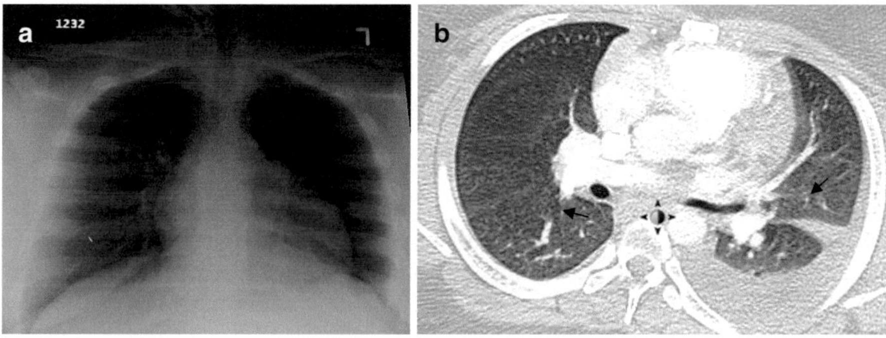

Fig. 13.4 (**a**) Chest x-ray shows small airway disease, with bilateral perihilar patchy opacities. (**b**) Axial CT with contrast of the chest showed multiple bilateral subsegmental filling defects (arrows) within the pulmonary arteries, including the right and left upper lobes. A pleural effusion is present on the left

Case 4

A 15-year-old morbidly obese female with a history of stage V lupus nephritis and hypertension presents to the emergency department with a chief complaint of fever and difficulty breathing. She began having pain in her left shoulder 1 week ago. On presentation, she complained of chest pain and "heavier than normal" breathing, preceded by 2 weeks of upper respiratory infection symptoms and a lingering dry cough. She had a T_{max} of 100.7 °F on the day of presentation. She also reports a migraine headache with vomiting 4 days ago. She is currently taking hydroxychloroquine, mycophenolate, prednisone, lisinopril, and nifedipine. On physical exam, breath sounds are clear and equal bilaterally, and respirations are non-labored. There is a regular rhythm, no murmurs or gallop is present, and the pulses are equal in all extremities with normal peripheral perfusion. The left thigh is markedly swollen compared to the right with no tenderness on palpation, but stretching of the left leg does cause pain.

Vital signs: BP 148/88, heart rate 92, respiratory rate 25, temperature 37.4 °C, and oxygen saturation 92% on room air.

Laboratory evaluation: Electrolyte panel normal, WBC $5.0 \times 10^3/\mu L$, hematocrit 32.5%, platelets $218 \times 10^3/\mu L$, PT 9.4, INR 0.89, aPTT 25.4, D-dimer 139.2, fibrinogen 610, negative viral respiratory panel, pregnancy screen negative.

Chest x-ray and chest CT with contrast (see Fig. 13.4).

What is the most likely etiology for this child's symptoms?

(a) Pulmonary embolism
(b) Pneumonia
(c) Myocardial infarction
(d) Lung abscess
(e) Anxiety

Clinical Presentation

Chronic thromboembolic pulmonary hypertension (CTEPH) is a specific subclass of pulmonary hypertension that represents the cumulative effect of acute pulmonary emboli (PE) that have not completely resolved. Each unresolved embolus eventually organizes into fibrotic material that occludes the proximal large-caliber pulmonary arteries and causes microvascular dysfunction in more distal small-caliber pulmonary arteries that remain patent [7]. Most of our understanding about the clinical presentation, therapy, and prognosis of CTEPH comes from large adult studies since there are no large studies of pediatric CTEPH to date. However, venous thromboembolism has become a more frequent diagnosis in the pediatric patient population [8]; thus, CTEPH should be an important diagnostic consideration in symptomatic children with a known hypercoagulable state, a history of thromboembolism or venous catheter placement, and/or a diagnosis of pulmonary hypertension [7, 9]. In the largest pediatric CTEPH cohort studied to date, the most common presenting symptom was exertional dyspnea and/or exercise intolerance (94%), followed by syncope or presyncope (47%), chest pain (35%), cough (29%), cyanosis (18%), edema (12%), and hemoptysis (12%) [10]. Only 35% of patients had a recognized history of a prior PE at the time of diagnosis, and up to 42% had a history or ultrasound findings consistent with a diagnosis of deep venous thrombosis. Idiopathic pulmonary arterial hypertension was the initial diagnosis in 29%. A few patients were initially diagnosed with atypical pneumonia ($n = 3$) or asthma ($n = 2$) [10].

Diagnostic Clues

It is critical to have a high index of suspicion for CTEPH in any child with risk factors for thromboembolic disease in the acute care setting. Timely initiation of definitive surgical or medical therapy can treat the underlying pathology and potentially be lifesaving. The simplest way to think about CTEPH risk is the time-honored Virchow's triad: Hypercoagulable state—endothelial injury–stasis of flow (Fig. 13.5).

A preexisting hypercoagulable state is the most commonly diagnosed risk factor for CTEPH in children. A recent study showed that over 70% of pediatric CTEPH cases necessitating pulmonary thromboendarterectomy also had an identifiable thrombophilic state such as lupus anticoagulant (30%), anticardiolipin antibody (24%), and protein C deficiency (18%) [10]. Over 30% of patients had a positive family history of thromboembolism and/or hypercoagulable state. While these numbers are not necessarily generalizable to other acute care settings, they do illustrate the importance of immediate pediatric hematology consultation to ensure the proper laboratory studies are obtained for diagnosis and that the patient receives the proper long-term follow-up upon discharge. It is also important to recognize the use

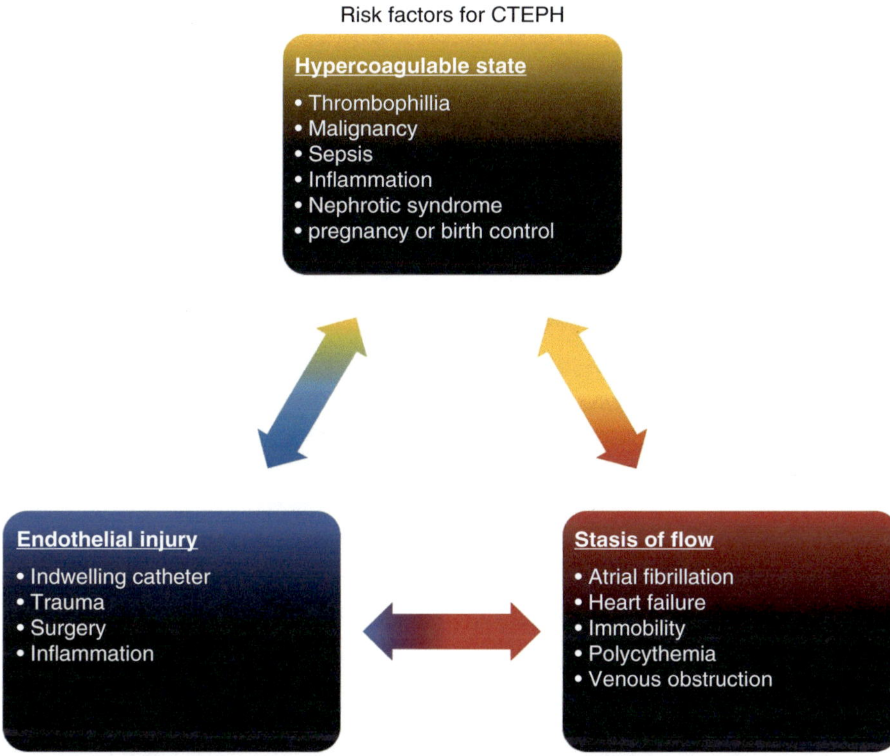

Fig. 13.5 Risk factors for chronic thromboembolic pulmonary hypertension

of oral contraceptives and pregnancy as risk factors for thrombotic disease, even in the pediatric population.

It is important to obtain a thorough history and physical exam to assess for obesity, sedentary habits, and injury-induced immobilization [10, 11] and history of cardiac disease/arrhythmias or signs/symptoms of cardiac dysfunction to assess for risk of blood flow stasis. Polycythemia, a commonly missed risk factor for venous stasis, causes increased blood viscosity and margination of platelets to the endothelial surface—further increasing the risk of thrombosis [12]. Polycythemia is common in the context of cyanotic congenital heart disease or chronic lung disease. Recent studies have cautioned against aggressive blood transfusions to achieve an arbitrary hematocrit in the absence of objective evidence of inadequate oxygen delivery [13–18]; thus, clinicians should avoid supraphysiologic hematocrit levels in the acute management of patients at risk for CTEPH.

Imaging to diagnose pulmonary thromboembolic disease and pulmonary veno-occlusive disease (PVOD) should be performed at the time of diagnosis (*class 1, Level of Evidence B*). Computed tomography pulmonary angiography (CTPA) is the most well-validated imaging modality for the diagnosis of pulmonary embolism [19, 20].

Emergency Management Principles

Once the clinician has recognized that CTEPH is the probable etiology for the child's acute presentation, stabilization and definitive surgical or medical therapy should be initiated as soon as possible and in parallel. Stabilization involves the basic ABCs of the PALS algorithm in the acute setting.

- *Airway patency*:
  - Hemoptysis:
    If severe, secure airway, isolate bleeding source (respiratory vs. GI), ventilate with high mean airway pressure to tamponade lower airway breathing, and administer appropriate blood products.
  - Loss of consciousness:
    Secure airway, determine etiology (history, examination, imaging), and treat.
  - Space-occupying tumor of the neck or mediastinum:
    Ensure anesthesia or advanced airway team available before attempting to secure airway.
- *Breathing*:
  - Infection (bacterial or viral pneumonia):
    CXR, antimicrobials, cultures, and respiratory support as needed
  - Hemoptysis-induced pneumonitis:
    See *airway*
  - Pulmonary edema:
    Deliver supplemental O_2 to maintain appropriate O_2 delivery and pulmonary vascular patency. Consider more invasive positive pressure delivery or nitric oxide in the context of persistent hypoxia.
  - Reactive airways disease/lower airway inflammation:
    Acute asthma management: Steroids
- *Circulation*:
  - Right ventricular dysfunction/cor pulmonale:
    Inotropic support for RV function and reduce RV afterload (see pulmonary vascular hypoperfusion)
  - Pulmonary vascular hypoperfusion:
    Correct hypoxia and hypercarbia, target neutral blood pH and nitric oxide, and consult cardiology for advanced PH therapy (sildenafil, bosentan, inhaled vs. IV prostacyclins).
  - Left ventricular failure:
    Echocardiogram to identify etiology (dilated, obstructive, tamponade, etc.). Treat underlying etiology (inotropes, diuresis, afterload reduction, drain effusion, etc.)
  - Sepsis:
    Antibiotics, intravascular volume expansion, and vasopressors
  - Dehydration:
    Identify source (GI loss, increased insensible loss, acute kidney injury, bleeding, etc.)
    Intravascular volume expansion

CTEPH is one of the few subclasses of pulmonary arterial hypertension that is potentially curable. Patients diagnosed with CTEPH should be rapidly transferred to a tertiary care center for consideration of surgical pulmonary thromboendarterectomy (PTE) or catheter-based removal or lysis of the acute and chronic thromboembolic material. PTE offers an effective treatment for this condition, significantly improving cardiopulmonary hemodynamics, gas exchange, functional status, and survival [7, 10]. Although there is controversy about many aspects of CTEPH management, it is generally accepted that PTE should be pursued if the patient is a candidate for the procedure.

Not all patients with CTEPH are surgical candidates, and there are emerging treatments—medical therapy and balloon pulmonary angioplasty—that have shown benefit in this patient population. In the acute setting, especially when the patient's candidacy for PTE is being evaluated, heparin is the anticoagulant of choice. Heparin can be titrated based on the individual institution's anticoagulation protocol, although a PTT range of 60–80 s is generally acceptable. Some institutions adjust heparin dose based on anti-Xa levels.

Recommendation from the American Heart Association and American Thoracic Society for management of pediatric pulmonary hypertension is to use warfarin for long-term anticoagulation. The guidelines state "Warfarin may be considered in patients with IPAH/HPAH, patients with low cardiac output, those with a long-term indwelling catheter, and those with hypercoagulable states (*Class IIb; Level of Evidence C*). Targeting the therapeutic range for an international normalized ratio (INR) between 1.5 and 2.0 is recommended for young children with PAH (*Class I; Level of Evidence C*). Anticoagulation beyond baby aspirin should not be used in young children with PAH because of concerns about harm from hemorrhagic complications (*Class III; Level of Evidence C*) [21]."

Without treatment, CTEPH can lead to progressive pulmonary vascular obstruction, right heart failure, and death. Thus, it is important for clinicians to recognize this subtype of PH.

Correct answer: a-Pulmonary embolism

Case 5

A 17-year-old boy with sickle cell disease presents to the emergency department with fatigue, tachypnea, chest pain, retractions, wheezing, hepatomegaly 3 cm below the costal margin, and pulse oximetry of 75%. He is afebrile and has a heart rate of 135, respiratory rate of 43, and BP of 110/72. Hemoglobin is 7.1 g/dL and reticulocytes 35%. Chest x-ray revealed clear lung fields and severe cardiomegaly. EKG showed biventricular hypertrophy. An echocardiogram showed mild bilateral, biventricular, and pulmonary artery dilation with an estimated right ventricular systolic pressure of 52 mmHg. Oxygen, red cell exchange transfusion, and bronchodilators were administered, and he continues to require 6 L oxygen via nasal cannula to maintain pulse oximetry >90%.

What mechanism of action best explains the presenting symptoms in this patient?

(a) Airway inflammation and bronchial smooth muscle constriction
(b) Fat emboli resulting from bone marrow infarction becoming lodged in the renal arteries
(c) Free hemoglobin scavenging endothelial nitric oxide, resulting in pulmonary vascular constriction
(d) Acute infarction of the left anterior descending coronary artery
(e) Referred pain from acute splenic infarction

Clinical Presentation

Sickle cell disease (SCD) is a monogenetic disease caused by a single point mutation in the gene for hemoglobin, resulting in a complex multimodal phenotype. Erythrocyte sickling in response to hypoxia and dehydration leads to hemolysis, highly adhesive erythrocytes, systemic inflammation, and baseline hypercoagulable state. All of these factors contribute to pulmonary vasculopathy and acute pulmonary vasoconstriction in patients with SCD.

Children with SCD most commonly present to the emergency setting with acute onset of vaso-occlusive pain requiring opiate analgesia for relief. It is important to remember that even in the case of isolated pain episodes, children with SCD can develop secondary pulmonary complications as a result of:

- Bone infarction ⇒ fat emboli ⇒ pulmonary artery embolus ⇒hypoxia
- Rib pain ⇒hypoventilation ⇒atelectasis ⇒ hypoxia and hypercarbia
- Opiate analgesia ⇒hypoventilation ⇒ hypoxia and hypercarbia

Both hypoxia and hypercarbia can predispose a child with SCD to acute chest syndrome and increased pulmonary vascular resistance in the acute setting.

Many children with SCD also present in a state of acute hemolysis, causing the release of cell-free hemoglobin in the plasma. Free hemoglobin can sequester endothelial nitric oxide, impairing the normal pulmonary artery vasoactive response [22]. Additionally, cell-free hemoglobin can also suppress arginase activity and initiate vascular inflammation through oxidant stress, all of which can further contribute to the acute impairment of normal pulmonary artery vasoactive functions [22]. This can all lead to refractory hypoxia and increase pulmonary arterial pressure.

Children presenting with acute chest syndrome are at very high risk for acute pulmonary hypertensive episodes. One study found that approximately 60% of adults presenting with severe acute chest syndrome have evidence of acute pulmonary hypertension on echocardiography, defined as a tricuspid regurgitant jet (TRJ) velocity > 2.5 m/s. Elevated TRJ velocity also positively correlated with B-type natriuretic peptide (rho = 0.54, $P < 0.01$) and cardiac troponin I (rho = 0.42, $P < 0.01$). Cor pulmonale occurred in 11 (13%) episodes [23].

Diagnogstic Clues

Mild steady-state pulmonary hypertension, with a TRV of 2.5 m/s or greater, is a major independent risk factor for death in adults with SCD [24]. It is important to remember that the relative anemia and hyperdynamic left ventricle characteristics of most individuals with SCD can lower the measured TRV. Moderate pulmonary artery pressure elevation may be poorly tolerated by patients with SCD, especially in the context of increased oxygen consumption (pain, increased work of breathing) and decreased oxygen delivery (acute on chronic anemia). These factors contribute to high risk of sudden death. Furthermore, acute pulmonary artery pressure elevation has been documented during vaso-occlusive pain crisis or exercise in patients with SCD [25]. While mild pulmonary hypertension is a risk factor for death in adults with sickle cell disease, this has not been proven in children. However, as acute PH has been reported during exercise and vaso-occlusive pain crisis in sickle cell patients [23], acute pulmonary hypertension should be suspected in any child with sickle cell disease presenting to the ED with difficulty breathing, chest pain, dyspnea on exertion, or any sign of low cardiac output.

The severity of anemia and the rate of hemolysis are risk factors for developing pulmonary hypertension in SCD [26]. Direct laboratory indicators of hemolysis include cell-free plasma hemoglobin and red blood cell microparticles, and indirect laboratory indicators include low plasma haptoglobin levels and elevated reticulocyte counts, bilirubin levels, RBC aspartate amino transferase, and lactate dehydrogenase enzymes [27]. Clinical manifestations of hemolysis—induced vascular disease in SCD—include low-oxygen saturations, pulmonary hypertension, increased systemic systolic artery pressures and pulse pressures, chronic kidney disease (proteinuria), cutaneous leg ulcerations, and stroke in children. In numerous clinical cohorts, the severity of both anemia and measured indexes of hemolytic rate is a risk factor for developing pulmonary hypertension in sickle cell patients [28–33]. Vaso-occlusive painful crisis and acute chest syndrome (ACS) are associated with higher steady-state free hemoglobin levels and high leukocyte counts [34].

Emergency Management Principles

Children with SCD who have symptoms suggestive of acute chest syndrome should be carefully managed given their unique risk for a vicious cycle of pulmonary arterial hypertension, hypoxia, and erythrocyte cycling. The following are the ABCs of emergency management:

1. *Airway patency*:
   (a) Opiate-induced loss of pharyngeal tone or preexisting obstructive sleep apnea:
      - Many patients require opiate analgesia to treat acute pain episodes.
      - Although opiate-induced hypoventilation is rare in SCD, impairment of ventilation and oxygenation can dramatically increase the risk of acute pulmonary hypertension in this population.

2. *Breathing*:
   (a) Pain-induced hypoventilation:
      - Treat pain aggressively.
      - Monitor response to opiate analgesia closely.
      - Administer supplemental oxygen to maintain $FiO_2 > 94\%$.
      - Obtain CXR if the patient requires supplemental O_2.
   (b) Opiate-induced hypoventilation:
      - Assist ventilation and administer supplemental O_2 to maintain $FiO_2 > 94\%$.
      - CXR to rule out acute chest syndrome or atelectasis.
      - Aggressively treat acute chest syndrome if suspected.
   (c) Reactive airways disease/lower airway inflammation:
      - Acute asthma management: Steroids.
      - Asthma is common in patients with SCD; wheezing in SCD can also be caused by pulmonary vascular disease or chronic lung disease.
3. *Circulation*:
   (a) Acute vaso-occlusive crises:
      - CBC, reticulocyte %, bilirubin, lactate dehydrogenase, and hemoglobin electrophoresis.
      - Simple or exchange transfusion for acute hemolysis.
      - Treat pain as needed (NSAIDs and opioids).
      - Encourage incentive spirometry while awake to reduce risk of ACS.
   (b) Acute chest syndrome:
      - CXR.
      - Treat pain as needed.
      - Supplemental O_2 to keep O_2 saturations >95%.
      - Intravenous cephalosporin and an oral macrolide antibiotic.
      - Urgent exchange transfusion in consultation with hematology, critical care, and/or apheresis subspecialists when there is rapid progression (O_2 saturation < 90% despite supplemental oxygen), respiratory distress, progressive pulmonary infiltrates on CXR, and/or decline in hemoglobin concentration despite simple transfusion
   (c) Pulmonary hypertension:
      - CXR (cardiomegaly, atelectasis, ACS)
      - EKG (right heart strain pattern)
      - Echo and cardiology consult:
         - Right heart catheterization may be useful if:
           TRJ >2.5 m/s and symptoms
           TRJ > 3.0
           No TRJ on echo to estimate pulmonary pressures
         - Consider PAH therapy for precapillary PH:
           mPAP >25 mmHg
           PAWP <15 mmHg
           PVR > 2 indexed Wood units or 160 dynes-s/cm^5
         - Outpatient evaluation when stable:
           Sleep study
           Lab evaluation: ANA, HIV, and LFTs

- Check NT-proBNP
- Supplemental O_2 for O_2 saturations <95%

Correct answer: **c**-Free hemoglobin scavenging endothelial nitric oxide, resulting in pulmonary vascular constriction

References

1. Ross RD, Daniels SR, Schwartz DC, Hannon DW, Shukla R, Kaplan S. Plasma norepinephrine levels in infants and children with congestive heart failure. Am J Cardiol. 1987;59(8):911–4.
2. Devaney EJ, Chang AC, Ohye RG, Bove EL. Management of congenital and acquired pulmonary vein stenosis. Ann Thorac Surg. 2006;81(3):992–5; discussion 995–996.
3. Gowda S, Bhat D, Feng Z, Chang CH, Ross RD. Pulmonary vein stenosis with Down syndrome: a rare and frequently fatal cause of pulmonary hypertension in infants and children. Congenit Heart Dis. 2014;9(3):E90–7.
4. McLaughlin VV, Archer SL, Badesch DB, Barst RJ, Farber HW, Lindner JR, et al. ACCF/AHA 2009 expert consensus document on pulmonary hypertension: a report of the American College of Cardiology Foundation Task Force on Expert Consensus Documents and the American Heart Association: developed in collaboration with the American College of Chest Physicians, American Thoracic Society, Inc., and the Pulmonary Hypertension Association. Circulation. 2009;119(16):2250–94.
5. Khemani E, McElhinney DB, Rhein L, Andrade O, Lacro RV, Thomas KC, et al. Pulmonary artery hypertension in formerly premature infants with bronchopulmonary dysplasia: clinical features and outcomes in the surfactant era. Pediatrics. 2007;120(6):1260–9.
6. Mourani PM, Ivy DD, Gao D, Abman SH. Pulmonary vascular effects of inhaled nitric oxide and oxygen tension in bronchopulmonary dysplasia. Am J Respir Crit Care Med. 2004;170(9):1006–13.
7. Klok FA, Mos IC, van Kralingen KW, Vahl JE, Huisman MV. Chronic pulmonary embolism and pulmonary hypertension. Semin Respir Crit Care Med. 2012;33(2):199–204.
8. Raffini L, Huang YS, Witmer C, Feudtner C. Dramatic increase in venous thromboembolism in children's hospitals in the United States from 2001 to 2007. Pediatrics. 2009;124(4):1001–8.
9. Tormene D, Gavasso S, Rossetto V, Simioni P. Thrombosis and thrombophilia in children: a systematic review. Semin Thromb Hemost. 2006;32(7):724–8.
10. Madani MM, Wittine LM, Auger WR, Fedullo PF, Kerr KM, Kim NH, et al. Chronic thromboembolic pulmonary hypertension in pediatric patients. J Thorac Cardiovasc Surg. 2011;141(3):624–30.
11. Kim JS, McSweeney J, Lee J, Ivy D. Pediatric Cardiac Intensive Care Society 2014 consensus statement: pharmacotherapies in cardiac critical care pulmonary hypertension. Pediatr Crit Care Med. 2016;17(3 Suppl 1):S89–100.
12. Walton BL, Lehmann M, Skorczewski T, Holle LA, Beckman JD, Cribb JA, et al. Elevated hematocrit enhances platelet accumulation following vascular injury. Blood. 2017;129(18):2537–46.
13. Guzzetta NA. Benefits and risks of red blood cell transfusion in pediatric patients undergoing cardiac surgery. Paediatr Anaesth. 2011;21(5):504–11.
14. Carter HF, Lau C, Juma D, Wells B, Applegate RL II. Intraoperative red blood cell transfusion in infant heart transplant patients is not associated with worsened outcomes. Anesth Anal. 2016;122(5):1567–77.
15. Cholette JM, Swartz MF, Rubenstein J, Henrichs KF, Wang H, Powers KS, et al. Outcomes using a conservative versus liberal red blood cell transfusion strategy in infants requiring cardiac operation. Ann Thorac Surg. 2017;103(1):206–14.
16. Lacroix J, Tucci M, Du Pont-Thibodeau G. Red blood cell transfusion decision making in critically ill children. Curr Opin Pediatr. 2015;27(3):286–91.

17. Kuo JA, Maher KO, Kirshbom PM, Mahle WT. Red blood cell transfusion for infants with single-ventricle physiology. Pediatr Cardiol. 2011;32(4):461–8.
18. de Gast-Bakker DH, de Wilde RB, Hazekamp MG, Sojak V, Zwaginga JJ, Wolterbeek R, et al. Safety and effects of two red blood cell transfusion strategies in pediatric cardiac surgery patients: a randomized controlled trial. Intensive Care Med. 2013;39(11):2011–9.
19. Linguraru MG, Orandi BJ, Van Uitert RL, Mukherjee N, Summers RM, Gladwin MT, et al. CT and image processing non-invasive indicators of sickle cell secondary pulmonary hypertension. Conf Proc IEEE Eng Med Biol Soc. 2008;2008:859–62.
20. Robert-Ebadi H, Le Gal G, Righini M. Evolving imaging techniques in diagnostic strategies of pulmonary embolism. Expert Rev Cardiovasc Ther. 2016;14(4):495–503.
21. Wilkes J. AHA/ATS release guidelines on the diagnosis and treatment of pediatric pulmonary hypertension. Am Fam Physician. 2016;93(7):605–14.
22. Potoka KP, Gladwin MT. Vasculopathy and pulmonary hypertension in sickle cell disease. Am J Physiol Lung Cell Mol Physiol. 2015;308(4):L314–24.
23. Mekontso Dessap A, Leon R, Habibi A, Nzouakou R, Roudot-Thoraval F, Adnot S, et al. Pulmonary hypertension and cor pulmonale during severe acute chest syndrome in sickle cell disease. Am J Respir Crit Care Med. 2008;177(6):646–53.
24. Gladwin MT, Sachdev V, Jison ML, Shizukuda Y, Plehn JF, Minter K, et al. Pulmonary hypertension as a risk factor for death in patients with sickle cell disease. N Engl J Med. 2004;350(9):886–95.
25. Machado RF, Mack AK, Martyr S, Barnett C, Macarthur P, Sachdev V, et al. Severity of pulmonary hypertension during vaso-occlusive pain crisis and exercise in patients with sickle cell disease. Br J Haematol. 2007;136(2):319–25.
26. Dham N, Ensing G, Minniti C, Campbell A, Arteta M, Rana S, et al. Prospective echocardiography assessment of pulmonary hypertension and its potential etiologies in children with sickle cell disease. Am J Cardiol. 2009;104(5):713–20.
27. Nouraie M, Lee JS, Zhang Y, Kanias T, Zhao X, Xiong Z, et al. The relationship between the severity of hemolysis, clinical manifestations and risk of death in 415 patients with sickle cell anemia in the US and Europe. Haematologica. 2013;98(3):464–72.
28. Vichinsky EP. Pulmonary hypertension in sickle cell disease. N Engl J Med. 2004;350(9):857–9.
29. De Castro LM, Jonassaint JC, Graham FL, Ashley-Koch A, Telen MJ. Pulmonary hypertension associated with sickle cell disease: clinical and laboratory endpoints and disease outcomes. Am J Hematol. 2008;83(1):19–25.
30. Gladwin MT, Sachdev V. Cardiovascular abnormalities in sickle cell disease. J Am Coll Cardiol. 2012;59(13):1123–33.
31. Kato GJ, McGowan V, Machado RF, Little JA, Taylor JT, Morris CR, et al. Lactate dehydrogenase as a biomarker of hemolysis-associated nitric oxide resistance, priapism, leg ulceration, pulmonary hypertension, and death in patients with sickle cell disease. Blood. 2006;107(6):2279–85.
32. Machado RF, Anthi A, Steinberg MH, Bonds D, Sachdev V, Kato GJ, et al. N-terminal pro-brain natriuretic peptide levels and risk of death in sickle cell disease. JAMA. 2006;296(3):310–8.
33. Minniti CP, Sable C, Campbell A, Rana S, Ensing G, Dham N, et al. Elevated tricuspid regurgitant jet velocity in children and adolescents with sickle cell disease: association with hemolysis and hemoglobin oxygen desaturation. Haematologica. 2009;94(3):340–7.
34. Platt OS, Brambilla DJ, Rosse WF, Milner PF, Castro O, Steinberg MH, et al. Mortality in sickle cell disease. Life expectancy and risk factors for early death. N Engl J Med. 1994;330(23):1639–44.

Emergency Interventional Cardiology in Children

14

Daisuke Kobayashi, Daniel R. Turner, and Thomas J. Forbes

Introduction

Though infrequent, the performance of an interventional cardiac procedure in an emergent setting can be lifesaving and indicated for various conditions. It is important for clinicians to assess the need to perform emergent catheterization procedures in infants and children in a timely fashion. Based on our experience and that reported in the literature, the seven most common procedures performed emergently on patients seen in the emergency department will be discussed. These procedures are pericardiocentesis, foreign body retrieval, transvenous pacing lead placement, recanalization of an acutely thrombosed modified Blalock-Taussig shunt, balloon valvuloplasty, balloon atrial septostomy, and intervention for an acute pulmonary embolism. Although most of these procedures require special technical skills, all clinicians need to be aware of their indications and treatment strategies. Timely recognition and subsequent mobilization of the interventional cardiology team are critical in achieving a successful outcome for emergent interventional procedures.

Case 1

A 4-year-old girl presents to the emergency department (ED) with complaints of chest discomfort and dyspnea for 1 day. By history, she underwent a device closure of atrial septal defect (ASD) a few weeks ago. She is tachycardic with a heart rate of 140 beats per minute with a blood pressure of 82/44 mmHg. Chest radiography

D. Kobayashi, M.D., F.A.A.P., F.A.C.C. (✉) • D. R. Turner, M.D. • T. J. Forbes, M.D.
Department of Pediatrics, Wayne State University School of Medicine, Detroit, MI, USA

Division of Cardiology, Children's Hospital of Michigan, Detroit, MI, USA

Chapel Hill, NC, USA
e-mail: dkobayas@dmc.org; dturner@dmc.org; TForbes@dmc.org

© Springer International Publishing AG, part of Springer Nature 2018
A. P. Sarnaik et al. (eds.), *Cardiac Emergencies in Children*,
https://doi.org/10.1007/978-3-319-73754-6_14

shows satisfactory position of the ASD device, but demonstrates cardiomegaly. On examination, she has muffled heart sounds.

What is the most appropriate next step in the ED?

A. ECG
B. Cardiac enzymes
C. Cardiac catheterization
D. Stat transthoracic echocardiogram
E. Bronchodilator treatment

Pericardiocentesis

A pericardial effusion is fluid accumulation in the pericardial space which can occur in various situations including post-pericardiotomy syndrome following heart surgery, infection (usually viral), malignancy, autoimmune disease, cardiac erosion caused by atrial septal defect occluder device, and metabolic syndrome. Patients often tolerate a gradual accumulation of a pericardial effusion due to gradual stretching of the pericardium. However, an acute or rapidly progressive pericardial effusion is likely to be a hemodynamic significant medical emergency from pericardial tamponade.

Typical findings of cardiac tamponade include muffled heart sounds, tachycardia, hypotension, distended neck veins, and pulsus paradoxus. Chest radiography often shows "cardiomegaly" from a large fluid collection around the heart. Electrocardiography may show low QRS voltage and electrical alternans in the presence of a large effusion. When a pericardial effusion is suspected, transthoracic echocardiography is the gold standard diagnostic test. Echocardiography shows the location (global versus localized), size (small, moderate, and large), and hemodynamic effect of the effusion. Signs of tamponade are right atrial and ventricular collapse with significant variations of tricuspid and mitral valve inflow Doppler patterns with the phases of respiration. Pericardiocentesis is an invasive procedure to aspirate pericardial fluid through needle drainage. For patients with a large pericardial effusion and cardiac tamponade physiology, pericardiocentesis is a lifesaving procedure. In non-emergent situations, pericardiocentesis occasionally is performed for diagnostic purposes.

Pericardiocentesis is mostly performed under transthoracic echocardiography guidance with or without fluoroscopy (Fig. 14.1). The procedure is usually straightforward for large global effusions. It can be challenging for smaller localized effusions. The puncture needle is advanced from the subxiphoid area or left lateral chest to the pericardial space, depending on the location and size of pericardial effusion. Positioning a patient upright on a wedge can be helpful to increase the target pericardial space for needle insertion. When coming from the subxiphoid location, it is extremely important to aim laterally, toward the left shoulder, rather than staying medial, to minimize the risk of puncturing the atrial wall. Puncturing the atrial wall is more likely to cause uncontrolled bleeding within the pericardial space than

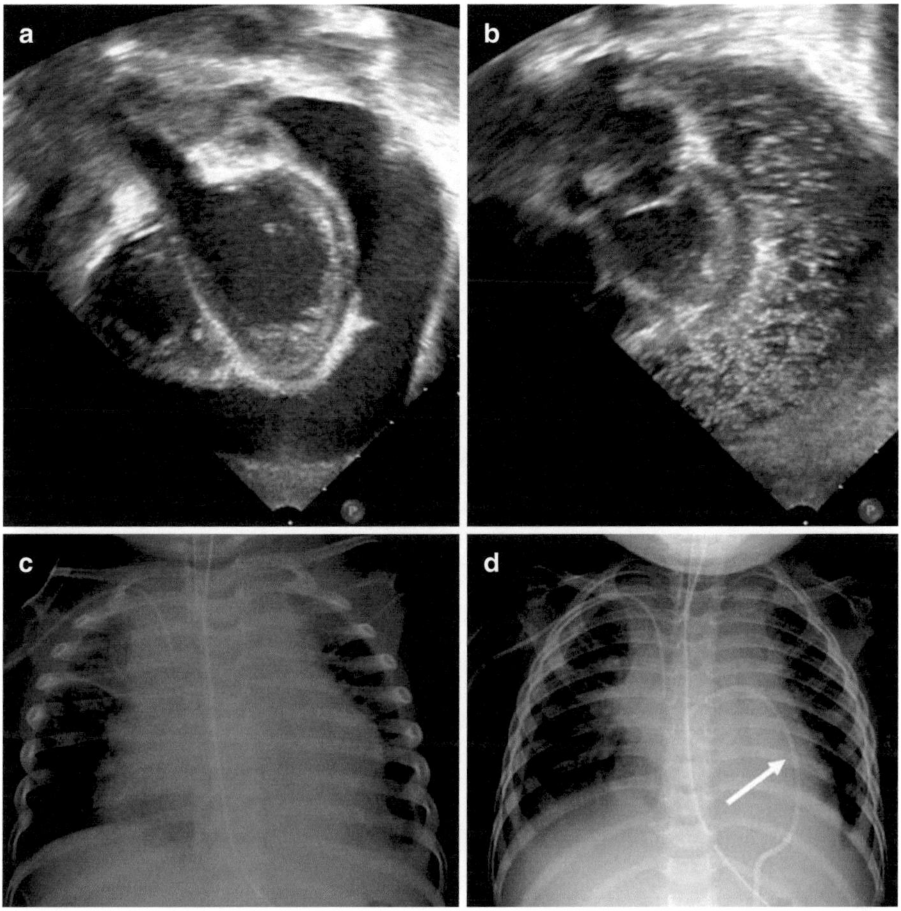

Fig. 14.1 Pericardiocentesis and pericardial drain placement in a 3-year-old girl with bacterial pericarditis and large pericardial effusion. (**a**) Baseline transthoracic echocardiography shows a large, global effusion. There is an echo-bright tissue at the visceral pericardium. (**b**) Bubble study in the pericardial space: agitated saline is injected through the needle to the pericardial space, confirming the needle position. (**c**) Baseline chest radiography shows a large cardiopericardial silhouette. (**d**) Post-pericardial drain placement, chest radiography shows smaller cardiac silhouette and placement of pericardial drain (arrow)

puncture of the ventricular free wall. Complications of pericardiocentesis are rare but include pneumothorax and accidental puncture of the myocardium [1]. When bloody fluid is withdrawn from the needle, it is of the utmost importance for the operator to confirm needle location. By advancing a wire through the puncture needle, the course of the wire can be seen as either in the pericardial space or in the heart under fluoroscopy. When ultrasound is used to assist in the pericardiocentesis, confirmation of the needle location can also be assisted with wire advancement or performance of a bubble study by injecting agitated saline via the puncture needle. Checking the hematocrit of aspirated fluid on a quick blood gas can also be extremely useful as a hematocrit the same as in the peripheral blood indicates cardiac perforation. Pericardial drain placement is often performed following the needle insertion due to the high likelihood of re-accumulation of the pericardial effusion. In the majority of cases, a pigtail catheter is advanced over a J-tipped wire and used as a pericardial drain.

Answer: D-Emergency transthoracic echocardiogram

This 4-year-old girl has an acutely developing pericardial effusion and cardiac tamponade due to cardiac erosion caused by the ASD device. Stat transthoracic echocardiography should be performed to confirm pericardial effusion, followed by emergent pericardiocentesis.

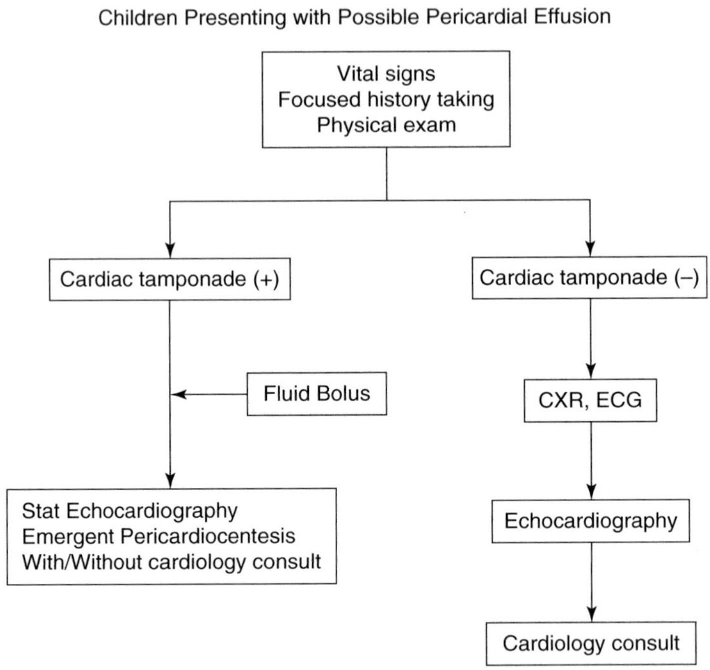

Flow Chart 1 Children presenting with possible pericardial effusion

Balloon Atrial Septostomy

Balloon atrial septostomy (BAS) is a well-established percutaneous procedure to enlarge or create an atrial septal communication. This procedure is to enhance mixing of the oxygenated and non-oxygenated blood at the atrial level. The most common reason to perform BAS is for patients with D-transposition of great arteries who are markedly cyanotic. BAS is performed under transthoracic echocardiography guidance at the bedside in the intensive care unit or in the cardiac catheterization laboratory. Although BAS can be performed through the umbilical vein, the femoral vein is the choice of venous access where a septostomy catheter

(5- or 6-Fr) is advanced from inferior vena cava to right atrium and left atrium. The balloon septostomy catheter is then fully inflated using diluted contrast in the left atrium. Under transthoracic echocardiography, the balloon is pulled against the atrial septum first. Then, the operator pulls the balloon through the atrial septum in a strong, quick, and short jerking motion of the wrist (Fig. 14.2). Echocardiography confirms both the pre-septostomy position of the balloon catheter and the efficacy of the BAS procedure (Fig. 14.3). Extra caution should be paid to avoid the injury to the mitral valve, left atrial appendage, and inferior vena cava. In newborns, BAS is usually safe and effective. In older infants and children with thicker atrial septal tissue, other techniques may be needed to enhance atrial mixing including static balloon dilation of the atrial communication, blade and

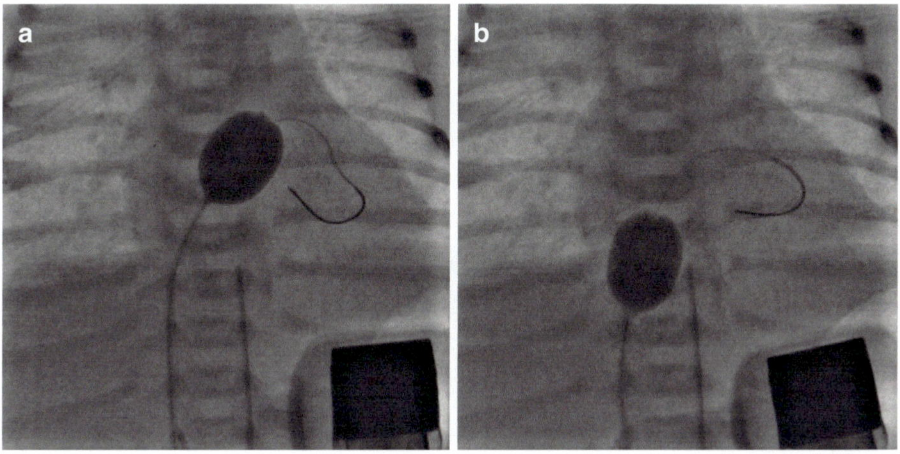

Fig. 14.2 Balloon atrial septostomy under transthoracic echocardiography and fluoroscopy. (**a**) A 6 Fr septostomy catheter (NuMED, Inc., Hopkinton, NY, USA) is advanced over a wire to the left atrium, where the balloon is fully inflated by diluted contrast. (**b**) The septostomy catheter is pulled through the atrial septum to the right atrium

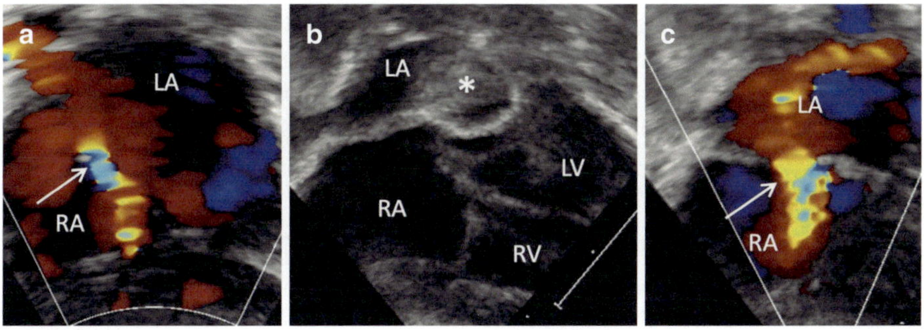

Fig. 14.3 Balloon atrial septostomy in the subcostal view of transthoracic echocardiography. (**a**) At baseline, color Doppler imaging shows a small restrictive atrial communication (arrow). (**b**) A balloon (*) of septostomy catheter is inflated in the left atrium (LA). (**c**) In post-balloon atrial septostomy, there is larger unrestrictive atrial communication (arrow)

then BAS, and stent placement across the atrial septum. Patients who have severe cyanosis require emergent evaluation by Pediatric Cardiology, and if BAS is required, then immediate transfer to an institution where this can be done should be arranged as the patient is stabilized in the ED. Prostaglandin E1 infusion can improve the saturation in the short term.

Case 2

A 10-year-old boy presents to the ED with a complaint of palpitations for 1 day. He has a past medical history of hydrocephalus, for which he underwent ventriculoatrial shunt 4 years before. On presentation, he is well-appearing with stable vital signs. ECG shows intermittent premature ventricular contractions.

What is the most appropriate next step in the ED?

A. Chest X-ray
B. Neurosurgery consult
C. Basic metabolic panel
D. Head CT scan
E. Cardiac enzymes

Foreign Body Retrieval

Transcatheter retrieval of embolized devices is usually a semi-emergent procedure. Embolized devices include transcatheter occluders (for atrial septal defect, ventricular septal defect, and patent ductus arteriosus), fractured segments of central intravenous indwelling catheters and ventriculoatrial shunt catheters. Foreign bodies potentially cause issues depending on their embolized location. Any retained foreign body increases the risk of infection, and those in an atrium and/or ventricle may cause an arrhythmia or cardiac perforation. Retained devices in a pulmonary artery can lead to pulmonary embolism and pulmonary hypertension. When a device embolizes to the arterial system, ischemic symptoms caused by acute arterial occlusion are a major concern. For these reasons, embolized devices are removed upon discovery. Transcatheter approach in the catheterization lab is the first choice of therapy and in most cases can be performed effectively and safely [2]. Various transcatheter techniques can be used to retrieve these embolized devices, with the GooseNeck snare being the most common (Figs. 14.4 and 14.5).

Answer: A-Chest X-ray

This patient has a fracture of the VP shunt that embolized into the right ventricle. This embolized shunt fragment causes ventricular ectopy. The appropriate test is chest X-ray to check the VP shunt. When chest x-ray demonstrates shunt embolization, an interventional cardiologist needs to be consulted for a foreign body retrieval procedure.

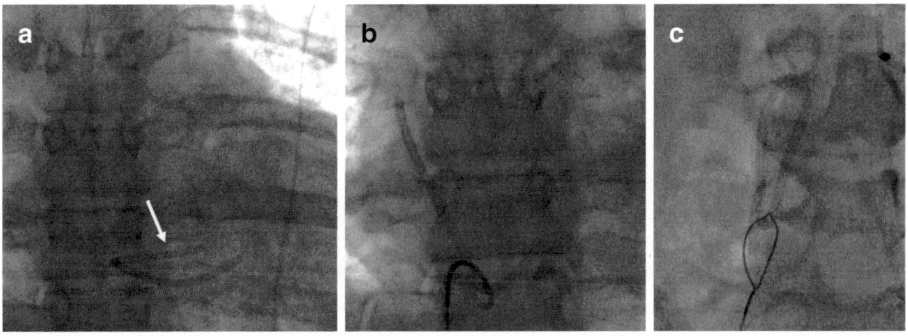

Fig. 14.4 Transcatheter retrieval of an embolized ventriculoatrial shunt. (**a**) An embolized shunt segment (arrow) is in the right ventricle. (**b**) Using a pigtail catheter, the shunt segment is pulled down from the right ventricle to the right atrium and inferior vena cava. (**c**) The shunt segment is captured by a snare and taken out from the femoral venous sheath

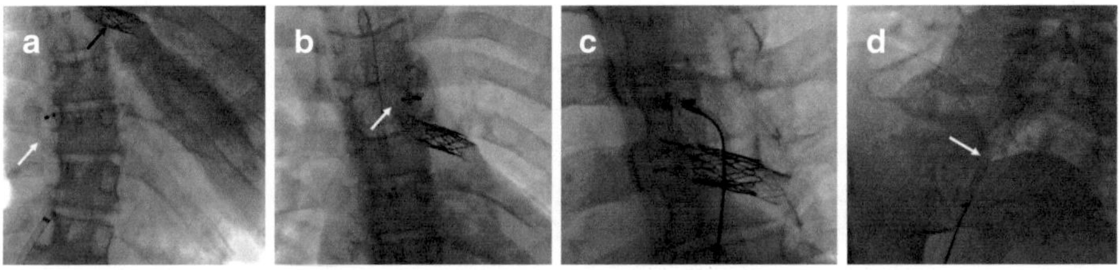

Fig. 14.5 Transcatheter retrieval of embolized atrial septal defect (ASD) occluder device in a 17-year-old boy with a moderate-sized ASD and history of a stented left pulmonary artery. (**a**) A 15 mm Amplatzer septal occluder (St. Jude Medical, Inc., St. Paul, MI; white arrow) is positioned at the atrial septum at the time of implantation. Previously implanted stents (black arrow) are in the proximal left pulmonary artery. (**b**) Device has embolized and caught in the transverse aortic arch. (**c**) The hub of the device is snared. (**d**) The snared device is withdrawn to a 12 Fr sheath in the right femoral artery. Arrow indicates the tip of the sheath

Case 3

A 7-month-old infant presents to the ED with a complaint of lethargy for 2 days. He underwent surgical repair of a ventricular septal defect at 6 months of life. Postoperatively, he required temporary pacing for complete heart block for 2 days. He was discharged 2 weeks before, and his discharge ECG showed sinus rhythm with right bundle branch block. On presentation, he appears ill with blood pressure of 75/35 mmHg and heart rate of 50 beats per minute. Arterial blood gas shows acidosis with pH of 7.15.

What is the most appropriate next step in the ED?

A. Echocardiography
B. ECG
C. Cardiac enzyme
D. Chest X-ray
E. Septic workup

Transvenous Pacing Lead Placement

New onset of complete heart block can be a life-threatening condition frequently causing hemodynamic instability. The etiology of complete heart block includes congenital heart disease (i.e., L-transposition of great arteries) and intrinsic conduction disease including congenital complete heart block from maternal Lupus, infection (i.e., Lyme disease), post device placement (perimembranous ventricular septal closure devices), pacemaker malfunction (lead fracture), and post-cardiac surgery. An urgent temporary pacing lead placement via transvenous approach is required for these conditions. Percutaneous pacing is available but not always effective. Although transvenous pacing catheter placement can be performed at the bedside under transthoracic echocardiographic guidance, fluoroscopic guidance is preferable in the cath lab. A pacing catheter is advanced from any systemic vein to the right atrium and right ventricle. The pacing catheter is secured at the venous access site when consistent pacing capture is obtained. This procedure can be performed via either right internal jugular (RIJ) vein or femoral vein, though the RIJ is a more straightforward and convenient approach (Fig. 14.6).

Answer: B-ECG

This patient has postsurgical complete heart block that requires emergent intervention. Past history of transient complete heart block post-cardiac surgery indicates that his conduction system was injured to some extent and at risk for future advanced heart block. The appropriate first step is an ECG which shows atrioventricular dissociation. After making a diagnosis of complete heart block, urgent cardiology consult should be made. Transvenous pacing catheter placement can improve and stabilize the patient prior to the elective permanent pacemaker insertion.

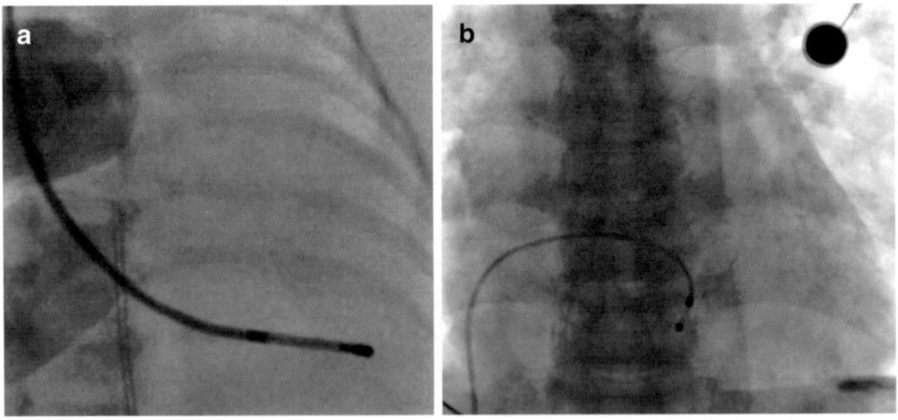

Fig. 14.6 Transvenous pacing lead placement. (**a**) Transjugular approach. A pacing lead is positioned at the right ventricle through the right internal jugular vein. (**b**) Transfemoral approach. A pacing lead is positioned at the right ventricle through the right femoral vein

Case 4

A 3-month-old girl infant presents to the ED after her parents note sudden onset of cyanosis. She was born with pulmonary atresia and ventricular septal defect. She underwent a right modified Blalock-Taussig shunt at 1 week of age and was discharged home on aspirin at 3 weeks of age. One day prior to the presentation, she started vomiting with decreased formula intake and urine output. On presentation, she is cyanotic with respiratory distress. Pulse oximetry reads 60% on room air. On auscultation, there was no shunt murmur. Arterial blood gas shows a pH of 7.1 with severe lactic acidosis. She required emergent intubation.

What is the most appropriate next step in the ED?

A. Stat echocardiography
B. Cardiology consult, fluid bolus, heparin administration
C. Chest X-ray
D. Septic workup
E. ECG

Recanalization of Acutely Thrombosed Modified Blalock-Taussig Shunt

The modified Blalock-Taussig shunt (mBTS) is a surgically created aortopulmonary communication. This is a palliative surgical procedure aimed at providing reliable pulmonary blood flow in patients with ductal-dependent or severely reduced pulmonary blood flow. Acute occlusion of this shunt leads to severe hypoxia and acidosis. This requires an emergent catheterization or surgical procedure. Early recognition of acute shunt thrombosis is vitally important, and upon arrival to the ED, the interventional team should be contacted even before any studies are obtained for any hypoxemic infant with a history of a mBTS. Disappearance of the shunt murmur is diagnostic with an acute drop in saturation and an unstable clinical status. Transthoracic echocardiography (TTE) is often done to confirm absent or diminished flow through the mBTS, though, at times, TTE can be misleading regarding the severity of obstruction. It is vital in this scenario to escalate care without delay if a patient presents with hypoxemia and history of pulmonary blood flow depending on a mBTS. While surgical revision of mBTS is an option, a transcatheter approach is the treatment of choice to recanalize the occluded shunt [3]. While activating the interventional cardiology team, it is important to optimize medical therapy by intubation, fluid boluses, possible red blood cell transfusion, and inotropic support. Pre-cath heparinization is another consideration to begin the anticoagulation process.

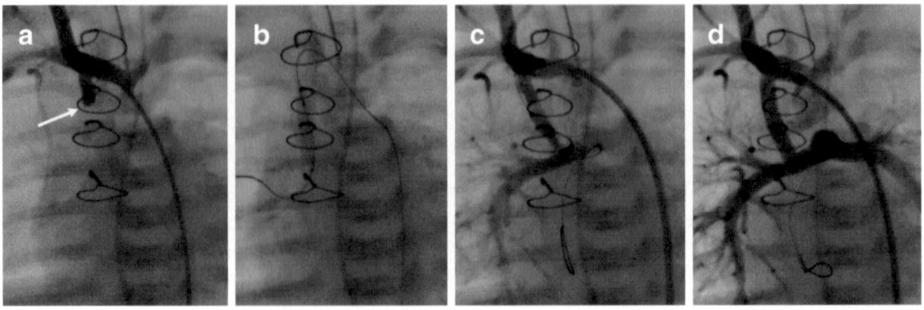

Fig. 14.7 Recanalization of a thrombosed right modified Black-Taussig shunt (rmBTS). (**a**) Complete occlusion of rmBTS (arrow). Contrast is injected at the base of right innominate artery. No flow is seen to the pulmonary artery system. (**b**) Balloon angioplasty of rmBTS. A coronary balloon catheter is inflated at the rmBTS. (**c**) Post-angioplasty: There is a better flow through the rmBTS to pulmonary artery system. However, there is still thrombus in the rmBTS, characterized by the irregular contour of shunt lumen. A coronary stent balloon catheter is positioned in the distal shunt. (**d**) Post-stent: Two coronary artery stents are placed in the rmBTS with abundant flow to the pulmonary arteries

Cardiac catheterization starts with femoral artery access. Shunt thrombosis is diagnosed with aortography and/or selective injection of brachiocephalic artery (Fig. 14.7). Recanalization of a thrombosed shunt often starts with balloon angioplasty, followed often by stent placement. For extensive thrombosis involving the proximal pulmonary artery, thrombolytic therapy may be necessary. In the setting of acute thrombosis, it is feasible to advance a wire through the occluded shunt to the branch pulmonary artery. A small balloon catheter is then advanced over the wire to the shunt, where serial inflations are performed along the entire length of shunt. Post-angioplasty selective angiography often shows improved shunt flow with residual thrombus. Therefore, stent placement is often performed to maintain long-term patency. Although this procedure is often performed via the femoral artery approach, the carotid artery approach provides a straight course to the mBTS for the wire positioning and stent placement. After transcatheter intervention, anticoagulation using intravenous heparin is necessary to prevent recurrent shunt thrombosis for 24–72 h. Anticoagulation is then maintained with antiplatelet therapy using aspirin and/or clopidogrel.

Answer: B-Cardiology consult, fluid bolus, heparin administration

This infant has a history of right modified Blalock-Taussig shunt and presents with acute cyanosis. In this circumstance, acute thrombosis of the shunt needs to be strongly suspected, and it is a true emergency. Escalation of care should not be delayed. While requesting stat cardiology consult and indicating the possible need for emergent cardiac catheterization, fluid bolus and inotropic support such as epinephrine to raise the blood pressure may be considered along with heparin administration.

Case 5

A 10-day-old boy infant presents to the ED after 911 was called when he stopped breathing. On presentation, the infant is very lethargic with poor perfusion. His extremities are cold with a capillary refill >3 s. His femoral pulses are barely palpable. He has grade 4/6 systolic ejection murmur at the right upper sternal border.

What is the most appropriate next step in the ED?

A. Chest X-ray
B. ECG
C. Septic workup
D. Fluid bolus and prostaglandin E infusion
E. Echocardiography

Balloon Valvuloplasty

Severe semilunar (aortic and pulmonary) valve stenosis in newborns is a serious condition. When antegrade flow through these valves is not sufficient to support systemic or pulmonary circulation, the stenosis is termed "critical," and prostaglandin E infusion is required to maintain or reopen the ductus arteriosus. Valvuloplasty is considered as the initial treatment of choice for severe or critical aortic or pulmonary valve stenosis. In critical aortic valve stenosis, left ventricular systolic dysfunction can develop, and it may be beneficial to treat with inotropes prior to catheterization.

Aortic valvuloplasty (Fig. 14.8) is indicated for critical (ductal-dependent) aortic valve stenosis or severe aortic stenosis with a resting peak systolic gradient

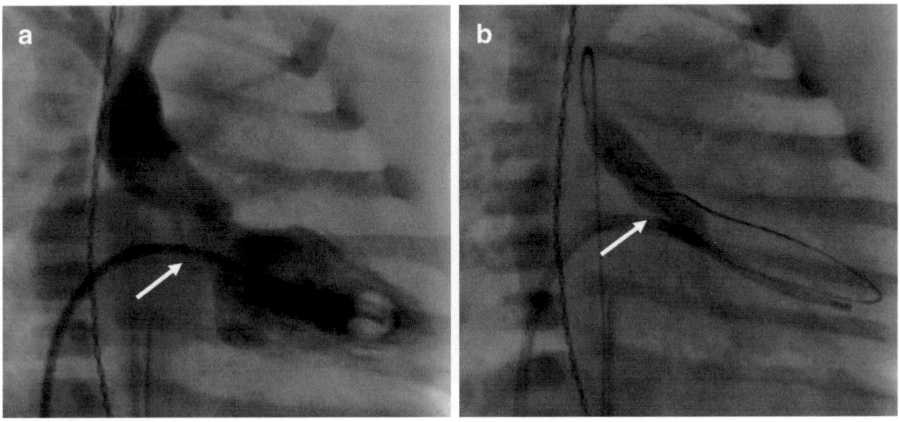

Fig. 14.8 Balloon aortic valvuloplasty for critical aortic valve stenosis in a newborn. (**a**) Left ventricular angiography shows dysplastic aortic valve leaflets (arrow) that dome in systole. (**b**) Balloon aortic valvuloplasty via a retrograde approach. A 6 mm × 2 cm Tyshak Mini balloon angioplasty catheter (NuMED, Hopkinton, NY) is advanced over a wire from a 3-Fr sheath (femoral artery) to the aortic valve. A waist in the balloon (arrow) is seen with inflation of balloon at the narrowed valve

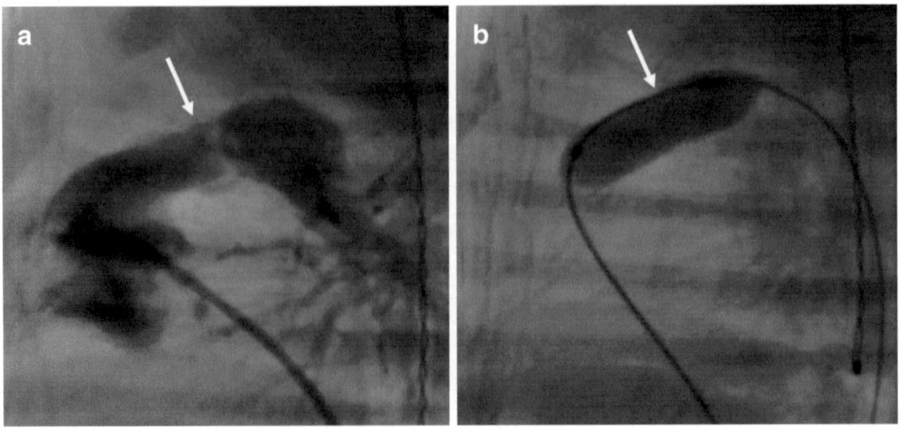

Fig. 14.9 Pulmonary balloon valvuloplasty for critical pulmonary valve stenosis in a newborn. (**a**) Lateral view: right ventricular angiography shows the dysplastic pulmonary valve leaflets (arrow) that dome in systole. (**b**) Balloon pulmonary valvuloplasty. A 6 mm × 2 cm Tyshak II balloon angioplasty catheter (NuMED, Hopkinton, NY) is advanced over a wire. A waist of the balloon (arrow) is seen with inflation of balloon

of ≥50 mmHg or ≥40 mmHg with evidence of left ventricular dysfunction or ischemia [4]. Complications of aortic valvuloplasty are a significant residual obstruction, aortic valve regurgitation, femoral vascular injury, thromboembolic stroke, injury to the mitral valve, and myocardial perforation. To avoid important aortic valve regurgitation, the balloon-to-valve annulus ratio is usually kept between 80–100%. Pulmonary valvuloplasty (Fig. 14.9) is indicated for critical (ductal-dependent) pulmonary valve stenosis, severe pulmonary valve stenosis with a resting peak gradient of ≥40 mmHg, or clinically significant stenosis with right ventricular dysfunction [4]. Complications of pulmonary valvuloplasty are perforation of the right ventricular outflow tract and pulmonary valve regurgitation. In the past, pulmonary valve insufficiency was thought not to be an important issue. However, more recently, closer attention to long-term RV dilation and subsequent dysfunction following pulmonary balloon valvuloplasty has led many centers to perform either surgical or transcatheter placement of a pulmonary valve in the RVOT position when significant RV dilation or dysfunction occurs.

Answer: D-Fluid bolus and prostaglandin E infusion

This 10-day-old infant has signs and symptoms of shock. Although septic and/or hypovolemic shock cannot be excluded, cariogenic shock with closure of the ductus arteriosus needs to be strongly suspected given this infant's age. Among the various ductal-dependent conditions, this infant has critical aortic valve stenosis. Along with ductal closure, cardiac output from a severely stenotic aortic valve becomes insufficient to maintain systemic circulation, leading to cariogenic shock. He has a significant heart murmur on examination, indicating the presence of congenital heart disease, although the murmur may be softer if there is poor left ventricular systolic function. Fluid bolus and prostaglandin E infusion is the most appropriate initial step in this clinical situation. Initiation of prostaglandin E infusion should not be delayed because it is lifesaving.

Case 6

A 15-year-old girl presents to the emergency department with a complaint of chest discomfort for 1 day. One month prior to the presentation, she underwent right hip replacement surgery and required bed rest for 2 weeks. She is on oral contraceptives for her dysmenorrhea. On presentation, she is mildly distressed and short of breath. Pulse oximetry is 88% on room air. Her blood pressure is 82/40 mmHg. Lung sounds are clear on auscultation. Her right lower leg is swollen and mildly erythematous with mild tenderness. D-dimer is mildly elevated.

What is the most appropriate next step in the ED?

A. Chest X-ray
B. Cardiac enzymes
C. Electrocardiography
D. Echocardiography
E. Chest CT angiography

Acute Pulmonary Embolism

Acute pulmonary embolism is a rare, life-threatening condition in the pediatric population. Significant risk factors are use of oral contraceptives, obesity, and immobility [5]. The severity of disease is classified into low-risk, intermediate-risk (submassive), and high-risk (massive) [6]. Anticoagulation should be started when acute pulmonary embolism is suspected, unless contraindicated. Computed tomography scan is diagnostic and delineates the extent of thrombus formation in the pulmonary artery system. Whereas anticoagulation therapy alone is used for low-risk patients, invasive treatment options should be considered for submassive and massive emboli due to the associated high mortality rates. Systemic fibrinolysis can be effective but has a higher risk of bleeding. Surgical thrombectomy can be performed but has been used only in extremis, resulting in poor outcomes. More recently, various catheter-based therapies have become available with the development of new devices [6]. The purpose of catheter-based therapy is immediate relief of obstruction and restoration of pulmonary blood flow. Mechanisms of action include clot fragmentation, manual or suction pump aspiration, and/or direct infusion of a low-dose fibrinolytic agent. The most common approach is a local and slow infusion of a fibrinolytic agent through an infusion catheter positioned in the target pulmonary artery (Fig. 14.10). Traditional methods of mechanical fragmentation of the clot to achieve partial relief of obstruction may be used, for example, balloon angioplasty and/or rotation of a pigtail catheter in the pulmonary artery. Active suction of thrombus can be performed using regular guide catheters or

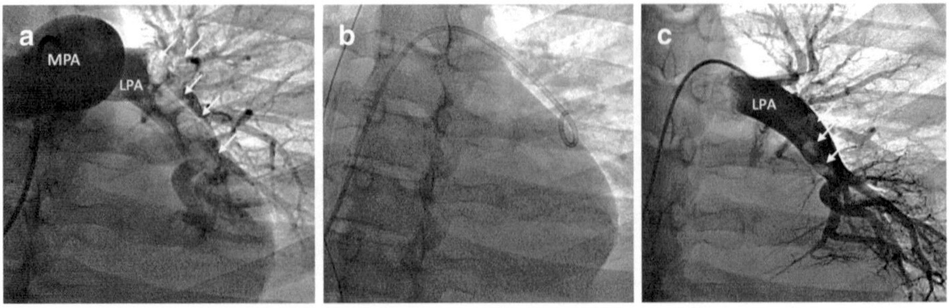

Fig. 14.10 Local infusion of a fibrinolytic agent for acute pulmonary embolism. (**a**) Multiple medium-sized thromboses (arrows) are in the left pulmonary artery (LPA). MPA = main pulmonary artery. (**b**) A 6-Fr Pigtail catheter is positioned in the LPA through which alteplase was infused. (**c**) Next day, repeat angiography shows better flow to distal LPA branches with significant reduction of thrombus size (arrows)

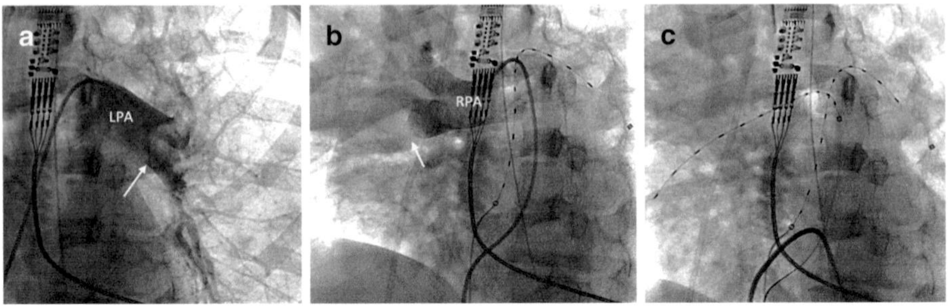

Fig. 14.11 Ultrasound accelerated fibrinolysis for acute pulmonary embolism. (**a**) Left pulmonary artery (LPA) angiography shows a large thrombus. (**b**) A EkoSonic endovascular device (EKOS Corp., Bothell, Washington, USA) is positioned in the LPA. Right pulmonary artery (RPA) angiography shows an occlusive thrombus (arrow) in the RPA lower lobe. (**c**) Another EkoSonic endovascular device is positioned in the RPA for thrombolysis

special aspiration catheter systems. Ultrasound accelerated fibrinolysis using an EkoSonic catheter (EKOS Corp., Bothell, Washington, USA) is a new technology that is promising for effective breakdown of a thrombus (Fig. 14.11). A special high-frequency, low-power ultrasound signal separates fibrin strands, allowing a fibrinolytic agent to penetrate into the thrombus.

Answer: E-Chest CT angiography

This adolescent girl has a classic presentation of acute pulmonary embolism. Significant risk factors are immobility due to surgery and use of oral contraceptives. Her leg finding is indicative of deep venous thrombosis. The diagnostic test is chest CT angiography that would be an appropriate next step. Once the diagnosis of acute pulmonary embolism is made, cardiac enzymes (troponin and NT-pro-BNP) and echocardiography (to evaluate right ventricular strain) are important tests. Depending on the severity of disease, the option of catheter-based therapies should be discussed with cardiology and hematology services.

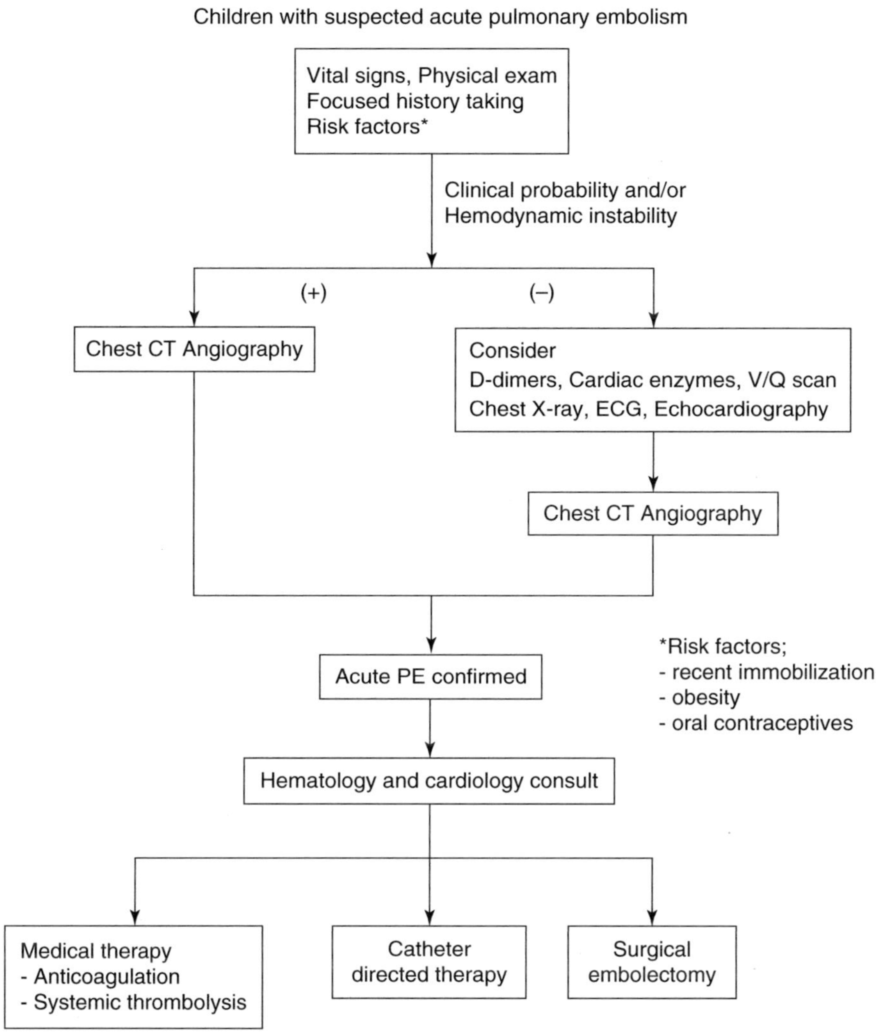

Flow Chart 2 Children with suspected acute pulmonary embolism

Percutaneous Approach for Mechanical Circulatory Support

Mechanical circulatory support is a lifesaving tool for cardiorespiratory failure resistant to maximal medical therapy. With recent improvement in technology, there are more devices available for mechanical circulatory support. Standard extracorporeal membrane oxygenation (ECMO) requires insertion of large arterial/venous cannulas into large-diameter vessels. Because ECMO cannulation is performed by surgeons via a cutdown approach in most centers, the timeliness of ECMO initiation remains a challenge. Recently, ECMO has been integrated into cardiopulmonary resuscitation (CPR), so called extracorporeal CPR (ECPR). In ECPR, ECMO is initiated during the resuscitation of a patient in cardiac arrest, requiring emergency cannulation. The 2015 international consensus recommends ECPR be considered for children with underlying cardiac conditions who have an in-house cardiac arrest [7]. In adults, emergency percutaneous ECMO cannulation can be used [8]; however, the option of percutaneous ECMO cannulation is currently limited in younger children (< 25 kg) due to small vessel size.

Percutaneous ventricular assist devices are another new modality utilized for circulatory support in the adult population. Impella® is a device that is inserted percutaneously from the femoral artery and advanced to left ventricle through the aortic valve, providing continuous blood flow. The use of Impella® device has been reported in children as young as 6.5 years [9]. Miniaturization and innovation of devices will be forthcoming to expand the availability of percutaneous interventions in younger children in the future.

In summary, emergent cardiac catheterization can lead to lifesaving intervention in a small group of patients seen in the emergency department. Knowledge of the type of patients who may be at risk is important. The greatest predictor for a successful outcome is early recognition of the problem and timely activation of the pediatric cardiology interventional team.

References

1. Tsang TS, El-Najdawi EK, Seward JB, Hagler DJ, Freeman WK, O'Leary PW. Percutaneous echocardiographically guided pericardiocentesis in pediatric patients: evaluation of safety and efficacy. J Am Soc Echocardiogr. 1998;11:1072–7.
2. Kudumula V, Stumper O, Noonan P, Mehta C, De Giovanni J, Stickley J, Dhillon R, Bhole V. Transcatheter retrieval of cardiovascular foreign bodies in children: a 15-year single centre experience. Pediatr Cardiol. 2017;38(6):1183–90. https://doi.org/10.1007/s00246-017-1639-0.
3. Gillespie MJ, Rome JJ. Transcatheter treatment for systemic-to-pulmonary artery shunt obstruction in infants and children. Catheter Cardiovasc Interv. 2008;71:928–35.
4. Feltes TF, Bacha E, Beekman RH III, Cheatham JP, Feinstein JA, Gomes AS, Hijazi ZM, Ing FF, de Moor M, Morrow WR, Mullins CE, Taubert KA, Zahn EM, American Heart Association Congenital Cardiac Defects Committee of the Council on Cardiovascular Disease in the Young; Council on Clinical Cardiology; Council on Cardiovascular Radiology and Intervention; American Heart Association. Indications for cardiac catheterization and intervention in pediatric cardiac disease: a scientific statement from the American Heart Association. Circulation. 2011;123(22):2607–52.
5. Wang CY, Ignjatovic V, Francis P, Cain T, Babl F, Kowalski R, Cochrane A, Monagle P. Risk factors and clinical features of acute pulmonary embolism in children from the community. Thromb Res. 2016;138:86–90.
6. Jaber WA, Fong PP, Weisz G, Lattouf O, Jenkins J, Rosenfield K, Rab T, Ramee S. Acute pulmonary embolism: with an emphasis on an interventional approach. J Am Coll Cardiol. 2016;67:991–1002.
7. de Caen AR, Maconochie IK, Aickin R, Atkins DL, Biarent D, Guerguerian AM, Kleinman ME, Kloeck DA, Meaney PA, Nadkarni VM, Ng KC, Nuthall G, Reis AG, Shimizu N, Tibballs J, Veliz Pintos R, Pediatric Basic Life Support and Pediatric Advanced Life Support Chapter Collaborators. Part 6: pediatric basic life support and pediatric advanced life support: 2015 international consensus on cardiopulmonary resuscitation and emergency cardiovascular care science with treatment recommendations. Circulation. 2015;132:S177–203.

8. Tonna JE, Johnson NJ, Greenwood J, Gaieski DF, Shinar Z, Bellezo JM, Becker L, Shah AP, Youngquist ST, Mallin MP, Fair JF III, Gunnerson KJ, Weng C, McKellar S, Extracorporeal REsuscitation ConsorTium (ERECT) Research Group. Practice characteristics of Emergency Department extracorporeal cardiopulmonary resuscitation (eCPR) programs in the United States: the current state of the art of Emergency Department extracorporeal membrane oxygenation (ED ECMO). Resuscitation. 2016;107:38–46.
9. Parekh D, Jeewa A, Tume SC, Dreyer WJ, Pignatelli R, Horne D, Justino H, Qureshi AM. Percutaneous mechanical circulatory support using Impella® Devices for decompensated cardiogenic shock: a pediatric heart center experience. ASAIO J. 2017;64(1):98–104.

Check for updates

Common Problems in the Emergency Department in a Child with Known Heart Disease

15

Syana Sarnaik, Nirupama Kannikeswaran, Prashant Mahajan, and Ashok P. Sarnaik

Introduction

Patients with known heart disease often present with illnesses not related to their underlying disease, and the interplay between their acute illness and underlying heart disease can be challenging to manage. Further, with the surgical repair of certain heart diseases at an earlier age and the improved outcomes of children with congenital heart diseases, it is expected that emergency department (ED) visits for acute illness in patients with heart disease would increase. Thus, the understanding of common ED presentations among patients with heart disease and their management is important.

Few studies have specifically addressed the reasons for ED visits among patients with underlying heart disease (CHD) [1, 2]. A retrospective study evaluated the common reasons for presentation to a tertiary care ED among 286 children with known heart disease [3]. The most common presenting complaints in these patients were respiratory tract infections (24.1%), dysrhythmia (16.4%), heart failure (14.3%), aggravated cyanosis (5.6%), protein-losing enteropathy (4.9%), hemoptysis (4.5%),

S. Sarnaik, M.D. (✉) • N. Kannikeswaran, M.D.
Division of Emergency Medicine, Department of Pediatrics, Children's Hospital of Michigan, Wayne State University School of Medicine, Detroit, MI, USA
e-mail: ssarnaik2@dmc.org; nkannike@dmc.org

P. Mahajan, M.D.
Department of Emergency Medicine, CS Mott Children's Hospital of Michigan, Ann Arbor, MI, USA

University of Michigan School of Medicine, Ann Arbor, MI, USA
e-mail: pmahajan@med.umich.edu

A. P. Sarnaik, M.D., F.A.A.P., F.C.C.M.
Division of Critical Care Medicine, Department of Pediatrics, Children's Hospital of Michigan, Wayne State University School of Medicine, Detroit, MI, USA
e-mail: asarnaik@med.wayne.edu

© Springer International Publishing AG, part of Springer Nature 2018

A. P. Sarnaik et al. (eds.), *Cardiac Emergencies in Children*,
https://doi.org/10.1007/978-3-319-73754-6_15

drug side effects (4.1%), and infective endocarditis (3.0%). The highest mortality (5.8%) in the study cohort was related to respiratory infections. Atrial flutter was the most frequent arrhythmia (70.2%), and 70% of these patients were post-Fontan surgery.

There is scant literature regarding the ED management of common pediatric illnesses in patients with underlying heart disease. The limited research, and consequently the lack of evidence, has precluded development of management guidelines that can aid the ED clinician. A recent study noted that children with functionally univentricular heart (single ventricle) physiology presented to the ED frequently and with high acuity during the tenuous period between the first and second stages of repair [4]. However, the ED physicians surveyed were unfamiliar with pathophysiology and the complex management concerns of these patients.

Children with CHD at any stage of repair are at an increased risk of suffering from complications from routine childhood infections [5]. It is important that the pediatric care providers be familiar with the pathophysiology of various types of cardiac diseases as the management of common pediatric medical complaints varies with the type of underlying heart disease. As the number of infants undergoing CHD repair increases, the ED physicians who are most likely to encounter them during an acute illness will need to be familiar with their unique physiology and potential complications [6]. Children with underlying heart disease tend to have a higher mortality and morbidity and a more complicated hospital course from common pediatric illness compared to children without heart disease.

Cardiopulmonary Interactions

While anatomically the heart is placed between the two lungs, physiologically the lungs could be considered as situated between the two sides (right and left) of the heart. The right side of the heart has to pump blood through the lungs before it returns to the left side of the heart. Changes in the function of one organ have significant effects on the function of the other. The heart and lungs share the intrathoracic cavity and are subjected to the same intrathoracic pressure changes during respiration or therapeutic interventions. The burden imposed by these pathophysiologic changes on an already compromised heart can be substantial. The clinician should recognize the unique challenges imposed on an already compromised heart and plan management accordingly.

Influence of Intrathoracic Pressure Changes on Cardiac Function: Fluctuations in intrathoracic pressure during respiration influence both the preload and afterload of the left ventricle (LV) but only the preload of the right ventricle (RV). This is because the entire pulmonary circulation (arterial, capillary, and venous) resides in the thoracic cage and is subjected to the same pressure change. Part of the systemic circulation, on the other hand, lies outside the thoracic cage and is not exposed to the same changes in pressure compared to the part within the thoracic cage (Fig. 15.1). Thus, during

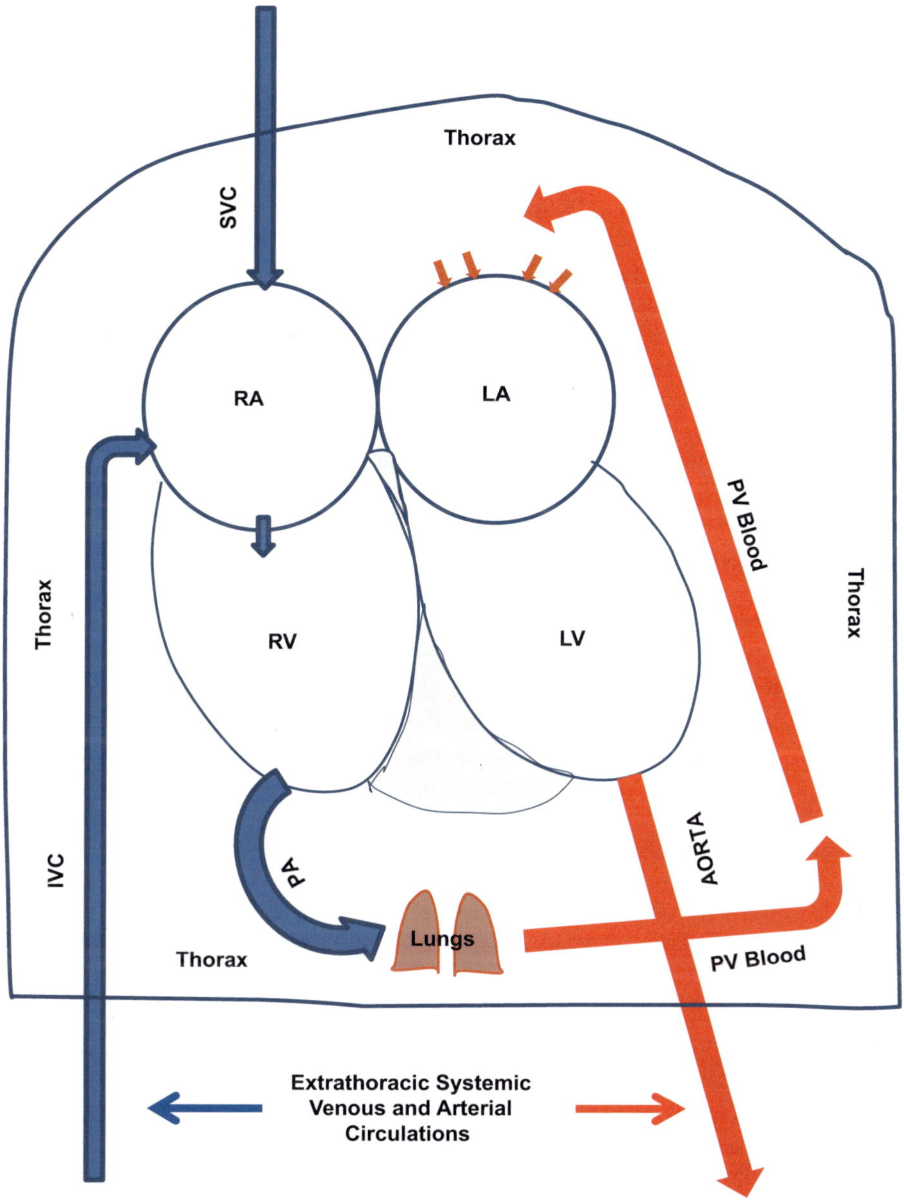

Fig. 15.1 Schematic representation of pulmonary and systemic circulations. While the entire pulmonary circulation (arterial, capillary, and venous) resides in the thoracic cavity, part of the systemic circulation (arterial, capillary, and venous) is outside the thorax. Pressure differences across circulatory bed due to respiratory effort are therefore experienced by LV but not RV. During inspiration, starting with negative pressure, LV must generate greater cavitary tension to eject its contents (increased afterload)

respiration, a pressure gradient is created between the intrathoracic and extrathoracic parts of the systemic circulation.

Preload is defined as the end-diastolic fiber length of the ventricle. Greater the preload, greater is the stroke volume until an optimum myocardial stretch has been attained. Afterload is the cavitary tension during isovolumic contraction where the ventricle must generate to begin emptying. The greater the afterload, the lower is the stroke volume. In spontaneous respiration, the negative intrathoracic pressure during inspiration lowers the pressure in the right atrial and the intrathoracic part of the systemic venous circulation resulting in increased venous return to the RV. The resultant RV distension shifts the interventricular septum to the left, thus diminishing LV compliance and therefore the LV preload. Also, the LV must generate greater cavitary tension during the isovolumic contraction phase to eject its stroke volume since it is surrounded by negative intrathoracic pressure. Both the increased LV afterload and decreased preload result in a decrease in stroke volume and a lower systolic pressure during inspiration. During expiration, the changes in intrathoracic pressure are reversed resulting in relatively greater stroke volume and higher systolic pressure. This difference in systolic pressure between inspiration and expiration does not exceed 5 mmHg during normal respiration.

In certain conditions, such as pericardial effusion and airway obstruction, the normal decline in systolic blood pressure during inspiration is exaggerated (>10 mmHg), termed pulsus paradoxus (PP). In extrathoracic airway obstruction (e.g., croup) and intrathoracic airway obstruction (e.g., asthma, bronchiolitis), the pressure changes associated with respiration are pronounced resulting in greater afterload and lower preload for LV. While a normal heart is capable of handling these pressure changes, a functionally challenged heart (myocarditis, patient after Norwood procedure, etc.) may rapidly decompensate. Positive-pressure breathing is beneficial in these situations as it will reduce the LV afterload.

Effect of Functional Residual Capacity (FRC) on Pulmonary Vascular Resistance PVR represents RV afterload. It is calculated as:

$$\begin{aligned}\text{PVR} = &\left[\text{mean pulmonary artery pressure} - \text{left atrial pressure}\right]\\ &\div \text{pulmonary blood flow}\end{aligned}$$

RV afterload increases with increasing PVR. In order to maintain the same pulmonary blood flow with rising afterload, the RV's work must increase. With increasing afterload, the RV's ability to compensate is overwhelmed resulting in decreased pulmonary blood flow and cardiac output. This is especially important in children with an already compromised heart or those with a functionally univentricular heart who have had a Fontan operation where pulmonary blood flow is passive without the benefit of a pumping chamber. FRC, the lung volume at the end of tidal expiration, significantly influences the PVR. At normal FRC, pulmonary capillaries are widely open and PVR is at its lowest. When FRC is "too low" or "too high," there is a rise in PVR resulting in an impediment to pulmonary blood flow (Fig. 15.2). A significantly decreased FRC may be encountered in viral or bacterial respiratory infections resulting in atelectasis. A high FRC may be a result of air trapping (e.g., asthma, bronchiolitis) or from excessive positive end-expiratory pressure (PEEP) delivered via mechanical ventilation.

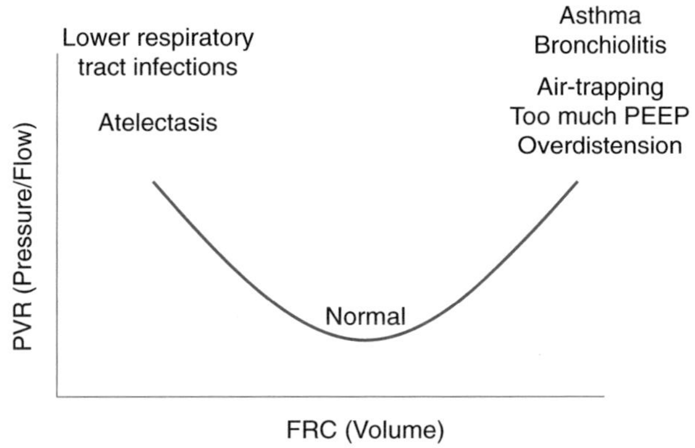

Fig. 15.2 At normal functional residual capacity, pulmonary vascular resistance (PVR) is the lowest. PVR rises at too low (atelectasis) and too high (overdistension) FRC

Effects of Abnormalities in Arterial Blood Gases and Acid-Base Balance on Cardiac Function: In addition to the negative inotropic effects of hypoxia and acidosis on the myocardium, arterial blood gas and the acid-base status have significant effects on PVR. Hypercarbia, hypoxia, and acidosis are potent pulmonary vasoconstrictors posing additional burden on the RV and also increasing resistance to passive pulmonary circulation in patients after Fontan operation. An increase in arterial PO2 on the other hand leads to pulmonary vasodilatation and decreased PVR. An excessively decreased PVR may result in increased left-to-right shunting in lesions with systemic to pulmonary communication or diversion of systemic blood flow to pulmonary circulation in a functionally univentricular heart.

Influence of Mean Systemic Venous Pressure on Pulmonary Blood Flow: In patients who have had bidirectional Glenn procedure or Fontan surgery, the pulmonary circulation flows passively from a higher mean systemic venous pressure (MSVP) to a lower intrathoracic pulmonary circulation. Such children are vulnerable to decreased pulmonary flow and therefore the cardiac output in three distinct situations: [1] a fall in MSVP; [2] a rise in pressure in the intrathoracic portion of systemic veins, pulmonary arteries, and pulmonary veins; and [3] a rise in intrathoracic pressure. A fall in MSVP occurs in any condition resulting in hypovolemia such as dehydration and sepsis. A rise in pressure in the intrathoracic systemic venous system and the pulmonary circulation may be associated with thromboembolic disease, myocardial dysfunction, or respiratory infection. A global rise in intrathoracic pressure may occur with abnormal fluid accumulation such as a pleural effusion, air trapping due to airway obstruction, or therapeutic intervention such as application of positive end-expiratory pressure (PEEP).

Objectives

1. Review the clinical presentation of common pediatric diseases such as bronchiolitis, croup, and acute gastroenteritis and their effects on the underlying pathophysiology of the heart lesion
2. Discuss the management of these common illnesses in a child with heart disease

3. Take-home points for management concerns in respiratory illness and gastroenteritis in a child with underlying heart disease

Bronchiolitis

Case Vignette: *A 4-month-old patient with unrepaired ventricular septal defect (VSD) presents to the ED with runny nose, congestion, and cough for the last 3 days. Mom states that he is taking longer to feed and is breathing "hard." She says that the baby chokes and gags with coughing but denies any color change or apnea. On physical examination, vital signs are as follows: temperature of 38.3 °C, heart rate of 180/min, respirations of 70/min, blood pressure of 82/50 mmHg, and oxygen saturation of 91% in room air. Child is tachypneic with moderate intercostal and subcostal retractions with bilateral wheezing. A grade 3/6 holosystolic murmur is heard along the left sternal border. Peripheral pulses are well felt and capillary refill is 2 s. Abdominal exam reveals a liver edge palpated 3 cm below right costal margin.*

Bronchiolitis is one of the leading causes of hospitalizations among infants and accounts for between 57,000 and 172,000 hospitalizations annually with healthcare costs for hospital admissions exceeding $1.7 billion in children less than 2 years of age. Although a diverse group of viruses can cause bronchiolitis, respiratory syncytial virus (RSV) and rhinovirus are the two most common pathogens. Typically, infants present with upper respiratory tract infection symptoms and signs of respiratory distress with crackles or wheezing. Infants less than 3 months of age are also prone to apnea.

Nearly one-half of hospital admissions related to acute respiratory tract infections in infants with heart disease are secondary to bronchiolitis. Children with heart disease and RSV bronchiolitis have been shown to have a higher rate of hospitalization, longer length of hospital stay, higher severity of illness as judged by the need for intensive care admission (63% vs. 14%) and invasive ventilation (22% vs. 0.5%), and a significantly higher mortality rate (37% vs. 1.5%) compared to those without heart disease [7, 8]. Patients with congestive heart failure, cyanosis, and pulmonary hypertension are particularly prone to higher morbidity and mortality from bronchiolitis.

Airway obstruction associated with bronchiolitis can result in wide intrathoracic pressure fluctuations during respiration and increased left ventricular afterload. Dynamic hyperinflation and auto-PEEP may result in a decrease in systemic venous return which in turn can lead to reduction in cardiac output. Further, hyperinflation can increase PVR resulting in increased RV afterload. Pulmonary hypertension can be worsened by hypoxia and acidosis which in turn impairs cardiac output.

Patients with single ventricle physiology after Norwood procedure present to the ED with worsening hypoxia secondary to respiratory infections. While providing supplemental oxygen to these patients, it is important to maintain the oxygen saturation between 75% and 80% to balance pulmonary and systemic blood flows. Patients with functionally univentricular heart physiology after Glenn procedure are more likely to present to the ED with cyanosis. Since the pulmonary blood flow is passive in these patients, a decrease in systemic venous return secondary to relative hypovolemia due to poor fluid intake or increase in pulmonary vascular resistance can result in oxygen desaturation. In such patients, supplemental oxygen will decrease the pulmonary vascular resistance promoting pulmonary blood flow.

Bronchiolitis is usually diagnosed clinically. Although there are no studies about work-up of fever specifically in children with heart disease and bronchiolitis, the risk of serious bacterial infections (such as bacteremia and meningitis) other than urinary tract infections has been shown to be low (about 1%) in children with bronchiolitis and fever. Serum B-natriuretic peptide (BNP) concentrations have been shown to be useful in diagnosing heart failure in children with heart disease who present with respiratory distress. In a prospective cohort study of children with heart disease and bronchiolitis, those children with heart failure had a higher level of BNP when compared to those who did not have heart failure [9].

Most of the patients with heart disease and bronchiolitis will require admission to the hospital for observation given their high-risk status and severe clinical course. Younger infants, those with heart failure and acyanotic heart disease requiring medications or surgery, tend to have a particularly more severe clinical course. Other risk factors for hospitalization in children with underlying heart disease include children with chromosomal abnormalities such as trisomy 21, cardiomyopathy, and hemodynamically significant heart disease.

The main treatment for bronchiolitis is supportive care with oxygen and hydration. Fluids should be used judiciously in children with congestive heart failure. Those children with underlying heart disease who are preload dependent for their cardiac output would benefit from cautious IV hydration with aliquots of 5 mL/kg normal saline with close monitoring of vital signs and clinical signs for heart failure. While oxygen administration is beneficial in children who are hypoxic secondary to a respiratory tract infection, it should be used with caution and only to maintain the oxygen saturation at the patient's baseline level. In those patients with left-sided obstructive lesions and parallel circulations (Norwood, Hybrid), achieving a high O_2 saturation (>85%) with supplemental oxygen can result in decrease in PVR with increased pulmonary blood flow at the expense of systemic perfusion and organ ischemia. In those patients with parallel circulations, the systemic (Qs) and pulmonary (Qp) blood flows must be balanced, with an optimal systemic oxygen saturation of 75–85% reflecting a Qp:Qs of 1.

There is no role for administration of bronchodilators in the ED in children with bronchiolitis. Use of bronchodilators, in addition to lack of beneficial effect, may be especially harmful in children with underlying heart disease as the tachycardia associated with such treatment may further increase myocardial oxygen consumption. Beta-agonist therapy has been associated with tachyarrhythmias, congestive heart failure, myocardial ischemia, and cardiac arrest. These risks are higher in children with heart disease. Nebulized hypertonic saline (3%) therapy has been suggested by some for its presumed effects of reduction in airway edema and mucus plugging and improved mucociliary clearance. However, there are currently no studies that have evaluated the effect of nebulized hypertonic saline specifically in children with heart disease and bronchiolitis.

Heated, humidified, high-flow nasal cannula (HFNC) therapy has emerged as an important noninvasive modality of respiratory support and has been shown to significantly reduce the need for mechanical ventilation in children with bronchiolitis [10]. HFNC allows for the delivery of high inspired gas flows, with or without an increased oxygen concentration providing continuous positive airway pressure which helps to overcome upper airway obstruction as well reduction of inspiratory resistance in the work of breathing. HFNC provides for washout of the nasopharyngeal dead space resulting in alveolar ventilation as a greater fraction of minute ventilation resulting in improvement in the work of breathing [11]. Furthermore, providing adequately warmed and humidified oxygen improves conductance and pulmonary compliance. HFNC is well tolerated when compared to nasal continuous positive airway pressure (CPAP). The optimal flow for HFNC therapy has not been established and varies from 4–8 l/min depending on the age, the weight, and the respiratory status of the child. Adverse events related to HFNC therapy are rare although pneumothorax, abdominal distention, and mucosal injury with nasal bleeding have been reported.

The need for mechanical ventilation has been shown to be two times higher in children with RSV infection and underlying heart disease than those without heart disease. Mechanical ventilation reduces the work of breathing and the metabolic demands while improving hypoxia and hypercarbia. In infants with left-to-right shunting, with excessive pulmonary blood flow, positive-pressure ventilation increases the pulmonary vascular resistance and decreases intracardiac shunting leading to an improvement in systemic blood flow. Further, in this group of patients, positive-pressure ventilation along with PEEP decreases alveolar water content and improves gas exchange. These beneficial effects should be weighed against the deleterious effects of decrease in systemic venous return which could result in a decrease in cardiac output. Patients who have had a Fontan or a bidirectional Glenn procedure are especially intolerant of decreases in preload associated with positive-pressure ventilation.

Croup

Case Vignette: A 2-year-old male with history of mild aortic stenosis with a bicuspid aortic valve presents to the ED with a new-onset barky cough, stridor, and fever. The child had a prodrome of coryzal symptoms for 2 days prior to presentation. Vital signs are as follows: temperature 38.4 °C, heart rate 154/min, respirations 54/min, and pulse oximetry of 89% on room air. Physical examination reveals an agitated, crying cyanotic child, with severe dyspnea and audible stridor. As the child is calmed, the cyanosis resolves but the stridor persists. His lung fields are clear. Cardiac examination reveals tachycardia with a II/VI systolic murmur at the left lower sternal border with good peripheral pulses and capillary refill less than 2 s. Abdominal examination is normal with no evidence of organomegaly.

Croup, or laryngotracheobronchitis, is a common viral illness responsible for up to 15% of ED visits for respiratory illness. A retrospective study of patients presenting to the ED with fever and underlying heart disease found that croup represented 1.2% of visits for respiratory illness [5]. Croup is caused by parainfluenza virus, adenovirus, influenza, and respiratory syncytial virus and presents with an upper respiratory tract infection, low-grade fever, and coryza followed by a barking cough. The degree of respiratory distress due to the subglottic narrowing can be variable, but the illness itself is usually self-limited with resolution of symptoms within a few days. Children aged 6–36 months are most severely affected.

Children with heart disease, either pre-repair or at any stage in their repair, are at an increased risk of compromised cardiac output due to the excessive increase in the negative intrathoracic pressure during inspiration. Adequate airway management and effective ventilation are important. Children with heart disease and croup may have worsened hypoxia, especially if they have an underlying cyanotic heart condition. In such patients, oxygen should be utilized to target their baseline oxygen saturations. The increase in negative intrathoracic pressure leads to an increase in afterload that imposes extra demands on a potentially poorly functioning ventricle or functionally univentricular heart. The dominant effects of mechanical ventilation are to decrease the left ventricular afterload. Thus, in a child with croup and airway obstruction, the use of judicious intubation and positive-pressure ventilation helps counteract the increased negative intrathoracic pressures seen with obstructed inspiration. The management of croup in a child with univentricular physiology necessitates close monitoring for potential hypoxia and worsening obstruction with a low threshold for early intubation. In children with heart disease, a history of prior intubations, prolonged neonatal ventilation, and genetic conditions such as Down syndrome, there may be an underlying subglottic narrowing. Thus, the use of dexamethasone, recommended in all children with croup, is especially useful in children with heart disease. The use of racemic epinephrine nebulization along with dexamethasone is recommended in children with croup who present with stridor at rest. Racemic epinephrine therapy should be closely monitored for its adverse effects such as tachycardia. Racemic epinephrine works twofold to cause mucosal vasoconstriction and beta-2 agonist activity leading to smooth bronchial muscle relaxation. Hospitalization is indicated for patients with (1) severe respiratory distress, (2) stridor at rest, and (3) hypoxia below baseline oxygen saturation and (4) those requiring repeated racemic epinephrine nebulizations.

Gastroenteritis

Case Vignette: Paramedics bring in a 16-year-old male with a history of Fontan surgery for tricuspid atresia. He has a 2-day history of nausea, vomiting, and diarrhea and feels weak and lightheaded. Upon arrival to the ED, his temperature is 36.7 °C, heart rate 127/min, respirations 16/min, BP 85/34 mmHg, and pulse oximetry 84% in room air. His baseline saturations are 93% on room air. On examination, the patient appears somnolent with dry mucous membranes and sunken eyes. He has clear breath sounds with no increased work of breathing. He has a well-healed sternotomy scar and a loud holosystolic murmur. He has poor perfusion and capillary refill at approximately 4 s. Abdominal exam is normal with no organomegaly.

This patient presents with acute dehydration noted by changes in mental status, with compromised perfusion as well as hypoxia. Dehydration can affect cardiac output by decreasing the preload or the diastolic loading of the heart. Cardiac output is further compromised in a child with poor cardiac contractility and ventricular compliance. With a Fontan procedure, the patient is particularly vulnerable to decreased cardiac output because of dehydration with predilection to hypoxia from compromised pulmonary blood flow. After a Fontan or a bidirectional Glenn procedure, the systemic venous blood flow is routed to the pulmonary circulation passively without the benefit of a contracting chamber. In such a situation, hypovolemia and decreased MSVP leads to a decreased driving force for the passive pulmonary circulation. Thus, increasing the MSVP with a normal saline fluid bolus is necessary to improve the pulmonary blood flow and increase oxygen saturation. While addressing dehydration with a fluid bolus is essential, close monitoring for signs of volume overload is necessary in a child with known heart disease due to potential for congestive heart failure. Rehydration should be conducted in frequent, small increments of 5–10 mL/kg of normal saline until clinical improvement in heart rate, oxygen saturation, perfusion, and mental status is noted.

In cyanotic heart disease or after a Norwood procedure, pulmonary circulation is dependent on a systemic to pulmonary shunt such as a Blalock-Taussig shunt. Dehydration and the resultant hyper viscosity may predispose to thrombosis within the shunt. Thus, acute dehydration should be promptly treated with volume resuscitation and further investigation, including an echocardiogram if a shunt obstruction is suspected.

Multiple Choice Questions

1. A 4-week-old infant with hypoplastic left heart syndrome (HLHS) s/p the Norwood procedure presents to the ED with poor feeding, easy fatigue, and nasal congestion noted over 3 days. Vital signs were as follows: temperature 38.9 °C, HR 174/min, RR 70/min, BP 74/40 mmHg, and SpO_2 65% on room air (base 75%). Physical examination reveals a tired, pale, cyanotic, listless infant with copious rhinorrhea, labored breathing, retractions, diffuse wheezing, and crackles. He is tachycardic and hypoxic with a continuous murmur and capillary refill time of 2 s. His respiratory syncytial virus (RSV) swab is positive. His CXR demonstrates mild stable cardiomegaly with stable minimal pulmonary vascular congestion. Most recent echocardiogram after his Norwood surgery demonstrated normal single right ventricular function. What is the next best step in management?
   (A) Oxygen therapy to maintain SpO_2 around 75%
   (B) Immediate intubation
   (C) Albuterol nebulization
   (D) IV fluid bolus
   (E) Dobutamine infusion

Answer: A. After stage 1 palliation for HLHS, there are three common causes of cyanosis: (a) blockage of the Blalock-Taussig shunt, (b) pulmonary parenchymal disease, and (c) acute increase in pulmonary vascular resistance. In this case, the baby with a stage 1 palliative repair has hypoxemia due to V/Q abnormalities from bronchiolitis.

Management considerations are primarily supportive in nature with the goal of maintaining the patient's baseline oxygen saturations with care taken to avoid pulmonary over-circulation from oxygen saturations that are higher than baseline (>80–85%). Hypoxia resulting from respiratory tract infections, such as bronchiolitis, results in pulmonary vasoconstriction, increased pulmonary vascular resistance, and reduction in pulmonary blood flow. Thus, hypoxemia needs to be corrected to improve oxygen delivery. The supplemental oxygen should however be titrated to keep SpO_2 around 75% to maintain an acceptable balance between pulmonary and systemic blood flows. Endotracheal intubation and mechanical ventilation would be appropriate if the child develops hypercarbia, exhaustion, or apnea. Careful fluid resuscitation with 5–10 mL/kg of normal saline over 10–15 min with frequent assessment of signs of systemic improvement in perfusion such as decrease in heart rate, improved pulses, and improved capillary refill time should be conducted. The use of inotropic support is not indicated as the infant is presenting with primary pulmonary disease with stable blood pressure and perfusion. However, institution of dobutamine (5–10 μg/kg/min) and afterload reduction with milrinone (0.3–0.7 μg/kg/min) infusions are appropriate with persistent signs of poor perfusion or cardiac function. Both inotropes can be safely administered even via peripheral intravenous access.

2. In the above patient, after providing supplemental oxygen, there is no improvement in oxygen saturation, and the continuous murmur is no longer audible. The child is no longer responsive. Vital signs are as follows: temperature 38.9 °C, HR 50/min, RR 6/min and shallow, BP 35/19 mmHg, and SpO_2 40% on HFNC. What is the most likely cause of the clinical deterioration?
   (A) Decreased pulmonary vascular resistance
   (B) Increased pulmonary blood flow
   (C) Thrombosed B-T shunt
   (D) Under resuscitated sepsis
   (E) Worsened V/Q mismatch

   Answer: C. In this scenario, severe cyanosis would indicate compromised pulmonary blood flow via either a narrow or partially thrombosed BT shunt. Management includes an urgent echocardiogram and immediate referral to interventional cardiology for opening the occluded BT shunt if diagnosed as such. The ED physician can also consider starting the patient on a heparin drip.

3. A 6-month-old child s/p hybrid repair for HLHS presents to the ED for respiratory distress. Mother notes a barky cough and noisy breathing. Vital signs: temperature 36.9 °C, HR 190/min, RR 56/min, BP 45/25 mmHg, and SpO_2 94% on 100% non-rebreather. Physical examination reveals a child who is tachycardic

with a continuous murmur and capillary refill of approximately 4 s with poor peripheral pulses. Lungs are noted to be clear. What is the most appropriate next step in management?
(A) Start inhaled nitric oxide
(B) Start dobutamine infusion
(C) Stop supplemental oxygen
(D) Administer broad-spectrum antibiotics
(E) Intubate and provide positive-pressure ventilation
Answer: C. This infant has viral laryngotracheobronchitis or croup. The most important first step would be to stop the use of supplemental oxygen as it causes pulmonary over-circulation leading to compromise of systemic perfusion which this child exhibits with poor peripheral pulses and hypotension. The use of inhaled nitric oxide would further increase pulmonary circulation by pulmonary vasodilatation and compromise systemic perfusion. Dobutamine infusion is not warranted as the underlying physiology of hypotension is due to pulmonary over-circulation and systemic under-perfusion rather than ventricular failure. The use of broad-spectrum antibiotics is not indicated in this scenario. Intubation may eventually be required; however, the first step should be to stop supplemental oxygen unless the child was presenting with hypoxia beyond baseline values. Intubation should be considered early in a child with severe obstruction or refractory hypoxia to alleviate the markedly increased negative intrathoracic pressures generated with upper airway obstruction as this increased afterload is poorly tolerated by a functionally univentricular heart.

4. A 16-year-old boy presents to the ED with cyanosis. He was in his usual state of health until he developed nausea, vomiting, and diarrhea on the day of presentation. He has a history of HLHS s/p three open heart surgeries, the last one occurring at 3 years of age. Parents report good ventricular function in the recent echocardiogram. His oxygen saturations are normally in the 90s. Vital signs: T 37.0 °C, HR 100/min, RR 24/min, BP 85/50 mmHg, and SpO_2 78% on room air. Physical examination reveals mild respiratory distress, good air entry, no crackles, and no hepatomegaly. He has cool extremities and capillary refill of 3 s. On 100% non-rebreather, saturations increase to 81%. What is next best step in management?
(A) Furosemide 0.5 mg/kg IVPB
(B) Normal saline 20 mL/kg bolus
(C) Dobutamine infusion
(D) Endotracheal intubation and mechanical ventilation
(E) Bi-level positive airway pressure
Answer: B. This patient has gastroenteritis with underlying Fontan repair. The correct therapy for this patient includes treatment with normal saline fluid bolus to increase mean systemic venous pressure and improve pulmonary blood flow. With a Fontan procedure, the patient is particularly vulnerable to dehydration and can develop significant hypoxia due to limited pulmonary blood flow. Thus, in this scenario, administering a fluid bolus will help increase his oxygen saturations by increasing the passive pulmonary blood flow. Intubation or providing

positive-pressure ventilation might exacerbate the underlying hypoxia by increasing the intrathoracic pressure, increasing pulmonary vascular resistance, and diminishing pulmonary circulation. IV furosemide would further exacerbate the dehydration. While the use of inotropes may be required, especially if the cardiac function is impaired, the utility of inotropic support is optimized after adequate hydration and intravascular repletion.

5. A 6-month-old boy presents to the ED with poor feeding, irritability, and weight loss. He was born at home with a midwife delivery. He is exclusively breastfed and mom reports progressively worsening easy fatigability with feeds, diaphoresis, and increased work of breathing. Vital signs: temperature 37.4 °C, HR 180/min, RR 64/min, BP 75/40 mmHg, and SpO_2 98% in room air. Physical examination reveals a pale and sweaty infant in moderate respiratory distress and good air entry without any crackles or wheezes. On cardiac examination, he is noted to be tachycardic, with a S3 gallop rhythm and a holosystolic murmur. He is noted to have hepatomegaly and cool, mottled extremities with a cap refill at 4 s. Chest x-ray demonstrates cardiomegaly and pulmonary edema. What is best next step in management?
   (A) High-flow nasal cannula with 40% oxygen
   (B) 0.9% sodium chloride 20 mL/kg bolus
   (C) Furosemide 0.5 mg/kg IV
   (D) Endotracheal intubation and mechanical ventilation
   (E) Epinephrine 0.05ug/kg/min

   Answer C. The physical examination suggests a left-to-right shunt and pulmonary over-circulation such as a ventricular septal defect (VSD). The patient has congestive heart failure, and diuretics such as furosemide will reduce preload and improve congestive symptoms. In this case, the use of a 20 mL/kg normal saline bolus would exacerbate the congestive heart failure and worsen respiratory failure and cardiogenic shock. The use of peripheral epinephrine as an adrenergic inotrope is generally reserved for infants who remain in severe cardiogenic shock despite the use of dopamine or dobutamine. While intubation and securing the airway may be necessary, at this point, the infant is maintaining his airway and optimizing the infant's hemodynamic status prior to any potential intubation is the preferred management option.

Conflicts of Interest *Disclosures*: The authors have not disclosed any potential conflicts of interest.

References

1. Abu-Harb M, Hey E, Wren C. Death in infancy from unrecognized congenital heart disease. Arch Dis Child. 1994;71:3–7.
2. Savitsky E, Alejos J, Votey S. Emergency department presentations of pediatric congenital heart disease. J Emerg Med. 2003;24:239–45.
3. Lee YS, Baek JS, Kwon BS, et al. Pediatric emergency room presentation of congenital heart disease. Korean Circ J. 2010;40(1):36–41.
4. Cashen K, Gupta P, Lieh-Lai M, et al. Infants with single ventricle physiology in the emergency department: are physicians prepared? J Pediatr. 2011;159(2):273–7.

5. Tibbles CD, Bouton M, Lucas JM, et al. Emergency department management of pediatric patients with cyanotic heart disease and fever. J Emerg Med. 2013;44(3):599–604.
6. Chauhan M, Mastropietro CW. Hypoplastic left heart syndrome in the emergency department: an update. J Emerg Med. 2014;46(2):51–4.
7. MacDonald NE, Hall CB, Suffin SC, et al. Respiratory syncytial viral infection in infants with congenital heart disease. N Engl J Med. 1982;307(7):397–400.
8. Thorburn K. Pre-existing disease is associated with a significantly higher risk of death in severe respiratory syncytial virus infection. Arch Dis Child. 2009;94(2):99–103.
9. Samuel N, Hershokovitz T, Brik R, et al. Diagnosing heart failure in children with congenital heart disease and respiratory syncytial virus bronchiolitis. Am J Emerg Med. 2014;32(12):1510–2.
10. Ganu SS, Gautam A, Wilkins B, Egan J. Increase in use of non-invasive ventilation for infants with severe bronchiolitis is associated with decline in intubation rates over a decade. Intensive Care Med. 2012;38(7):1177–83.
11. Dysart K, Miller TL, Wolfson MR, Shaffer TH. Research in high flow therapy: mechanisms of action. Respir Med. 2009;103(10):1400–5.

Recognizing and Managing Cardiogenic Shock

16

Saurabh Chiwane, Usha Sethuraman, and Ajit Sarnaik

Vignette 1: A 7-Year-Old Boy with Influenza
A 7-year-old boy presented to the ED with a 3-day history of fever, difficulty breathing, and muscle pain. Influenza A had been diagnosed at another hospital the day before. He was started on oseltamivir. His vital signs in the ED were: temperature, 39.2 °C; pulse, 180 bpm; respirations, 30/min; blood pressure, 88/67; and oxygen saturation, 100% in room air. After 2 h and two bolus infusions of fluids of 1 l each, his vital signs in the ED were: temperature, 36.5 °C; pulse, 150 bpm; respirations, 48/min; blood pressure, 91/52; and oxygen saturation, 100% in room air. He now has bibasilar fine crackles and wheezing. He is alert and still in moderate respiratory distress, with a capillary refill time of 4 s.

Concepts and Mechanisms of Cardiogenic Shock

Shock

Shock is an acute failure of the cardiovascular system to meet the metabolic demands of the tissues, namely, delivery of substrate and removal of metabolic waste. Inadequate tissue oxygenation leads to anaerobic metabolism and acidosis and eventually loss of cellular function [1].

S. Chiwane, M.B.B.S., M.D. (✉) • A. Sarnaik, M.D.
Critical Care Medicine, Children's Hospital of Michigan, Wayne State University School of Medicine, Detroit, MI, USA
e-mail: asarnai@med.wayne.edu

U. Sethuraman, M.D.
Pediatric Emergency Medicine, Children's Hospital of Michigan, Wayne State University School of Medicine, Detroit, MI, USA
e-mail: USethura@dmc.org

© Springer International Publishing AG, part of Springer Nature 2018
A. P. Sarnaik et al. (eds.), *Cardiac Emergencies in Children*,
https://doi.org/10.1007/978-3-319-73754-6_16

Table 16.1 Causes of cardiogenic shock, by typical age of occurrence

Age	Causes of cardiogenic shock	
Day 1 of life	• Birth asphyxia congenital heart disease – TAPVR with obstruction – TGA with IVS with restricted atrial septum – HLHS with restricted atrial septum	• Sepsis • Fetal/neonatal myocarditis • Hypocalcemia • Hypoglycemia • Brady/tachyarrhythmia
First week of life	• Ductal-dependent systemic circulation – HLHS – Critical aortic stenosis – Interrupted aortic arch	• Congenital adrenal insufficiency and inborn errors of metabolism • Sepsis
2–6 weeks	• Ventricular septal defects • Complete AV canal defects • Aortopulmonary window • Truncus arteriosus • Unobstructed TAPVR • Persistent PDA	• ALCAPA • Coarctation of Aorta • Pompe's disease • Sepsis • Myocarditis/cardiomyopathy
6 weeks to 1 year	• Coarctation of aorta, Aortic stenosis, sepsis • Kawasaki disease	• Dysfunction of repaired/palliated congenital heart disease • Infective endocarditis
Older children and adolescents	• Arrhythmias • Acute rheumatic fever • Infective endocarditis • Acute aortic insufficiency • Cardiomyopathy • Drug ingestions: calcium channel and beta-blockers • Hypertensive emergency	• Dysfunction of repaired/palliated congenital heart disease – Fontan baffle obstruction – Atrioventricular valve regurgitation – Aortic arch obstruction

TAPVR total anomalous pulmonary venous return, *TGA* transposition of the great arteries, *IVS* intact ventricular septum, *HLHS* hypoplastic left heart syndrome, *AV* atrioventricular, *PDA* patent ductus arteriosus, *ALCAPA* anomalous left coronary artery from the pulmonary artery
N.B. Arrhythmias, myocarditis, cardiomyopathies, sepsis, and electrolyte disturbances can cause cardiogenic shock at all ages

Cardiogenic Shock

Cardiogenic shock is an acute state of end-organ hypoperfusion following cardiac failure [2]. It occurs from various etiologies leading to primary pump failure, with or without contributions from inadequate preload or afterload (Table 16.1).

Oxygen Demand

Oxygen demand is the amount of oxygen necessary to meet the metabolic requirements of all body tissues. Tissues and organs demand oxygen, but they are unable to store it.

Oxygen Consumption

Oxygen consumption is the amount of oxygen used by the tissues. It is the difference between the oxygen delivered by the arterial system and the amount of oxygen returned to the heart by the venous system. In healthy individuals, oxygen consumption is equal to oxygen demand.

Oxygen Delivery (Fig. 16.1)

Oxygen delivery is the product of

Cardiac output (**CO**) × **arterial oxygen content** (**CaO$_2$**),where cardiac output is the product of **heart rate** × **stroke volume**. Any imbalance between oxygen delivery and oxygen demand may lead to shock.

Causes of Decreased Oxygen Delivery

A. Decreased cardiac output: Cardiac output can be reduced by decreased preload (e.g., hypovolemia), decreased contractility (e.g., of myocarditis), increased afterload (e.g., coarctation of the aorta), and atrioventricular asynchrony (e.g., complete heart block) (Fig. 16.2).

Causes of Decreased Arterial Oxygen Content

B. Arterial oxygen content can be decreased by anemia, abnormal hemoglobin concentrations (carboxyhemoglobin, methemoglobin), shifts in oxygen hemoglobin dissociation curve, and acute hypoxemic respiratory failure.

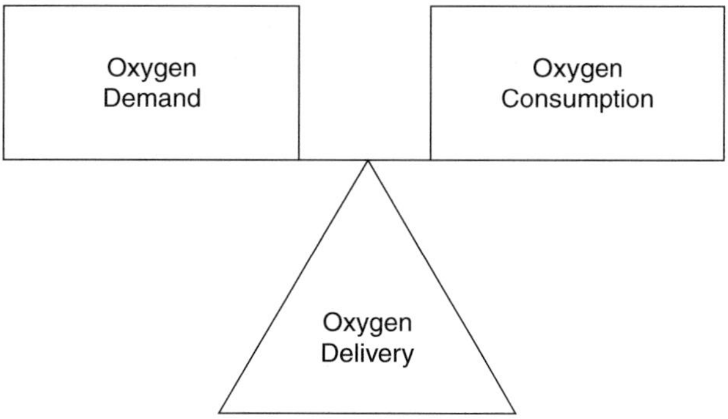

Fig. 16.1 Oxygen delivery balances oxygen demand and oxygen consumption

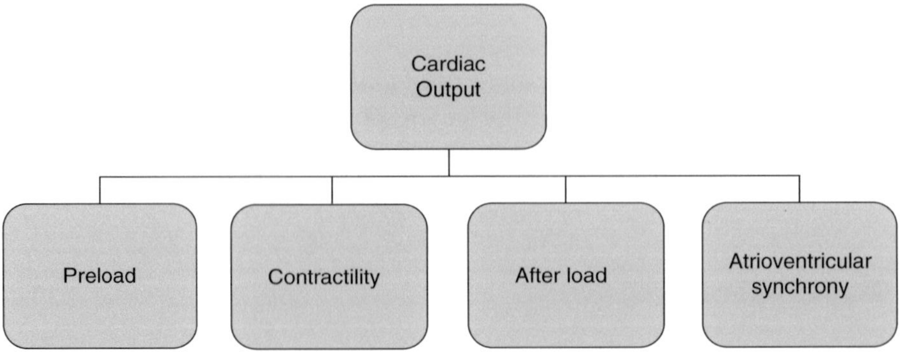

Fig. 16.2 Factors affecting cardiac output. Cardiac output depends on preload, afterload, myocardial contractility, and atrioventricular synchrony. Any disease affecting any of these determinants can reduce cardiac output

Differences in the Myocardia of Neonates and Children

Neonates tend to have a limited ability to increase stroke volume in response to a fluid bolus (preload). Myocardial contractility is already maximized; hence, cardiac output is predominantly rate-dependent. In contrast, children and adolescents have a greater ability to increase myocardial contractility and stroke volume in response to a fluid bolus. Several histopathological features that make the neonatal myocardium less compliant and less responsive to preload [4] explain these physiologic differences.

In neonates:

1. The myocardium is relatively deficient in mitochondria.
2. The cellular densities of actin, myosin, and ATPase are decreased.
3. Intracellular water is excessive.
4. Cardiac myocytes tend to be spherical instead of the normal bullet shape, which is a mechanical disadvantage in contractility.
5. Contractile filaments are disorganized.
6. The myocardium has less compact connective tissue.

Diagnosing Cardiogenic Shock

A thorough history and physical examination, close attention to vital signs and response to therapies such as fluid challenges, and frequent clinical assessments will help make the diagnosis of cardiogenic shock. No single diagnostic laboratory test or imaging modality will confirm the diagnosis; the diagnosis is based on a high clinical index of suspicion (Tables 16.2 and 16.3).

Table 16.2 Symptoms and causes of cardiogenic shock

Symptom	Pathophysiology
Feeding difficulty	• Fatigue from low stroke volume • Pulmonary congestion from increased LVEDP
Failure to thrive	• Poor calorie intake from feeding difficulty • Increased myocardial and respiratory muscle caloric demand
Irritability or lethargy	• Decreased oxygen delivery to the brain • Myocardial ischemia
Dyspnea	• Pulmonary congestion
Palpitations	• Tachycardia, bradycardia, or arrhythmias
Sweating	• Increased sympathetic activity
Abdominal pain, vomiting	• Congestive hepatomegaly • Bowel ischemia

LVEDP left ventricular end-diastolic pressure

Table 16.3 Signs and pathophysiologic mechanisms of cardiogenic shock

Sign	Pathophysiology
Cold extremities weak distal pulses prolonged capillary refill	• Vasoconstriction • Tissue hypoperfusion
Disproportionate tachycardia	• Sympathetic overactivity • Rate-dependent cardiac output
Tachypnea	• Lung tissue J receptor stimulation in response to increased pulmonary venous pressures leading to interstitial congestion
Narrow pulse pressure	• Systemic vasoconstriction, decreased stroke volume
Crepitations	• Increased pulmonary venous pressures leading to alveolar edema
Dependent edema and hepatomegaly	• Elevated right atrial pressure leading to passive venous congestion
Gallop rhythm	• S3: Ventricular dilatation from volume overload • S4: Ventricular hypertrophy from pressure overload

Disproportionate Tachycardia

In Vignette 1, the boy has a heart rate of 180 bpm, which is significantly elevated for a 7-year-old child. He also has fever of 39.2 °C, and tachycardia is often attributed to fever. However, for every 1 °C rise in temperature, the heart rate increases by 10 bpm. Hence, this child's heart rate is elevated disproportionately to the degree of fever. Indeed, sinus tachycardia in cardiogenic shock is often disproportionate to the degree of fever, pain, activity, or anxiety. When in doubt, one should always confirm sinus tachycardia with an electrocardiogram. Arrhythmias are also a frequent cause of disproportionate tachycardia and may be the sole cause of cardiogenic shock.

Blood Pressure

Blood pressure is often maintained until late in the development of any kind of shock in children:

$$\textbf{Blood pressure} = \textbf{cardiac output} \times \textbf{systemic vascular resistance}$$

Although cardiac output declines in cardiogenic shock, blood pressure is often maintained because systemic vascular resistance is increased. Marked tissue hypoxia can occur in the setting of normal blood pressure. The boy in Vignette 1 is normotensive, with a BP of 88/67 mmHg, yet he is in shock. The 5th percentile for systolic blood pressure for a 7-year old is 84 mmHg [70 + (2 × age in years)].

Pulse Pressure

Pulse pressure is the difference between systolic and diastolic blood pressure.

Pulse pressure depends on stroke volume and arterial compliance and so is better defined as [5]:

$$\textbf{Pulse pressure} = \textbf{stroke volume} / \textbf{artery compliance}$$

Hence, as stroke volume drops in cardiogenic shock, pulse pressure narrows. In Vignette 1, the boy has a narrow pulse pressure (88–67 mmHg = 21 mmHg), which can be seen in hypovolemic or cardiogenic shock. In distributive shock, pulse pressure is usually wide.

Wheezing

Wheezing is a very common sign in the ED, especially during winter when EDs see large numbers of children with bronchiolitis. Monophonic left lung wheezing in cardiogenic shock is often caused by a large left atrium compressing the left mainstem bronchus. Polyphonic wheezing is usually caused by bronchioles that are narrowed from engorged capillaries or by interstitial edema secondary to elevated left atrial pressures. Wheezing can be a sign of left ventricular dysfunction. Failure to recognize wheezing as a sign of LV dysfunction can inadvertently lead to the administration of albuterol, which can often worsen LV dysfunction by inducing tachycardia and increasing myocardial oxygen consumption without increasing global and myocardial oxygen delivery (Figs. 16.3 and 16.4).

Vignette 1: Response to Therapy

After 2 h and two fluid boluses, the boy was reassessed in the ED. He was normothermic, normotensive, and tachycardic (although his pulse rate improved, from 180 to 150 bpm). His pulse pressure had improved, but his tachypnea had worsened. After fluid administration, signs of pulmonary congestion developed, which is a detrimental response to fluid therapy and could have been avoided by careful

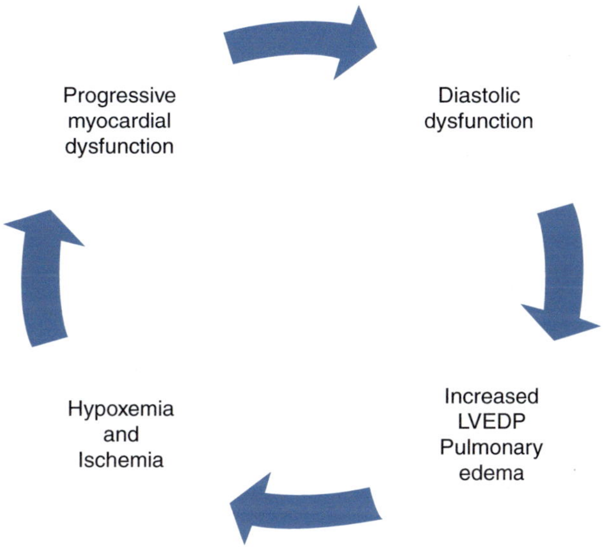

Fig. 16.3 Diastolic dysfunction can increase ventricular end-diastolic pressure. Increased left ventricular end-diastolic pressure (LVEDP) can in turn lead to pulmonary edema, causing hypoxemia. Increased right ventricular end-diastolic pressure will in turn decrease coronary perfusion pressure. A combination of myocardial and end-organ ischemia and hypoxia will lead to multi-organ dysfunction [3]

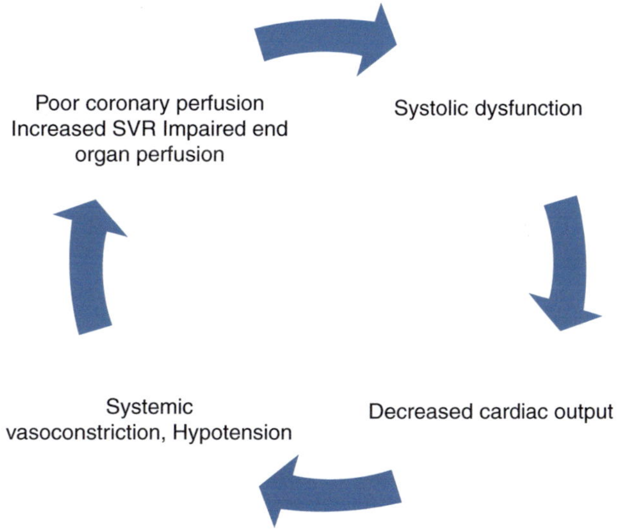

Fig. 16.4 Systolic dysfunction reduces cardiac output, which in turn leads to poor coronary perfusion and systemic vasoconstriction. The combination of myocardial ischemia and increased systemic vascular resistance (SVR) leads to further systolic dysfunction [3]

attention to his admission vital signs. Such attention could have resulted in an earlier diagnosis. Frequent reassessments are critical to determining the response to therapy.

Treating Cardiogenic Shock

The basic tenet of treating any kind of shock is to optimize (not maximize) oxygen delivery to meet oxygen demand. Two principles should be followed: improving oxygen delivery and decreasing oxygen demand.

Oxygen Delivery

Oxygen delivery can be increased by optimizing preload with diuretics or judicious fluid administration, improving contractility with inotropic agents or by optimizing electrolyte balance, gently reducing afterload with vasodilators or positive pressure ventilation (PPV), and improving AV synchrony with anti-arrhythmic therapy. These measures improve oxygen delivery by improving cardiac output. **Arterial oxygen carrying capacity** can be increased by improving oxygenation in the lungs or by improving hemoglobin concentrations.

Oxygen Demand

Oxygen demand can be decreased by reducing the work of the respiratory muscles with PPV, decreasing or preventing fever or pain, or by sedating (including induced paralysis) an agitated intubated patient.

Optimizing Preload

Children with right ventricular dysfunction or hypertrophy may need a higher preload to restore optimum contractility. These patients may benefit from a fluid challenge, which should be given slowly and in small aliquots of 5 mL/kg. One needs to watch for increasing liver size, crackles, increased jugular venous pressure, and worsening capillary refill and perfusion. Children with left ventricular dysfunction benefit from decreasing preload and thus may need diuretics.

Improving Contractility

Cardiac contractility can be improved with various inotropic medications, such as catecholamines, phosphodiesterase inhibitors, and calcium sensitizers. All inotropic agents, except milrinone, increase myocardial oxygen consumption. All inotropic agents are also potentially arrhythmogenic. (More details of these medications can be found in the chapter, "Pharmacologic Support of Circulation.") All electrolyte concentrations (e.g., potassium, ionized calcium, and magnesium) should be optimized because they all affect myocardial function.

Reducing Afterload

In children with left ventricular dysfunction, in addition to optimizing inotropy, mildly reducing afterload can help increase stroke volume. This is the only intervention that improves stroke volume without increasing end-diastolic pressure. Positive-pressure ventilation greatly reduces afterload for the left ventricle.

Selective vasodilator infusions, such as sodium nitroprusside, esmolol, and nicardipine, can also reduce afterload. In patients with severe aortic insufficiency or AV valve regurgitation, reducing systemic vascular resistance with antihypertensive agents can improve stroke volume as long as objective values of oxygen delivery are maintained.

Milrinone is a unique inotrope because it also reduces systemic and pulmonary afterload, although it is a weak antihypertensive. In children with right ventricular dysfunction, pulmonary vasodilators, such as inhaled nitric oxide and milrinone, should be considered. Prostaglandin can also reduce afterload in children with coarctation of the aorta.

Improving Atrioventricular Synchrony

Optimizing electrolyte concentrations should prevent arrhythmias. Avoidance of catecholaminergic inotropic agents or using the lowest possible doses is important in conditions in which arrhythmias are common, such as acute myocarditis, cardiomyopathy, or coronary ischemia. Aggressively treating arrhythmias with pharmacotherapy, pacing, cardioversion, or defibrillation is warranted. Patients with single-ventricle physiology rely heavily on active atrial contractions ("atrial kick") to fill the involved ventricle. Hence, in these patients otherwise well-tolerated arrhythmias, such as supraventricular or junctional tachyarrhythmias, need aggressive therapy.

Increasing Arterial Oxygen Carrying Capacity

Increasing arterial oxygen carrying capacity not only improves systemic oxygen delivery but also myocardial oxygen delivery and thus improves myocardial function. Oxygenation of the lungs can be improved with PPV. Optimum positive end-expiratory pressure can recruit alveoli and establish functional residual capacity, thus improving oxygenation of the lungs. Judicious use of packed red blood cell transfusions can also improve oxygen carrying capacity, but transfusions should be used only after maximizing myocardial contractility or in the event of blood loss or severe anemia. These transfusions carry the risk of volume overload and increasing viscosity (which in turn can increase afterload) and hence should be given with caution and in small aliquots.

When attempting to increase oxygen delivery, oxygen demands should be kept to a minimum. Simple measures, such as aggressive treatment of fever and pain, can be helpful. Positive-pressure ventilation reduces oxygen demand by decreasing the work of the respiratory muscles. It also decreases left ventricular work by reducing afterload. In intubated patients with severe myocardial dysfunction, pain and agitation should be treated aggressively with sedatives, analgesics, or paralytics.

These principles of treatment will be illustrated in the following vignettes.

Vignette 2: A 2-Day-Old Neonate with Difficulty Breathing
A 2-day-old term neonate presents to the ED with difficulty breathing. He had an unremarkable prenatal course and was discharged home from the nursery after 24 h. Vital signs at triage were: temperature, 36 °C; pulse, 160 bpm; respirations, 50/min; blood pressure, 60/40; and oxygen saturation, 90% on room air. He has cool extremities and mottling, bibasilar fine crackles, mild intercostal retractions, and hepatomegaly, and capillary refill time is 3 s.
After being placed on 100% oxygen with a nonrebreather face mask, his vital signs were: temperature, 36 °C; pulse, 180 bpm; respirations, 60/min; blood pressure, 50/35; and oxygen saturation, 95% on room air. Capillary refill time increased to 4 s, and his skin is grayer than before.
Two hours later, an IV is placed and a bolus of 10 mL/kg of normal saline, ampicillin, and gentamicin is administered, oxygen is discontinued, and a prostaglandin infusion of 0.05 μg/kg/min is started. Vital signs are: temperature, 36 °C; pulse, 150 bpm; respirations, 50/min; blood pressure, 70/30; and oxygen saturation, 85% on room air.

Differential Diagnosis of Shock in Neonates

As mentioned above, shock is the failure of circulation to meet the metabolic demands of organs. The differential diagnoses of a newborn in shock include hypovolemic shock, cardiogenic shock, septic shock, neurogenic shock or abusive head trauma, and inborn errors of metabolism (Table 16.4).

Hypovolemic shock is characterized by inadequate cardiac output caused by reductions in intravascular volume. The most common type of shock worldwide, hypovolemic shock is most often caused by infectious diarrhea. In the newborn, hypovolemic shock can be caused by poor feeding or from sepsis. Decreased oral intake can be caused by sepsis, central nervous system pathology, gastrointestinal malformations, delayed milk letdown in exclusively breastfed infants, inborn errors of metabolism, and respiratory problems. Hypovolemic shock is unlikely for the neonate in Vignette 2, given the presence of rales and hepatomegaly.

Septic shock is characterized by intravascular depletion caused by decreased oral intake, increased capillary permeability, and increased arteriolar capacitance, resulting in diastolic runoff of intravascular volume. Cardiac dysfunction is often present in septic shock because of direct myocardial depression from bacterial endotoxins and inflammatory mediators.

Table 16.4 Types of shock and associated hemodynamic changes

Types of shock	Central venous pressure	Cardiac output	Exam findings	Pulse pressure
Obstructive	High	Low	Cold	Narrow
Hypovolemic	Low	Low	Cold	Narrow
Cardiogenic	High	Low	Cold	Narrow
Distributive	Low	High or normal	Early: Warm Late: Cold	Wide

Neurogenic shock is caused by vasodilation from neurologically mediated vasoplegia. The most common cause in infants and neonates is abusive head trauma, but it can also be caused by spinal cord injuries (birth trauma).

Treating Shock in Neonates

Treating septic, hypovolemic, and neurogenic shock in the neonate should focus on restoring adequate intravascular volume. However, compared to older infants, children, and adults, neonates have less ability to handle fluid load during resuscitation. Inotropic agents should be considered earlier in the course than in the older age groups. The diagnosis of septic shock could be considered for the child in this vignette, given the presence of hypotension, tachycardia, and poor perfusion. However, deterioration after oxygen administration is unlikely. A history of peripartum risk factors for sepsis is common and includes maternal group B *Streptococcus* colonization, maternal fever, or prolonged rupture of membranes.

Inborn errors of metabolism, which can also cause neonatal shock, include urea cycle defects, fatty acid oxidation defects, congenital adrenal hyperplasia, and organic acidemia. In addition to cardiovascular decompensation, the hallmark of these disorders in neonates is severe lethargy. Immediate treatment includes administering dextrose-containing fluids to prevent hypoglycemia early in the disease course, providing an energy substrate, and preventing catabolism of proteins and lipids.

Ductal-Dependent Systemic Blood Flow Lesions

In fetal circulation, most of the deoxygenated blood ejected from the right ventricle bypasses the lungs by way of the ductus arteriosus to the distal aortic arch. Oxygenated blood from the placenta is baffled across the right atrium and through the foramen ovale to the left atrium. Oxygenated blood ejected from the left ventricle supplies the head and neck and mixes with the deoxygenated blood from the ductus arteriosus to supply the lower body before returning to the placenta.

In a healthy neonate, placental circulation is removed from the circuit, as the first breath causes a rapid increase of blood flow to the lungs, closure of the atrial septum, and functional closure of the ductus arteriosus. In congenital anatomic conditions in which ejection from the left ventricle into the aorta is critically limited, the right ventricle supplies both the pulmonary circulation and the systemic circulation at birth through the ductus arteriosus. These conditions, known as "ductal-dependent systemic blood flow lesions," include hypoplastic left heart syndrome, critical coarctation of the aorta, critical aortic stenosis, and interrupted aortic arch. In these conditions, pulmonary venous return to the left atrium mixes with deoxygenated systemic venous blood through an obligate atrial septal defect. Mixed blood from the right ventricle reaches the systemic circulation through the ductus arteriosus. Despite the mixing, cyanosis is not always evident. In fact, cyanosis may not be diagnosed, and neonates with cyanosis may even be discharged from the nursery, only to develop the symptoms of shock at home.

Survival of a neonate with a ductal-dependent systemic blood flow lesion depends on the patency of the ductus arteriosus. In humans, however, the structure has evolved to close shortly after birth. In neonates with these lesions, flow through the ductus arteriosus continues longer than in unaffected neonates, so patency may be maintained slightly longer. When the ductus arteriosus does close, systemic circulation decreases and shock ensues. Signs include gray skin, poor perfusion, tachypnea, rales, and hepatomegaly. The treatment for a neonate with a ductal-dependent lesion is a prostaglandin infusion. This should be started immediately, even before the diagnosis is confirmed, unless an alternative diagnosis is certain. Side effects of a prostaglandin infusion include apnea, vasodilation, fever, irritability, and leukocytosis. The risk of developing apnea is greatest in the first hour of the infusion, especially in children weighing less than 2 kg. However, these side effects are not as severe as those of a closed ductus.

Oxygen can be a dangerous therapy for ductal-dependent systemic blood flow lesions. Oxygen decreases pulmonary vascular resistance, which increases pulmonary blood flow by stealing it from the systemic circulation. To balance the pulmonary and systemic circulations, oxygen delivery should be adjusted to provide arterial saturation levels of between 75% and 85%. If a ductal-dependent lesion is suspected in a neonate, a STAT echocardiogram should be obtained, and consultation with a pediatric cardiologist should be sought. Correcting electrolyte imbalances and hypoglycemia are imperative.

Vignette 3: A 9-Year-Old Girl with Mid-sternal Chest Pain

A 9-year-old girl presented to the ED reporting mid-sternal chest pain, fever, and a slight cough for 3 days. She had no history of difficulty breathing. She reported that her chest pain was worse with deep breathing and improved when sitting up and leaning forward. She had been evaluated in the ED a day earlier for similar symptoms, received a diagnosis of costochondritis, and was discharged to home on analgesics. However, her symptoms worsened, prompting the second visit to the ED.

On this second visit, she appeared mildly tachypneic and uncomfortable from chest pain. Her vital signs during this visit were: temperature, 38.3 °C; pulse, 120 bpm; respirations, 36/min; blood pressure, 112/90 mmHg; and oxygen saturation, 98% on room air. Her capillary refill was 2 s. Her lungs were clear to auscultation, and an abdominal examination was unremarkable. For tachycardia, she was given a bolus of fluids, and the chest radiograph was repeated, which revealed a left-sided pneumonia versus atelectasis. After a 40 mL/kg fluid bolus, her heart rate decreased to 105 bpm, and her respiration rate was 36. She was admitted to the floor on antibiotics for pneumonia. Persistent tachycardia prompted an electrocardiogram (Fig. 16.5) and an echocardiogram (Fig. 16.7a, b). The ECG revealed T wave and ST segment changes in Leads II and III, and the echocardiogram showed a large pericardial effusion with cardiac tamponade.

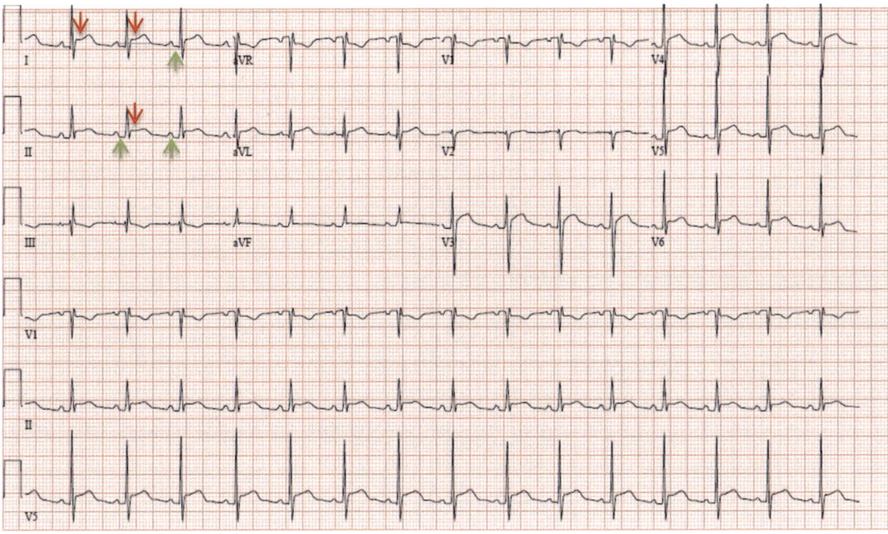

Fig. 16.5 Widespread concave ST elevation and PR depression throughout most of the limb leads (I, II, III, aVL, aVF) and precordial leads (V2–6). Blue line, baseline T-P segment; Green arrows, PR segment; Red arrows, ST segment

Pericardial Tamponade

Pericardial tamponade is characterized by the accumulation of fluid in the pericardial space that reduces ventricular filling and compromises cardiac output. Pericardial tamponade is a medical emergency that, if untreated, can result in shock and death.

The pericardial sac has two layers: a fibrous layer bound to the diaphragm and a serous layer. The serous layer consists of a parietal layer that adheres to the outer fibrous layer and a visceral layer that is reflected on the heart. Between the parietal and visceral layers is the pericardial cavity, which contains between 30 and 50 mL of a plasma ultrafiltrate similar to pleural fluid. The pericardium lubricates, anchors, stabilizes, and protects the heart and maintains the negative intrathoracic pressure needed for atrial filling. Excessive accumulation of fluid results in tamponade, which occurs in three stages:

1. The accumulating fluid in effect reduces ventricular compliance. Ventricles require higher diastolic pressure in order to exceed pericardial pressure and for filling to occur.
2. As fluid continues to accumulate, the rising pericardial pressure approaches ventricular end-diastolic pressure, resulting in decreased ventricular inflow and output.
3. The equilibration of ventricular filling pressure and pericardial pressure causes acute deterioration and shock.

Increased intrapericardial pressure causes right atrial collapse, and a marked reduction in systemic venous return and right ventricular diastolic filling. The amount of pericardial fluid required to reduce cardiac output depends on the compliance of the heart and the rate of fluid accumulation. A rapid accumulation of a small amount of fluid can markedly lower cardiac output. Conversely, a liter of fluid accumulated over time may not affect diastolic filling because of the slow stretching of fibers.

Causes of Pericardial Tamponade

Pericardial effusions and tamponade can be caused by hemopericardium, infections, rheumatologic disease, uremia, postcardiotomy syndrome, malignancy, or idiopathic causes. The most common cause of pericardial tamponade has shifted from viral infections to postcardiotomy syndromes in recent years. In a large retrospective study of hospitalized children with pericarditis and pericardial effusion, the causes included postcardiotomy syndromes (54%), neoplasia (13%), renal disease (13%), idiopathic or viral infections (5%), and rheumatologic disease (5%) [6].

Postcardiotomy syndromes occur most commonly after atrial septal defect closures (28% of cases). Pericardial effusions seen in the ED are more likely to be either postcardiotomy syndromes, systemic illness, or viral infections [7]. Viral causes are more common in adolescents and in males. Commonly implicated viruses include Coxsackie virus, adenovirus, echovirus, Epstein-Barr virus, influenza virus, and human immunodeficiency virus. Bacterial causes (*Staphylococcus* and *Haemophilus influenzae*) although less common, are also possible.

Pericardial effusions from tuberculosis are seen in developing countries where the infection is endemic. Pericardial effusions after bone marrow transplantation are increasing in frequency. Graft-versus-host disease and transplant-associated thrombotic microangiopathy are risk factors for pericardial effusion after bone marrow transplant [8]. Penetrating trauma, including gunshot and stab wounds, can be a common cause of cardiac tamponade. Tamponade should be suspected in children who present with penetrating trauma and shock. In the setting of a noisy environment, clinical features, such as muffled heart sounds, may be difficult to discern and hence a high index of suspicion should be maintained.

Clinical Findings in Pericardial Tamponade

Chest pain is a common presenting symptom, although it may be absent in children with bacterial pericardial effusion. The pain is substernal, sharp, may be referred to the left shoulder, and may worsen when the patient is supine or takes a deep breath. The pain may also radiate to the scapula if the phrenic nerve is irritated. Infants may present with fussiness and tachycardia. Postpericardiotomy syndromes tend to appear between 1 and 2 weeks after surgery.

Other symptoms and signs may include fever, difficulty breathing, and tachycardia out of proportion to the fever. Severe cases may present as hypotension and shock. In the absence of tamponade, physical signs may be subtle and easily missed. A "pericardial rub" caused by friction between the two pericardial layers may occur but can be altered in quality by changing the patient's position and may be absent in the presence of a large effusion. Conversely, with large pericardial effusions, heart sounds appear distant and may accompany cool extremities, hypotension, and narrow pulse pressures. Signs of venous congestion, including distended neck veins and hepatomegaly, can occur but are often difficult to assess in a small infant. In some children, abdominal pain may be the first manifestation and is caused by hepatic venous congestion.

Pulsus paradoxus is an exaggerated (>10 mmHg) drop in systolic blood pressure with inspiration. During inspiration, venous return to the right ventricle increases because of negative intrathoracic pressure. However, there is not an associated increase in pulmonary venous return to the left ventricle. Consequently, the interventricular septum bows to the left, thereby decreasing left ventricular end-diastolic volume and stroke volume. Also, negative intrathoracic pressure during inspiration increases left ventricular afterload. Overall, this process decreases left ventricular stroke volume during inspiration. These changes are reversed during expiration. With cardiac tamponade, tension pneumothorax, severe airway obstruction, and hypovolemia, these changes may be exaggerated and lead to pulsus paradoxus [9]. Importantly, the classic Beck's triad (muffled heart sounds, hypotension, and venous distension) occurs in only 30% of all patients with cardiac tampondade.

Diagnosing Pericardial Tamponade

Characteristic chest pain, distant heart sounds, and shock should suggest the diagnosis. Laboratory findings are nonspecific but may include an elevated white blood cell count, C-reactive protein, and erythrocyte sedimentation rate. An ECG may show low-voltage complexes (the amplitude of the QRS complex in every limb lead <5 mm; Fig. 16.5) and tachycardia. Electrical alternans can be seen with pericardial tamponade and consists of cyclical changes in the amplitude of the QRS complex resulting from excessive motion of the heart inside the fluid-filled pericardial sac. A chest radiograph may reveal a "water bottle-shaped heart" (Erlenmeyer flask) (Fig. 16.6), but the cardiac silhouette may be normal in the initial stage. Bedside ultrasound is sensitive and specific for diagnosing pericardial tamponade and can quickly confirm the diagnosis, especially when performed by trained ED physicians [10] (Fig. 16.7). Features suggesting tamponade on ultrasound include a circumferential pericardial effusion with a hyperdynamic heart and "scalloping" (right atrial compression during late diastole and right ventricular collapse during early diastole). Other findings may include abnormal mitral valve motion, a dilated inferior vena cava that does not collapse with inspiration, and a counterclockwise rotation of the heart ("swinging heart"). An echocardiogram can confirm the diagnosis.

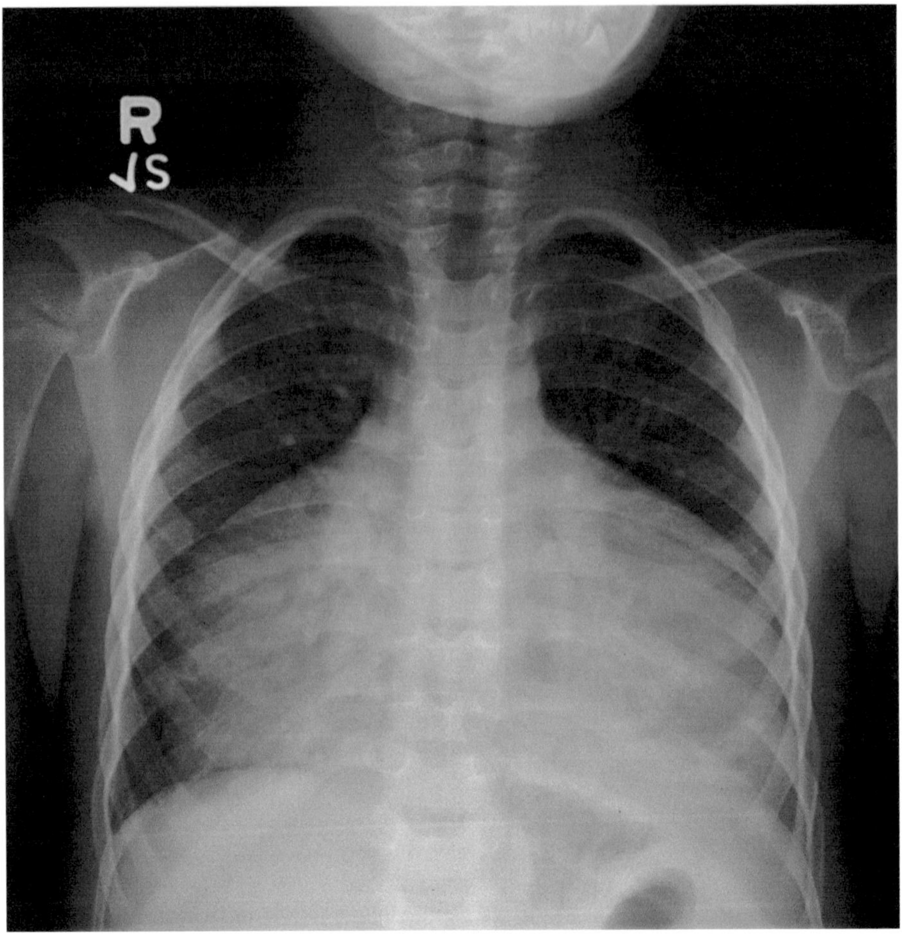

Fig. 16.6 Chest radiograph showing globular enlargement of the cardiac silhouette

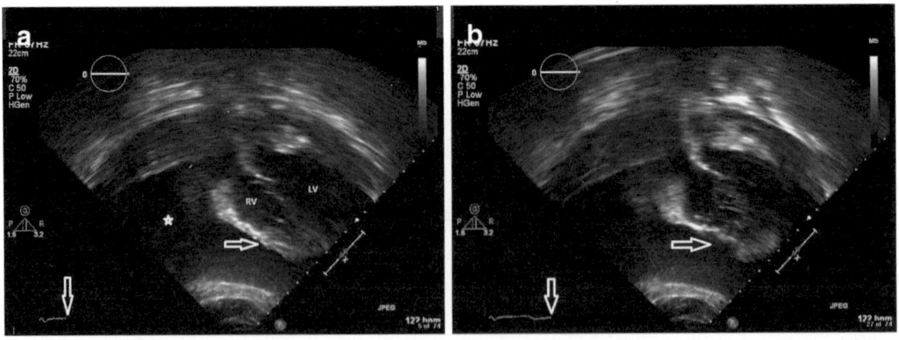

Fig. 16.7 An asterisk marks a large pericardial effusion. (**a**) Horizontal arrow shows right ventricular wall at the beginning of diastole. . (**b**) Horizontal arrow shows right ventricular wall collapse during diastole

Treating Pericardial Tamponade

Pericardial tamponade is an emergency and, if untreated, can lead to death. Immediate pericardiocentesis with a blind or ultrasound-guided technique is indicated. A subxiphoid or left parasternal approach between the 4th and 5th ribs may be used for blind drainage. A spinal needle can be advanced 5 cm through the identified area until either fluid is obtained or an injury pattern is noted on the ECG. If the injury pattern is an ST elevation, the needle should be carefully withdrawn until the pattern is no longer noted. The complication rate with this approach is 10–50% and can be reduced substantially by using ultrasound-guided pericardial aspiration, for which reported rates of major complications are as low as 1%.

Bacterial pericardial effusions should be treated with broad-spectrum antibiotics. In penetrating trauma cases with shock, pericardiocentesis may be both diagnostic and therapeutic. Recurrent cases of effusion may need to be treated with pericardiectomy or by creating a pericardial window.

Bibliography

1. Sinha R, Nadel S, Kissoon NT, Ranjit S, et al. Chapter 28. Recognition and initial management of shock. In: Roger's textbook of pediatric intensive care. 5th ed. Philadelphia: Lippincott Williams & Wilkins; 2016. p. 380–93.
2. Reynolds HR, Hochman JS. Cardiogenic shock. Current concepts and improving outcomes. Circulation. 2008;117(5):686–97.
3. Hochman JS. Cardiogenic shock complicating acute myocardial infarction: expanding the paradigm. Circulation. 2003;107(24):2998–3002.
4. Nichols DG, Ungerleider RM, Spevak PJ, et al. Critical heart disease in infants and children. 2nd ed. Amsterdam: Elsevier; 2006. p. 18–29.
5. Dart AM, DPhil BA, Kingwell BA. Pulse pressure-a review of mechanisms and clinical relevance. J Am Coll Cardiol. 2001;37(4):975–84.
6. Shakti D, Hehn R, Gauvreau K, et al. Idiopathic pericarditis and pericardial effusion in children: contemporary epidemiology and management. J Am Heart Assoc. 2014;3:e001483.
7. Roodpeyma S, Sadeghian N. Acute pericarditis in childhood: a 10-year experience. Pediatr Cardiol. 2000;21:363–7.
8. Lerner D, Dandoy C, Hirsch R, et al. Pericardial effusion in pediatric SCT recipients with thrombotic microangiopathy. Bone Marrow Transplant. 2014;49:862–3.
9. Clark JA, Lieh-Lai M, Thomas R, et al. Comparison of traditional and plethysmographic methods for measuring pulsus paradoxus. Arch Pediatr Adolesc Med. 2004;158(1):48–51.
10. Mandavia DP, Hoffner RJ, Mahaney K, et al. Bedside echocardiography by emergency physicians. Ann Emerg Med. 2001;38:377–82.

17 Point-of-Care Cardiac Ultrasound in the Emergency Department

Yamuna Sanil, Marjorie Gayanilo, and Curt Stankovic

Ultrasound can be a powerful tool when used as an accessory to the physical examination. This benefit is especially apparent in the emergency department (ED), where undiagnosed, acutely ill patients progress rapidly. Point-of-care ultrasound has been available to general emergency physicians since the 1980s, and it is now routinely used in the ED. The two primary applications of ultrasound in the ED are to aid in diagnosis and to guide procedures. Ultrasound can improve procedural success and safety by reducing attempts, procedural time, and placement failures [1–6].

The introduction of ultrasound into pediatric emergency medicine has been slower, but it has increased over the past decade, especially at academic medical centers. Pediatric emergency medicine physicians are now expected to use ultrasound, and it has been required in fellowship training since 2010 [7]. Specifically, the American Board of Pediatrics Pediatric Emergency Medicine Content Specifications require that candidates be proficient in using ultrasound to rapidly evaluate blunt abdominal trauma, ectopic pregnancy, foreign bodies and their removal, and emergency cardiac ultrasound [8]. Expert consensus educational guidelines affirmed the Board's goals and include the focused cardiovascular ultrasound (FOCUS) examination as a core application. The principal use of a FOCUS examination is to rapidly assess symptomatic patients. In particular, these guidelines identify four cardiovascular ultrasound applications: identifying pericardial

Y. Sanil, M.D. • M. Gayanilo, M.D.
Wayne State University, Detroit, MI, USA

Division of Pediatric Cardiology, Children's Hospital of Michigan, Detroit, MI, USA
e-mail: ysanil@dmc.org; mgayanil@dmc.org

C. Stankovic, M.D. (✉)
Division of Emergency Medicine, Children's Hospital of Michigan, Detroit, MI, USA

Wayne State University, Detroit, MI, USA
e-mail: cstankov@dmc.org

© Springer International Publishing AG, part of Springer Nature 2018

A. P. Sarnaik et al. (eds.), *Cardiac Emergencies in Children*,
https://doi.org/10.1007/978-3-319-73754-6_17

effusion, identifying cardiac standstill, evaluating function, and assessing the volume status of the inferior vena cava [9].

Comprehensive cardiac ultrasound is clearly different from FOCUS, which is not meant to replace it. Rather, FOCUS is an extension of the physical examination, and its goal is to answer specific questions. A comprehensive review reported a remarkable increase in diagnostic accuracy when a cardiac ultrasound was added to the physical examination [10]. However, evaluating the cardiovascular system with FOCUS remains underutilized despite the potential to improve the care of these critically ill patients [11]. Identifying cardiac pathology is essential because many patients with cardiac disease often report only vague respiratory or gastrointestinal symptoms. The FOCUS examination can quickly narrow the differential diagnosis and efficiently guide care for these critically ill patients.

This chapter describes how to perform a FOCUS examination and explains common emergency situations in which it is most impactful.

Image Acquisition

Phased-array or curvilinear transducers can be used to perform cardiac ultrasound (Fig. 17.1). Phased-array probes are preferred because they better delineate moving structures, such as the heart. The transducer footprint is an important consideration in children, given their small intercostal spaces. Multiple transducers with varying frequencies are usually chosen according to the age and size of the child. A high-frequency probe has higher image resolution but at the expense of lower depth penetrance. A rough guide for probe selection would be to use a probe with 8–12 MHz for neonates, 6–8 MHz for small children, and 2–5 MHz for older children and adults. A lower-frequency probe should be used when more depth is required to view the structure of interest.

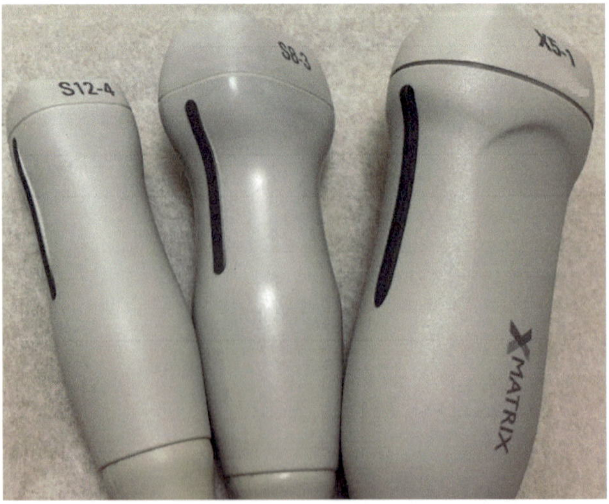

Fig. 17.1 Ultrasonic probes used for a focused cardiovascular ultrasound (FOCUS) examination. The black line on each probe helps identify the image orientation on the screen. The number is the frequency of the transducer in megahertz, i.e., S12–4 is 12–14 megahertz. A smaller probe with higher frequency has a smaller footprint, which is useful in infants

By convention, structures are depicted in the anatomically correct orientation in pediatric echocardiography. The configuration of the machine must be understood because many ultrasound machines in the ED are preset to display structures with the radiology settings. Image orientation in FOCUS has been a topic of much debate. However, with the probe placements as described below, the final image will be similar to standard cardiology conventions. The transducer has a "marker" or "notch" that corresponds to a "dot or symbol" on the screen which helps guide images on the monitor. Structures on the side of the notch are shown on the same side of the screen as the dot. Also, structures closest to the probe appear at the top of the monitor, and deeper structures appear lower on the monitor.

A FOCUS examination should use both two-dimensional and M-mode imaging. The standard views of the heart provided by 2D imaging are:

1. Subxiphoid view
2. Parasternal long-axis view
3. Parasternal short-axis view
4. Apical view

Throughout the examination, the child should be comfortably positioned. Parents should be involved because they can usually calm the child and encourage cooperation, especially in infants and smaller children. To obtain the parasternal and apical views, placing the child in the left lateral decubitus position brings the heart anteriorly, in direct contact with the chest wall and decreases the interference from the lung fields. Subxiphoid images should be obtained, while the patient is in the supine position. Having a supine child bend both knees often helps relax the abdominal muscles and makes proper images easier to obtain. If the study is being performed while the patient is actively being resuscitated, subxiphoid imaging windows are preferred as it does not interfere with the resuscitation.

Subxiphoid View: This view looks at the heart from the subxiphoid or subcostal area. The transducer should be placed just below the xiphoid, with the marker pointing to 9 o'clock. The transducer should also be angled superiorly at a 20° angle from the abdominal surface. Moving the probe slightly to the right while directing the ultrasound beam superiorly and leftward can improve image quality because the liver acts as an acoustic window. The depth must be adjusted in the subxiphoid view to visualize the entire heart. Novice sonographers often do not use the entire screen space, which displays the image in an unnecessary smaller area. In pediatric cardiac ultrasound, the heart should occupy most of the screen so that the details of the structure are easily visualized, which is best done by optimizing depth.

The appearance of all four cardiac chambers in the subxiphoid view is excellent, particularly in young children (Fig. 17.2). This view is often the preferred initial view in the FOCUS examination because it does not interfere with concurrent resuscitation efforts. In the subxiphoid four-chamber view, the liver is closest to the apex of the image sector. This view is useful for measuring global ventricular function and to evaluate pericardial effusion.

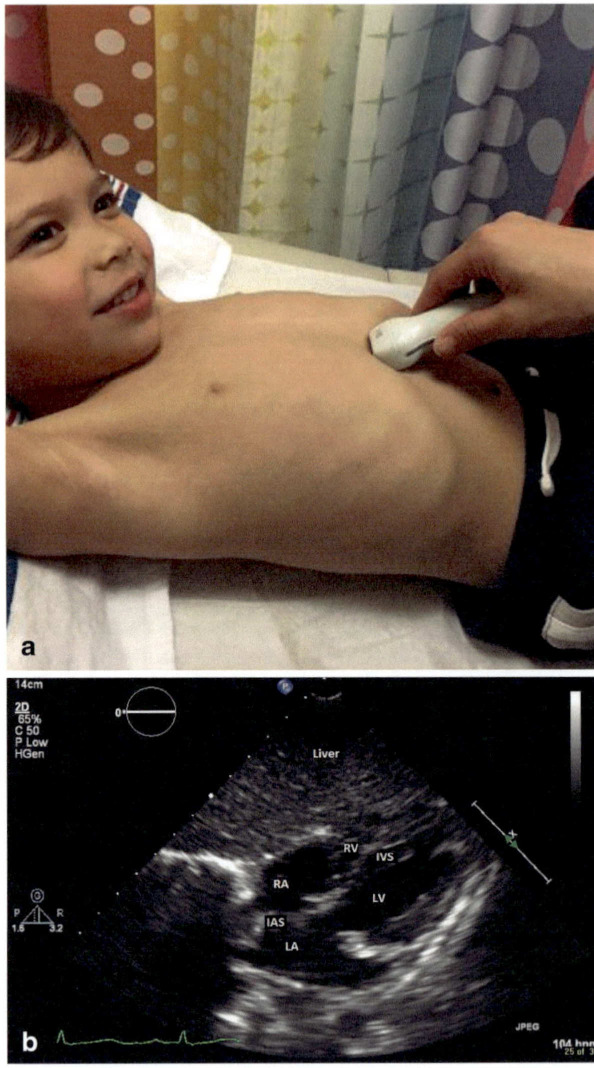

Fig. 17.2 (**a**) The subxiphoid or subcostal four-chamber view is obtained by placing the probe over the xiphoid with the marker at 9 o'clock, angled superiorly. (**b**) The subxiphoid or subcostal four-chamber view of the heart. The image sector is shown on the screen with the sector apex corresponding to the area nearest to the probe. The dot with the P is the area imaged by the beam at the probe marker. *RA* right atrium, *RV* right ventricle, *IVS* interventricular septum, *IAS* interatrial septum, *LA* left atrium, *LV* left ventricle

Parasternal Long-Axis View: This view depicts the heart in its long axis. The transducer should be placed in the left third intercostal space close to the sternal border, perpendicular to the chest wall, with the marker pointing at 4 o'clock and angled toward the patient's left hip. This view shows the right ventricle, interventricular septum, left ventricle, aortic valve, mitral valve, and left atrium (Fig. 17.3). In this view, both qualitative and quantitative global ventricular systolic function can be assessed. A pericardial effusion can be also identified in this view. The aforementioned probe positions are only guidelines. Often, moving between adjacent rib spaces is required to obtain an appropriate imaging window.

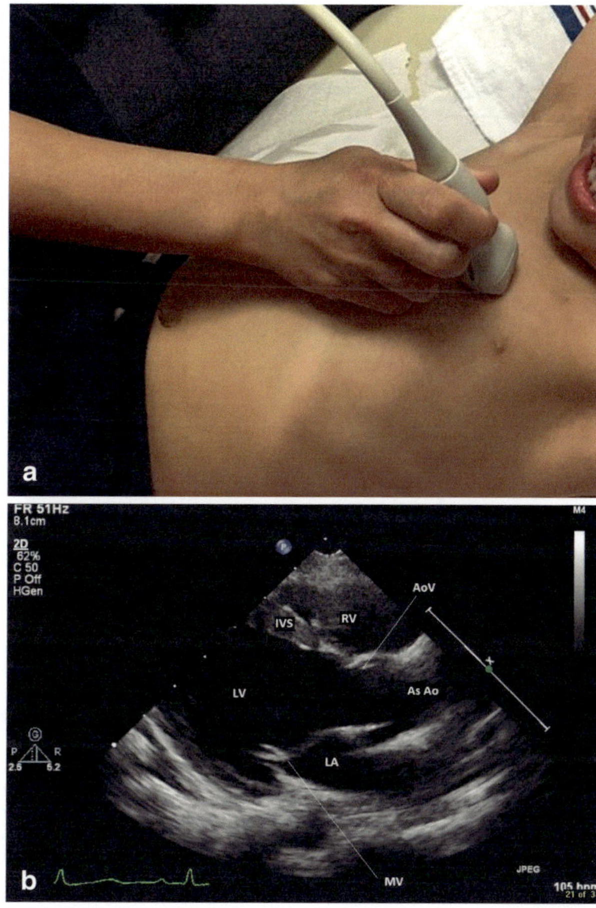

Fig. 17.3 (**a**) The parasternal long-axis view is obtained by placing the probe in third left intercostal space with the marker at 4 o'clock. (**b**) The parasternal long-axis view of the heart. *RV* right ventricle, *IVS* interventricular septum, *LV* left ventricle, *AoV* aortic valve, *As Ao* ascending aorta, *MV* mitral valve, *LA* left atrium

Parasternal Short-Axis View: This view corresponds to the cross-sectional plane of the heart. With the probe at the parasternal long-axis position, it should be rotated 90° clockwise, until the marker is at 7 o'clock, pointing to the patient's right hip. The probe should be perpendicular to the chest wall, and the right and left ventricles should be visualized. Changing the probe angle by manipulating or fanning the transducer allows various cross sections of the heart to be viewed. This allows the aortic valve, mitral valve, mitral papillary muscles, and cardiac apex to be visualized. Global ventricular function is measured by identifying the mitral papillary muscle. Structures seen with this technique include cross-sectional views of the left ventricle, the papillary muscles of the mitral valve, the ventricular septum, and the right ventricle (Fig. 17.4).

Apical View: This view images the coronal plane of the heart. All four cardiac chambers are visualized, and the relative sizes of each chamber can be appreciated in this view. The transducer should be placed at or just lateral to the cardiac apex, usually in the left fifth intercostal space on the midclavicular line. The marker

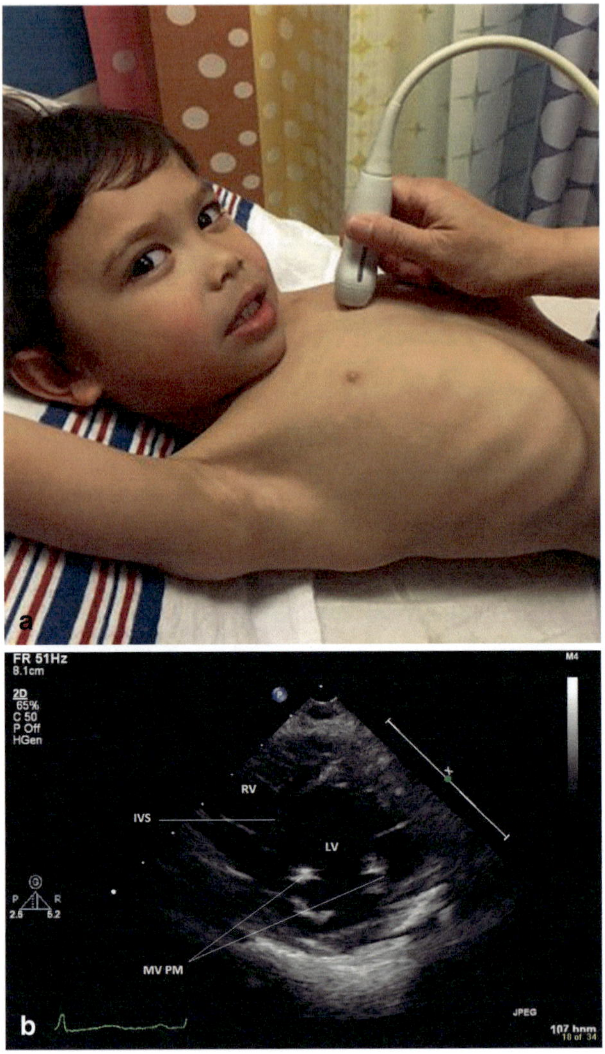

Fig. 17.4 (**a**) The parasternal short-axis view is obtained by placing the probe at the 3rd left intercostal space with the marker at 7 o'clock. (**b**) The parasternal short-axis view at the level of the mitral papillary muscle. *RV* right ventricle, *IVS* interventricular septum, *LV* left ventricle, *MV PM* mitral valve papillary muscles

should be pointed toward the 9 o'clock position and angled superiorly to view the cardiac chambers (Fig. 17.5). This view aids in assessing global ventricular function and pericardial effusion.

M-Mode Echocardiography

"Motion-mode" or M-mode echocardiography uses a single line of sound waves to plot changes in the position of the wall over time. In either the parasternal short-axis or the parasternal long-axis views, M-mode echocardiography can evaluate left ventricular function. Once the image is obtained, the M-mode option is selected, and

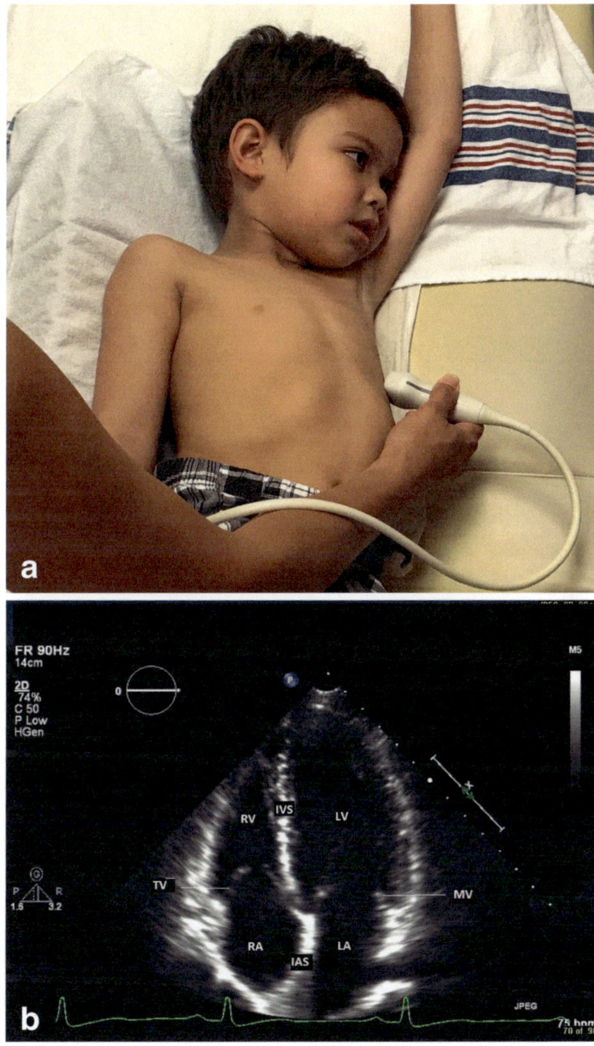

Fig. 17.5 (**a**) The apical four-chamber view is obtained by positioning the probe just lateral to the apical impulse with the marker at 9 o'clock, angled superiorly. (**b**) The apical four-chamber view. *RA* right atrium, *RV* right ventricle, *LA* left atrium, *LV* left ventricle, *IVS* interventricular septum, *IAS* interatrial septum, *MV* mitral valve, *TV* tricuspid valve

the M-line is directed to cross the left ventricle at the level of the papillary muscle (Fig. 17.6). The 2D image above the M-mode tracing shows the level at which the image was obtained. When the left ventricular systolic function is normal, both the septal wall and the posterior left ventricular wall should move well (Fig. 17.6). Decreased movement of the ventricular walls suggests decreased systolic function.

Measurement of the distance between the ventricular septum and the left ventricular posterior wall at the level of the papillary muscle in systole and diastole quantifies ventricular systolic function. This is called the shortening fraction. The shortening fraction is calculated as:

$$\textit{Shortening fraction} = (\text{LVIDd} - \text{LVIDs}) \div \text{LVIDd}.$$

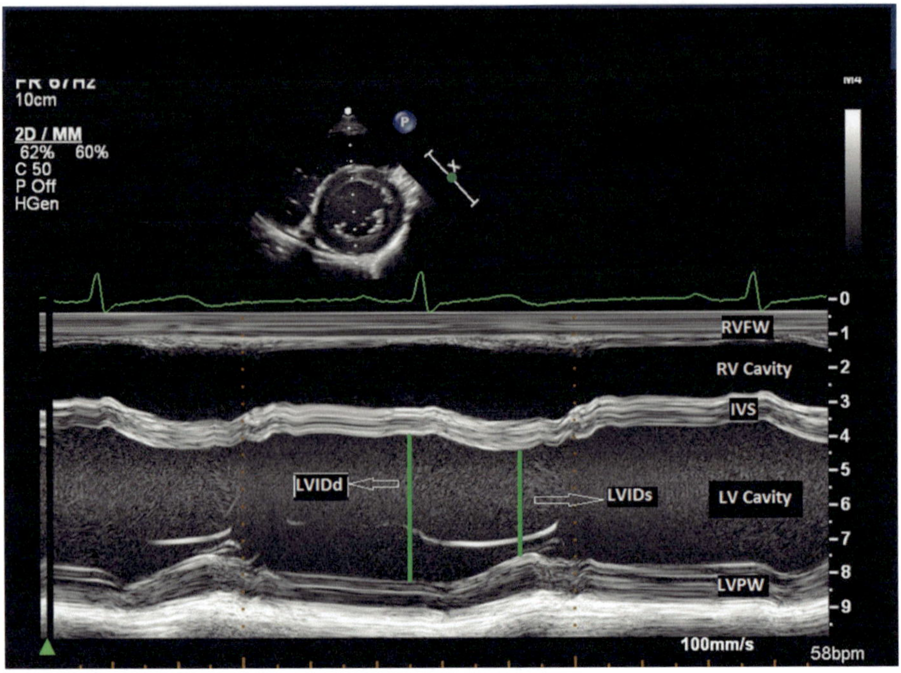

Fig. 17.6 M-mode image obtained at the parasternal short axis at the level of the mitral papillary muscle. The shortening fraction is calculated by dividing the left ventricular internal diameter in diastole dimension by the left ventricular internal diameter in systole as measured by M-mode echocardiography. *RV FW* right ventricular free wall, *RV* cavity, *IVS* interventricular septum, *LV* cavity, *LV PW* left ventricular posterior wall, *LVIDd* left ventricular internal dimension in diastole, *LVIDs* left ventricular internal dimension in systole

where LVIDd is the left ventricular internal dimension in diastole and LVIDs is the left ventricular internal dimension in systole. A shortening fraction of more than 28% is normal. Often qualitative assessment of ventricular function is sufficient to initiate appropriate management. However, quantitative measurement of ventricular function can further guide therapy for patients in cardiogenic shock.

Clinical Applications of FOCUS

Case 1: Pericardial Effusion

A 5-month-old girl presents with a 2-day history of reduced feeding and a 1-day history of shortness of breath. She presents 9 days after surgical repair of pulmonary stenosis and angioplasty of the left pulmonary artery. Over the past 2 days, her activity had been reduced, and she has been sleeping more than usual. On presentation, she is breathing faster and harder than usual, and her urine output is decreased. She is not febrile and does not have a cough. She had been discharged after surgery on Lasix, which caused vomiting. Her temperature is 36.5 °C; pulse, 152 bpm; respiration, 56; blood pressure, 116/53; and oxygen saturation, 97%. She appears tired and has nasal flaring as well as intercostal retractions, but her lungs are clear, without wheezing, stridor, or crackles. A cardiac examination reveals a 2/6 systolic ejection murmur with muffled S1 and S2 heart sounds. Her capillary refill is brisk. There is no edema. Her liver is palpable 2 cm below the costal margin. Otherwise, her examination is unremarkable.

How can a point-of-care cardiac ultrasound guide care in this patient?

A FOCUS examination can immediately identify a pericardial effusion, which has reduced the time to diagnosis from 42.4 to 15.5 min and has increased survival rates from 57% up to 100% [12]. The clinical diagnosis of a pericardial effusion can be elusive because many patients present with normal chest radiographic findings and vague reports of symptoms, such as tachypnea, dyspnea, and chest pain. Emergency physicians can detect a pericardial effusion with a sensitivity of 96% and a specificity of 98% [13]. In trauma patients, a FOCUS examination can detect pericardial effusion with a sensitivity of 100%, a specificity of 99%, and a diagnostic accuracy of 99% [14].

The view most often used in the ED to identify pericardial effusion is the subxiphoid view. However, pericardial effusions can be identified in any of the four views described above. A pericardial effusion will appear as a lucent separation of the parietal and visceral pericardium. Depending on the extent of fluid collection around the heart, a pericardial effusion can be described as small, moderate, or large. The hemodynamic impact of a pericardial effusion depends on the amount of accumulated fluid, as well as the speed of accumulation. Both acute accumulation of a moderate amount of fluid and a chronic accumulation of a large amount of fluid in the pericardial space can cause hemodynamic compromise and cardiac tamponade. Findings suggesting impending cardiac tamponade include diastolic collapse of the right ventricle and atrium. Diastolic collapse of the right atrium is more sensitive, while diastolic collapse of the right ventricle is more specific for tamponade [15]. A small posterior pericardial effusion is shown in Fig. 17.7. The patient described in the above clinical scenario had a large pericardial effusion as shown in Fig. 17.8.

Cardiac ultrasound can also guide pericardiocentesis, which is typically performed through a subxiphoid or an apical approach. When one of these approaches is used to access the pericardial space, the other view can guide the procedure. The sonographer should monitor the needle tip as it is moved from the skin into the pericardial space. Ultrasound-guided pericardiocentesis has been associated with improved successes rates and has decreased the rate of complications [16]. In the child described above, the large pericardial effusion was drained under ultrasound guidance (Fig. 17.9).

Case 2: Shock

A 6-year-old girl presents to the emergency department with a 3-day history of decreased activity. She has no history of fever, vomiting, or diarrhea, although she is nauseous, and during the past 24 h, her oral intake was poor and urine output had

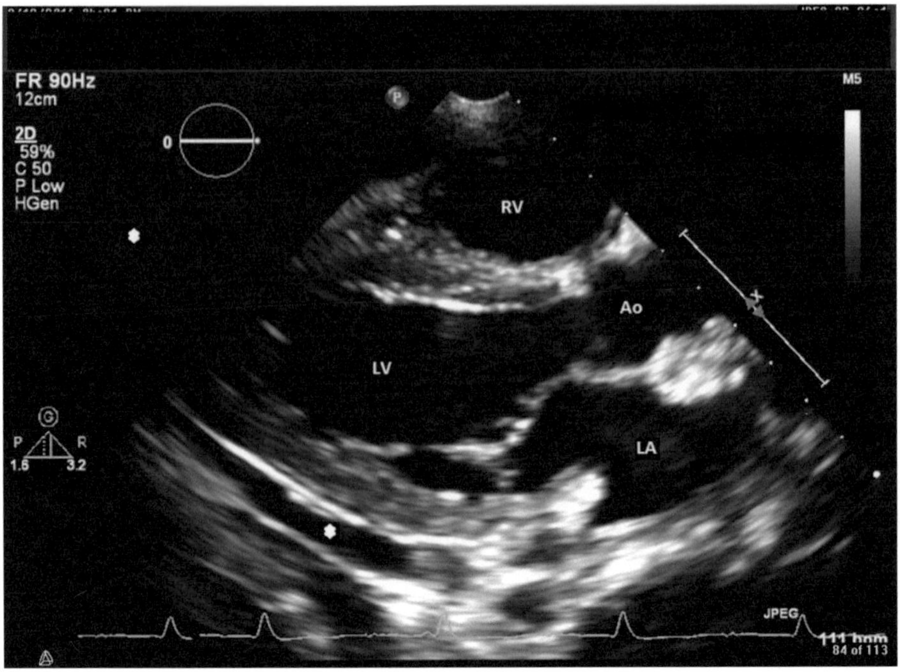

Fig. 17.7 A small posterior pericardial effusion (asterisk) behind the left ventricle as visualized from the parasternal long-axis view showing

decreased. She had come back from a family vacation 3 weeks ago, during which she had a cough and nasal congestion. Her temperature is 37.2 °C; pulse, 178 bpm; respirations, 42; blood pressure, 80/38; and oxygen saturation, 96%. She is sluggish and slow to respond. Her pupils are equal and reactive, and there are no signs of trauma. Her lungs are clear, and her examination reveals regular S1 and S2 heart sounds. Her capillary refill is 3 s. Her abdomen is soft and not tender, and the liver tip is palpable just below the costal margin. The ED team is establishing intravenous access to obtain samples for baseline lab tests and to begin appropriate management.

How can a point-of-care cardiac ultrasound help manage this patient?

Obtaining a global impression of cardiac function is vital when managing patients in shock, which requires early, aggressive intervention. The FOCUS examination provides a sense of endocardial excursion and myocardial thickening, which helps identify the cause of shock. This data help clinical decision-making especially in children whose presentation is often unclear and complicated by shock and respiratory distress. A poorly functioning left ventricle (LV) suggests a need for inotropic drugs or mechanical support (Fig. 17.10). Alternatively, a hyperdynamic LV suggests hypovolemia or sepsis, which must be managed differently. With FOCUS training, emergency physicians can accurately determine LV function in patients with hypotension [17].

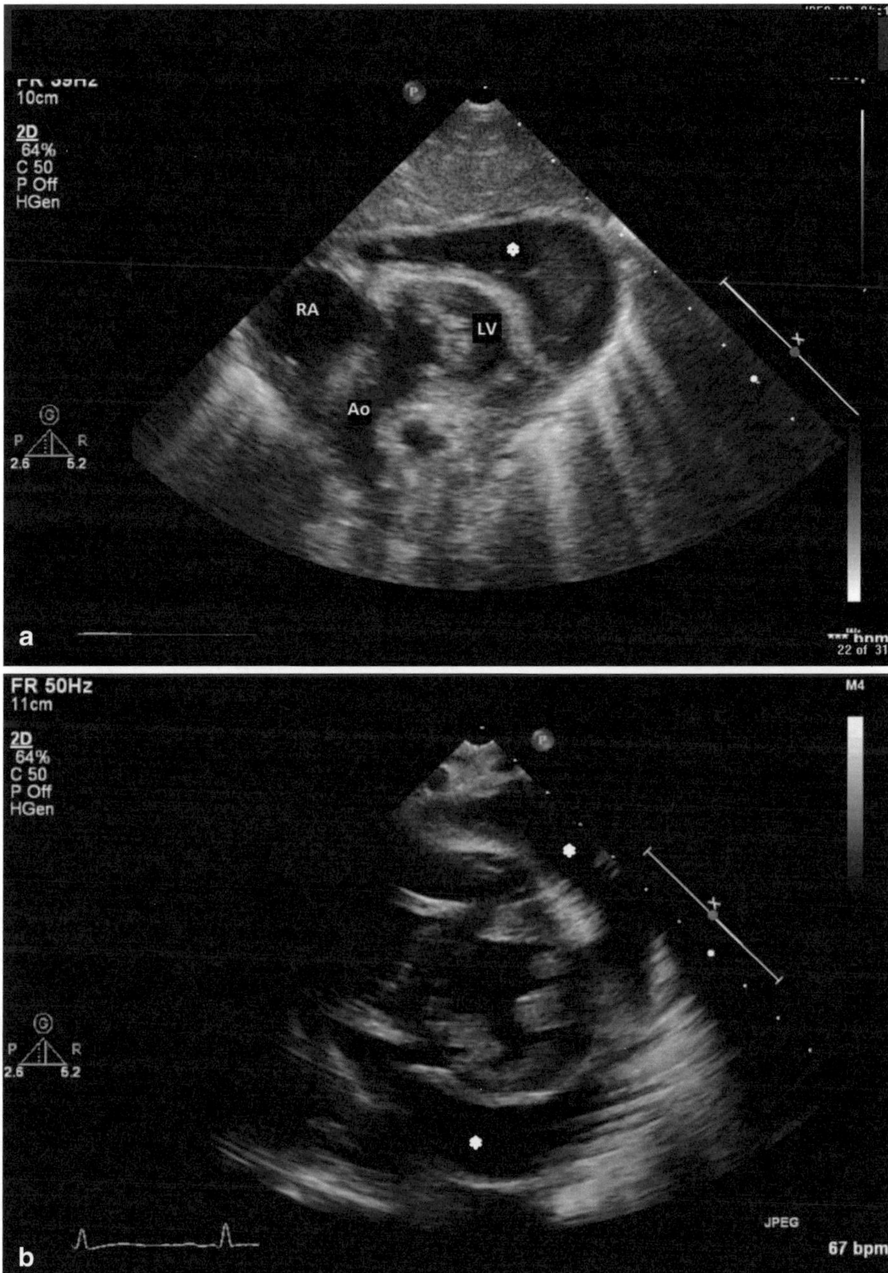

Fig. 17.8 A large pericardial effusion (asterisk) as seen from (**a**) the subxiphoid view and (**b**) the parasternal short-axis view. The echogenic area in the pericardial space is fibrinous material, as seen in the subxiphoid view

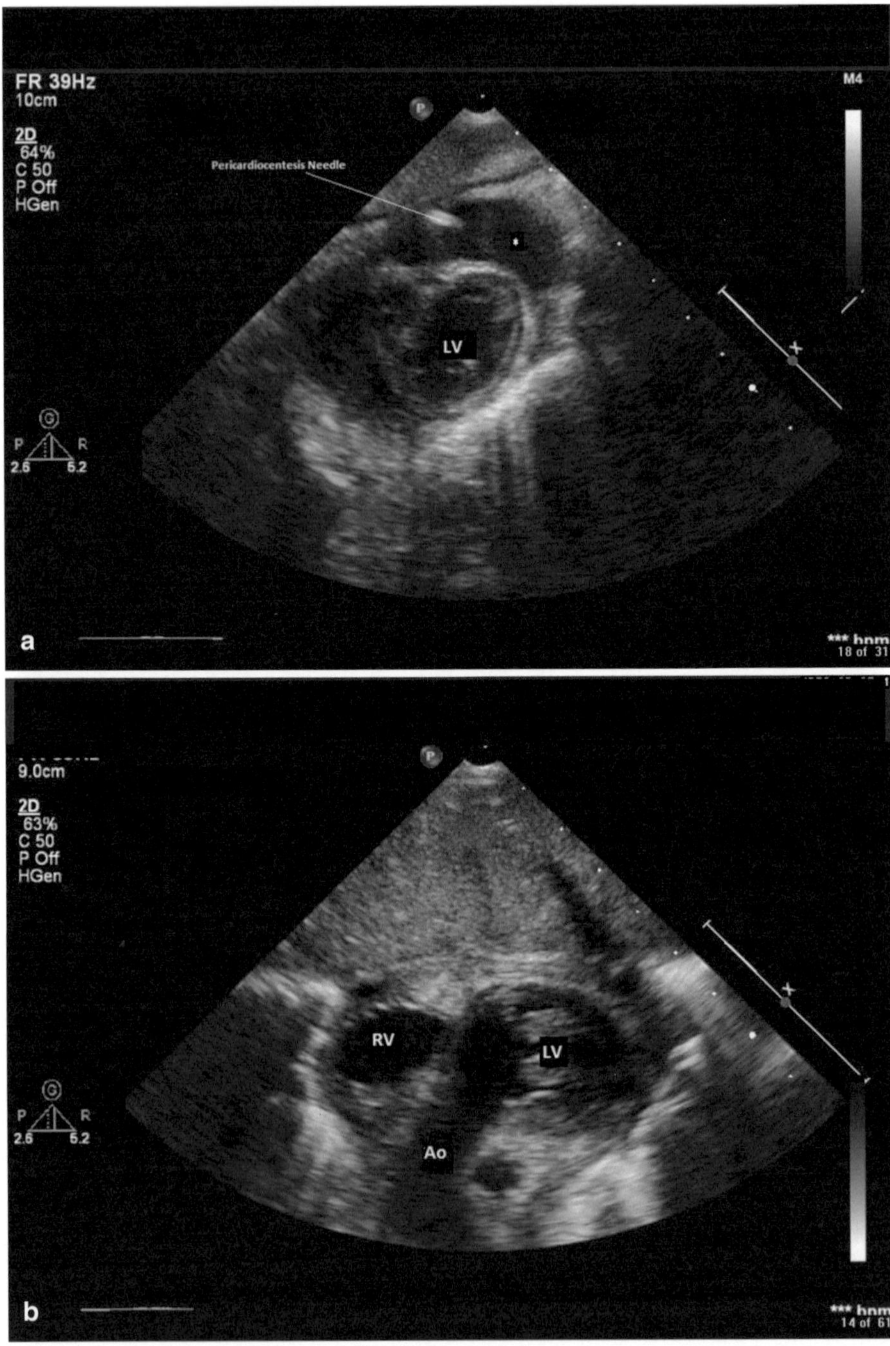

Fig. 17.9 Pericardial effusion (asterisk) in a 5-month-old girl in the subxiphoid view (**a**) during pericardiocentesis (the needle is visible) and (**b**) after pericardiocentesis, without the effusion. *LV* left ventricle

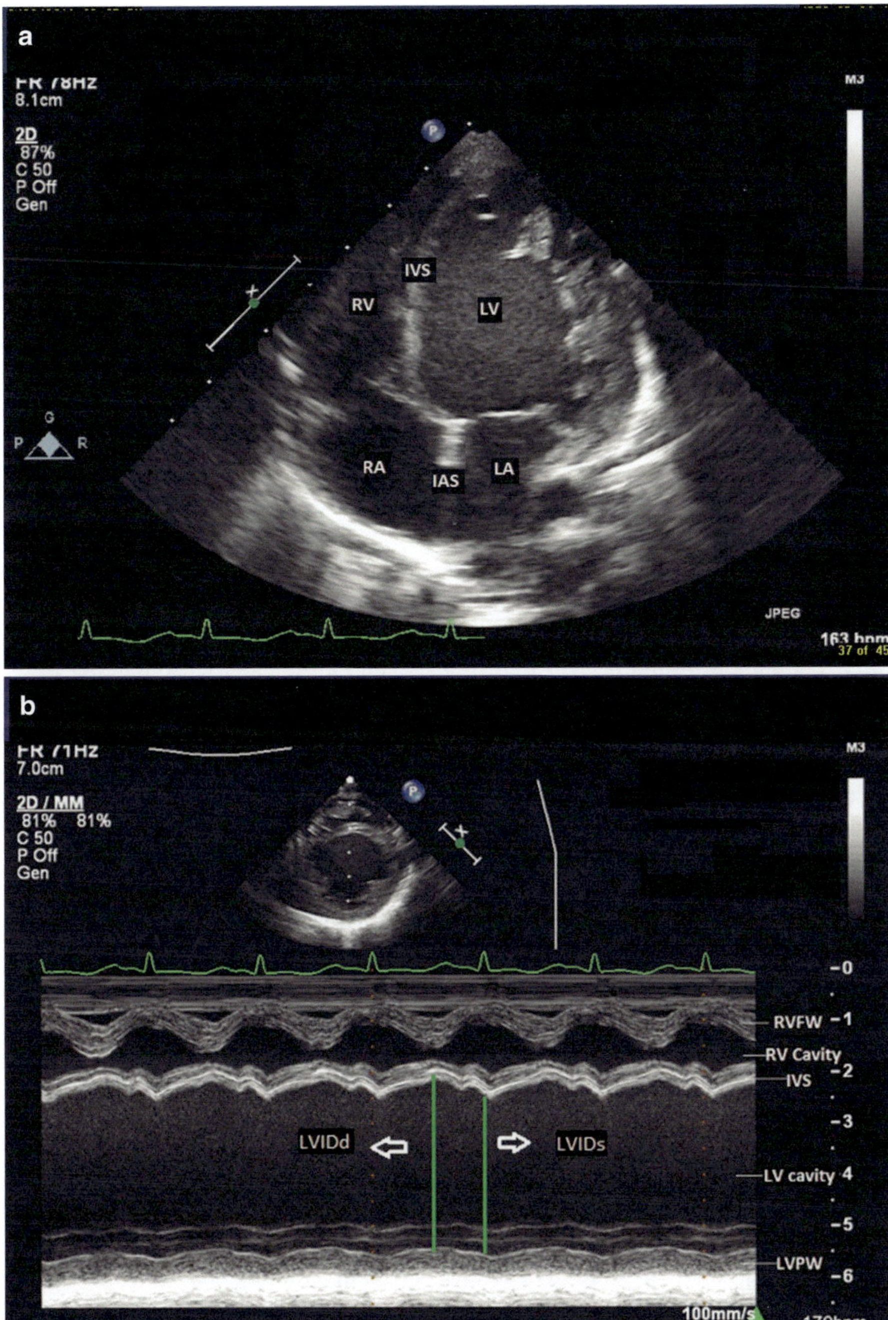

Fig. 17.10 A severely dilated left ventricle with decreased systolic excursion of the ventricular walls in a 6-year-old girl in shock. (**a**) Apical four-chamber view (**b**) parasternal short-axis view, as seen in M-mode echocardiography. The left ventricle is dilated; the ventricular walls show minimal contraction during systole, so function is severely decreased. *RA* right atrium, *RV* right ventricle, *IAS* interatrial septum, *IVS* interventricular septum, *LA* left atrium, *LV* left ventricle, *RVFW* right ventricular free wall, *RV cavity* right ventricular cavity, *LVFW cavity* left ventricular free wall cavity, *LVPW* left ventricular posterior wall

Global cardiac function can be assessed through the various imaging windows described above. Decreased global LV function is seen as decreased excursion of the ventricular walls during the cardiac cycle. Often, the left ventricle is dilated. Qualitative assessment of ventricular function is usually sufficient to guide initial management. Depending on the case, the shortening fraction can also be determined by M-mode from the parasternal long- or short-axis views. In the 6-year-old patient described above, an apical four-chamber view showed a severely dilated left ventricle with decreased systolic excursion of the ventricular walls (Fig. 17.10). M-mode images (Fig. 17.10b) obtained in the parasternal short axis show minimal contraction of the left ventricular walls in systole. The ventricular function in this patient was severely decreased. She was given a dose of IV diuretics, started on inotropic support, and admitted to the intensive care unit for further management.

Case 3: Cardiac Standstill

A previous well, 6-month-old girl presents to the ED unresponsive and without a pulse. The mother reports that she last fed the child 3 h ago, and the girl fed well, without fever, vomiting, color changes, or vomiting. She had gone to sleep uneventfully. The mother found the girl unresponsive and immediately brought her to the ED. In the ED, the patient is unresponsive. Her temperature is 36.5 °C, she has no pulse and is not breathing, and her oxygen saturation is 42%. The monitor shows a sinus rhythm. She has no radial or femoral pulses but has some heart sounds on auscultation. There is no spontaneous movement or breathing. The lung fields are clear. There are no signs of trauma. Cardiac resuscitation and positive-pressure ventilation are immediately started. Intraosseous infusion of fluids is immediately initiated.

How can point-of-care cardiac ultrasound help this patient?

Children are more likely than adults to survive an out-of-hospital cardiac arrest, with more than 10% surviving to hospital discharge. For inhospital cardiac arrests, 25% survive to hospital discharge [18]. Therefore, the emergency physician must differentiate cardiac standstill from correctable causes of pulseless electrical activity. In 10 s, a FOCUS examination can reliably distinguish cardiac activity from standstill, which is the recommended time period for a pulse check [19]. Additionally, determining a child's pulse is often difficult and in some studies was only 78% accurate [20]. A focused cardiac ultrasound can be a reliable alternative to a pulse check and can help diagnose correctible causes of pulseless electrical activity, such as cardiac tamponade and tension pneumothorax. A subxiphoid or parasternal view will show no ventricular wall motion in cardiac standstill. Although rare in children, pulmonary embolism, another cause of pulseless electrical activity, can be diagnosed with ultrasound.

Other Applications of the FOCUS Examination

In adults, the FOCUS examination has also been used to evaluate hydration and the response to fluid resuscitation. This response is usually determined by evaluating the size of inferior vena cava as it enters the right atrium and the extent of collapsibility with respiration. Inferior vena cava volume collapsibility is a marker for central venous pressure, and its collapse may predict hydration status [21]. The marker has not been widely employed in children. The pressure applied to the child's abdomen can compress the inferior vena cava, which can result in underestimation of its diameter on a subxiphoid long-axis image. Additionally, the normal range of IVC diameters in healthy children has not been determined. The vena cava aorta diameter ratio has been used to guide fluid management [22], but results are conflicting, and more research is needed to better measure hydration status with ultrasound.

Limitations

The FOCUS examination aims to diagnose pericardial effusion and cardiogenic shock. However, it cannot assess the heart comprehensively. Many children, especially infants, can present to the ED with undiagnosed congenital heart disease. Shock is often the presenting feature of critical left-sided obstructive lesions, such as coarctation of aorta. The closure of the ductus arteriosus in the first few weeks of life causes cardiogenic shock in infants with certain cardiac lesions, a situation in which administering prostaglandin E1 could be life-saving. Once any abnormal finding is seen during a FOCUS examination, or when a cardiac condition is still a concern despite a normal examination, a complete confirmatory echocardiographic examination should be performed.

When FOCUS is performed during cardiopulmonary resuscitative efforts, it is very important to be cognizant of possible interference with CPR. Chest compressions should not be stopped while attempting to obtain ultrasonographic images.

Conclusion

Timely recognition of pericardial effusion, cardiogenic shock, and cardiac standstill is a critical. A focused cardiac ultrasound, acting as an adjunct to physical examination, is a valuable tool that can be used by emergency physicians to guide clinical management.

Board Question

1. A 15-year-old girl presents after a first syncopal episode, which lasted 2 min. She has had an upper respiratory tract infection for the past 4 days but has no fever. She reports having had intermittent, vague, left-sided sharp chest pain for the past 3 days, although she has not had any chest pain since yesterday. There are no other symptoms and she has no history of trauma or seizures.

Her temperature is 37.0 °C; pulse is 140 bpm; respiration is 45, blood pressure is 112/88, and oxygen saturation is 99%. On examination, she is in respiratory distress, but her lungs are clear. She is tachycardic, and her heart sounds are difficult to hear. She has good peripheral perfusion, and there is no hepatomegaly. Which point-of-care cardiac ultrasound finding can explain her condition?

(A) A 25% collapse in the diameter of the inferior vena cava during inspiration
(B) Collapse of the right ventricle during diastole
(C) Hyperdynamic left ventricular function
(D) The presence of a ventricular septal defect
(E) An enlarged right ventricle with tricuspid regurgitation

References

1. Nomura JT, Leech SJ, Shenbagamurthi S, Sierzenski PR, O'Connor RE, Bollinger M, Gukhool JA. A randomized controlled trial of ultrasound-assisted lumbar puncture. J Ultrasound Med. 2007;26(10):1341–8.
2. Doniger SJ, Ishimine P, Fox JC, Kanegaye JT. Randomized controlled trial of ultrasound-guided peripheral intravenous catheter placement versus traditional techniques in difficult-access pediatric patients. Pediatr Emerg Care. 2009;25(3):154–9.
3. Galicinao J, Bush AJ, Godambe SA. Use of bedside ultrasonography for endotracheal tube placement in pediatric patients: a feasibility study. Pediatrics. 2007;120(6):1297–303.
4. Teichgraber UK, Benter T, Gebel M, Manns MP. A sonographically guided technique for central venous access. Am J Roentgenol. 1997;169:731–3.
5. Randolph AG, Cook DJ, Gonzales CA, Pribble CG. Ultrasound guidance for placement of central venous catheters: a meta-analysis of the literature. Crit Care Med. 1996;24:2053–8.
6. Froehlich CD, Rigby MR, Rosenberg ES, Li R, Roerig PL, Easley KA, Stockwell JA. Ultrasound-guided central venous catheter placement decreases complications and decreases placement attempts compared with the landmark technique in patients in a pediatric intensive care unit. Crit Care Med. 2009;37(3):1090–6.
7. Marin JR, Lewiss RE. Point-of-care ultrasonography by pediatric emergency physicians. Policy statement. Ann Emerg Med. 2015;65(4):472–8.
8. The American Board of Pediatrics. Content outline: pediatric emergency medicine. Subspecialty In-Training, Certification, and Maintenance of Certification (MOC) Exams. p. 135–6. Retrieved on 1/24/2018 from: https://www.abp.org/sites/abp/files/pdf/pediatric_emergency_medicine_content_outline.pdf
9. Vieira RL, Hsu D, Nagler J, Chen L, Gallagher R, Levy JA. Pediatric emergency medicine fellow training in ultrasound: consensus educational guidelines. Acad Emerg Med. 2013;20(3):300–6.
10. Kobal SL, Atar S, Siegel RJ. Hand-carried ultrasound improves the bedside cardiovascular examination. Chest. 2004;126(3):693–701.
11. Doniger SJ. Bedside emergency cardiac ultrasound in children. J Emerg Trauma Shock. 2010;3(3):282–91.
12. Plummer D, Brunette D, Asinger R, Ruiz E. Emergency department echocardiography improves outcome in penetrating cardiac injury. Ann Emerg Med. 1992;21(6):709–12.
13. Mandavia DP, Hoffner RJ, Mahaney K, Henderson SO. Bedside echocardiography by emergency physicians. Ann Emerg Med. 2001;38(4):377–82.

14. Ma OJ, Mateer JR, Ogata M, Kefer MP, Wittmann D, Aprahamian C. Prospective analysis of a rapid trauma ultrasound examination performed by emergency physicians. J Trauma. 1995;38(6):879–85.
15. Singh S, Wann LS, Schuchard GH, Klopfenstein HS, Leimgruber PP, Keelan MH Jr, Brooks HL. Right ventricular and right atrial collapse in patients with cardiac tamponade—a combined echocardiographic and hemodynamic study. Circulation. 1984;70(6):966–71.
16. Akyuz S, Zengin A, Arugaslan E, Yazici S, Onuk T, Ceylan US, Gungor B, Gurkan U, Kemaloglu OT, Kasikcioglu H, Cam N. Echo-guided pericardiocentesis in patients with clinically significant pericardial effusion. Outcomes over a 10-year period. Herz. 2015;40(Suppl 2):153–9.
17. Moore CL, Rose GA, Tayal VS, Sullivan DM, Arrowood JA, Kline JA. Determination of left ventricular function by emergency physician echocardiography of hypotensive patients. Acad Emerg Med. 2002;9(3):186–93.
18. Topjian AA, Nadkarni VM, Berg RA. Cardiopulmonary resuscitation in children. Cur Opin Crit Care. 2009;15(3):203–8.
19. Tsung JW, Blaivas M. Feasibility of correlating the pulse check with focused point-of-care echocardiography during pediatric cardiac arrest: a case series. Resuscitation. 2008;77(2):264–9.
20. Tibballs J, Russell P. Reliability of pulse palpation by healthcare personnel to diagnose paediatric cardiac arrest. Resuscitation. 2009;80(1):61–4.
21. Ayvazyan S, Dickman E, Likourezos A, Wu S, Hannan H, Fromm C, Marshall J. Ultrasound of the inferior vena cava can assess volume status in pediatric patients. J Emerg Med. 2009;37(2):219.
22. Randazzo MR, Snoey ER, Levitt MA, Binder K. Accuracy of emergency physician assessment of left ventricular ejection fraction and central venous pressure using echocardiography. Acad Emerg Med. 2003;10(9):973–7.

Infective Endocarditis

18

Harbir Arora, Eric McGrath, and Basim I. Asmar

Case Vignette

A 13-year-old previously healthy male presented to the emergency department with a 4-day history of fever, neck pain, headache, and vomiting with severe myalgia for 1 day. He had no history of sick contacts or upper respiratory symptoms. On physical examination he appeared tired, and his temperature was 39.5 °C, BP 110/50 mmHg, respiratory rate 20–40/min, and heart rate 90–120/min. He had diffuse muscle tenderness in his arms and legs, a soft grade 2/6 systolic murmur, and hepatosplenomegaly, which was confirmed with abdominal ultrasound. His white blood cell count was 2800/mm^3, hemoglobin 12.0 gm/dL, hematocrit 33.8%, and platelet count 70,000/mm^3, and C-reactive protein was elevated at 133 mg/L. Three separate blood cultures were drawn. He was started on IV vancomycin and ceftriaxone and admitted for further management.

A transthoracic echocardiogram revealed a bicuspid aortic valve, mild to moderate aortic valve insufficiency, and a small vegetation on the mitral valve where an aortic regurgitation jet hits the anterior leaflet. An MRI of the cervical spine obtained to investigate neck pain instead revealed a left cerebellar enhancing lesion that on further imaging was thought to be a brain microabscess. All three blood cultures subsequently grew *Staphylococcus aureus* sensitive to oxacillin. Treatment was changed to IV oxacillin plus gentamicin (for 5 subsequent days to achieve synergistic effect). Follow up two-dimensional transthoracic echocardiography confirmed the presence of an enlarging vegetation at least 10 mm in diameter. Subsequently he had acute mental changes including loss of short-term memory and disorientation. The following day, the vegetation was surgically removed, and the mitral valve was

H. Arora, M.D. (✉) • E. McGrath, M.D. • B. I. Asmar, M.D.
Department of Pediatrics, Wayne State University School of Medicine, Detroit, MI, USA

Division of Infectious Diseases, Children's Hospital of Michigan, Detroit, MI, USA
e-mail: harora@dmc.org; emcgrath@med.wayne.edu; basmar@med.wayne.edu

© Springer International Publishing AG, part of Springer Nature 2018

A. P. Sarnaik et al. (eds.), *Cardiac Emergencies in Children*,
https://doi.org/10.1007/978-3-319-73754-6_18

repaired with a bovine patch without resection of the native valve. He improved with a 6-week course of IV oxacillin. Patient returned to normal health.

Epidemiology of Infective Endocarditis

Infective endocarditis (IE) is seen less frequently in children than in adults, although over the last few decades, the incidence among children has increased in developed countries. This increase is attributed to the improved survival of patients with congenital heart diseases (CHD), the use of prosthetic devices for correction or palliation of heart defects, and more frequent and prolonged use of central venous catheters for medication infusion and blood drawing [1–5]. A recent analysis of the Healthcare Cost and Utilization Project's National Inpatient Sample (NIS) for 2000–2011 showed that the incidence of IE in the USA increased from 11 per 100,000 population to 15 per 100,000 across all age groups [6]. In another recent analysis of pediatric admissions in the same database for 2000–2010, the incidence of IE in pediatric patients was steady at 0.43 per 100,000 children throughout the study period [7].

Rheumatic heart disease was the underlying risk factor of IE in 30–50% of patients before the 1970s [9, 10]; however, recent reports show that this association has decreased to 1–5% [4, 11]. The incidence of IE is much higher in children with CHD, reaching up to 6.1 per 1000 children [12]. Children with cyanotic CHD are at higher risk [8, 11, 12]. Surgery for CHD is a major risk factor for IE. In a cohort of children with IE seen between 1980 and 2011, IE developed in 50% (24/47) of children with CHD after surgical repair. Similar rates of IE (~50%) were found in post-surgical patients with CHD in another case series [11]. In a large cohort study, aortic valve stenosis was the most common underlying CHD of IE, which developed after repair with a prosthetic valve [13]. However, between 18 and 31% of children with IE have no underlying cardiac defect [4, 8, 11]. In about 7% of children, IE is diagnosed within the first month of life, [3] and most patients in this age group (~70%) do not have an underlying CHD. Extreme prematurity, prolonged use of central venous catheters, and major surgeries are the notable risk factors in this age group [14–16].

Pathophysiology of Infective Endocarditis

Turbulent blood flow in the heart from an area of high pressure to an area of low pressure damages the endothelium on the down-pressure side, which becomes a nidus for infection and subsequent vegetation. Such turbulent blood flow can be generated by blood flowing across congenital atrial or ventricular defects, regurgitant or stenotic valves, or the endocardial cushion defect. The endothelium can also be injured by a foreign body, such as palliative shunts, conduits, and central venous catheters. The site of damaged endothelium and the exposed collagen underneath is the site of thrombogenesis where platelets, fibrin, and RBCs attach leading to the formation of sterile vegetation called nonbacterial thrombotic endocarditis (NBTE) [2, 9]. Transient bacteremia occurring because of daily activities such as tooth brushing, flossing, or chewing food seeds the NBTE nidus. Tooth extraction, periodontal surgery, and tonsillectomy are also particularly likely to cause bacteremia. Right-sided endocarditis occurs as a result of bacteremia due to intravenous drug abuse and cardiovascular electronic leads implanted in the right side of the heart [9]. Gram-positive pathogens including *Staphylococcus aureus*, *Streptococcus* species, and *Enterococcus* species express surface molecules called adhesins that are important in attaching the pathogen to the denuded endothelium and sterile vegetations [17]. Subsequently, the formation of vegetation which is composed of bacteria, fibrinogen, and platelets traps the organisms inside which help evade the phagocytes in the circulating blood. Endocarditis in neonates often involves the right side of the heart because of the disruption of endothelium by and concomitant bacteremia caused by central venous catheter contamination. Other possible sources of transient bacteremia in neonates are parenteral nutrition, umbilical catheters, vigorous endotracheal suctioning, and trauma to skin and mucous membranes [2].

Microbiology of Infective Endocarditis

Viridans group *Streptococcus* (VGS) such as *S. sanguis*, *S. mitis*, and *S. mutans* are frequent causes of IE. *Staphylococcus* species including *S. aureus* and coagulase-negative *Staphylococcus* (CONS) are more common than streptococci in causing IE in pediatric patients. *S. aureus*, CONS, and *Candida* species are more commonly isolated from newborns with IE [9].

Historically VGS has been the most common causative agent in children with underlying heart disease after the first year of life [2, 9]. However, recent reviews indicate that *S. aureus* has become the most common pathogen in patients with underlying heart disease after the first year of life [3, 7, 18]. This change was caused by the advanced surgical care and prolonged use of central venous catheters (CVC) in patients with CHD. *S. aureus* is also the most common cause of acute onset rapidly progressing IE.

Enterococci are less commonly found in children with IE than in adults. Gram-negative oropharyngeal flora, the so-called AACEK organisms (formerly HACEK) comprising of *Aggregatibacter* (formerly *Haemophilus*) *parainfluenzae*, *Aggregatibacter* (formerly *Actinobacillus*) *actinomycetemcomitans*, *Cardiobacterium hominis*, *Eikenella corrodens*, and *Kingella kingae*, are other less common causes of endocarditis in children. Among this group *K. kingae* and *A. parainfluenzae* are the more common ones causing IE in children [19]. Enteric gram-negative bacteremia associated with central venous catheters is common, but it generally does not lead to IE, because these gram-negative bacteria cannot adhere to the denuded valves.

Rarely IE is caused by fastidious pathogens previously referred to as nutritionally variant streptococci (NVS) comprised of *Abiotrophia* and *Granulicatella* sp. These pathogens depend on nutrients (L-cysteine and pyridoxal) for their growth and are difficult to grow in regular blood culture medium.

Table 18.1 Organisms isolated in children with infective endocarditis by study and period

	Stockheim et al. [20] (1978–1996) (*n* 134)	Johnson et al. [5] (1980–2011) (*n* 47)	Alshammary et al. [18] (1985–2004) (*n* 37)	Day et al. [3] (2000–2003) (*n* 632)
Organism				
VGS	35 (26%)	17 (36%)	5 (12.5%)	124 (20%)
S. aureus	30 (22%)	12 (25%)	16 (40%)	362 (57%)
Non-VGS (not *S. pneumoniae*)	7 (5%)	2 (4%)	4 (10%)	29 (5%)
S. pneumoniae	8 (6%)	2 (4%)	3 (7.5%)	≤10 (1%)
NVS	1 (0.7%)	3 (6%)	1 (2.5%)	
CONS	13 (10%)	3 (6%)	3 (7.5%)	91 (14%)
AACEK	5 (4%)	4 (8%)		≤10 (1%)
Enterococcus sp.	4 (3%)	1 (2%)	3 (7.5%)	
Other gram-negative	12 (9%)	1 (2%)	2 (5%)	12 (2%)
Candida sp.	4 (3%)	1 (2%)		
Others	15 (11%)	1 (2%)		

VGS Viridans group *Streptococcus*, *CONS* Coagulase-negative *Staphylococcus*, *NVS* Nutritionally variant *Streptococcus*, *AACEK Aggregatibacter parainfluenzae*, *Aggregatibacter actinomycetemcomitans*, *Cardiobacterium hominis*, *Eikenella corrodens*, and *Kingella kingae*, *n* number of culture-positive cases

Culture-negative endocarditis is seen in up to 10% of the cases, which is likely the result of previous antibiotic treatment or caused by fastidious pathogens such as *Coxiella burnetii*, *NVS*, *Bartonella* sp., *Brucella* sp., *or Legionella* species [2, 9].

Organisms isolated in children with infective endocarditis from four recent reviews at large North American centers are listed in Table 18.1.

Clinical Presentation of Infective Endocarditis

Infective endocarditis can present as a subacute illness progressing over a period of a few weeks or as an acute illness with short prodrome and sepsis-like presentation. Subacute presentation is marked by a generally persistent prodrome period of nonspecific symptoms such as low-grade fever (75–100%), malaise (50–75%), anorexia/weight loss (25–50%), arthralgia (17–50%), and chest pain (0–25%) that are generally persistent over a prolonged period of time [20].

Physical signs of IE are mainly the manifestations of valvular damage, embolic phenomena, or immune complex-mediated involvement of different body systems. Cardiac manifestations of IE from valve damage such as murmurs are variable and dependent on preexisting underlying heart disease. New or changed murmurs are found in 21–50% of children with IE. Immune complex deposition in the subcutaneous tissues of extremities leads to the development of small painful Osler nodes (0–10%). Embolic phenomenon in the skin of palms and soles produces Janeway lesions (0–10%) which are painless macules. Splinter hemorrhages in the nail beds (0–10%) and Roth spots with central pallor in the retina (0–10%) are manifestations of small hemorrhagic phenomenon. Embolization of vegetation (25–50%) from the left side of the heart to the abdominal viscera can cause sharp abdominal pain and visceral abscesses; and embolization to the brain may result in mycotic aneurysms and infarcts. Petechiae are seen in 21–50% and splenomegaly in 50–75% of patients. Glomerulonephritis due to immune complex deposition or renal infarcts due to embolization can manifest as hematuria [9, 20, 21].

Diagnosis of Infective Endocarditis

Laboratory Tests

The prompt evaluation and diagnosis of IE are critical to appropriate treatment. The hallmark for diagnosis of IE is serial positive blood cultures. Serial blood cultures (three to five specimens) should be obtained from different venipuncture sites over a period of time, at least 1 hour apart, to optimize recovery of a pathogen in the hemodynamically stable patient before beginning antimicrobial treatment [9, 22]. Modern blood culture technologies can detect nutritionally variant *Streptococcus* (*Abiotrophia* species) and AACEK group organisms. All other laboratory tests other than serial positive blood cultures are nonspecific for IE. A complete blood count may show anemia with thombocytopenia [21]. The erythrocyte sedimentation rate (ESR) is typically elevated, and the rheumatoid factor (RF) is characteristically positive especially in subacute endocarditis. Urinalysis may reveal hematuria, and serum complement levels may be low, suggestive of consumption [21].

Echocardiographic Changes

Echocardiography is paramount to evaluating IE in children and should be performed early to rapidly confirm the diagnosis. Two-dimensional imaging can detect vegetations as small as 2 mm, intracardiac abscesses, and other perivalvular abnormalities. Negative echocardiograms should be interpreted cautiously because images acquired early in the course of IE may miss small vegetations. Echocardiography should be repeated in 7–10 days if concern for IE continues. Transthoracic echocardiography (TTE) is usually adequate for initial rapid imaging and has a higher sensitivity in pediatric patients (≥80%) compared to adults (40–63%) [9, 21–23]. In IE, transesophageal echocardiograph (TEE) can be useful in evaluating patients with congenital heart disease or with complex cardiac anatomy, especially patients with indwelling foreign bodies, including prosthetic valves or post-cardiac surgery patients [2, 21].

Modified Duke Criteria

In the initial emergency department or critical care evaluation of a patient with possible endocarditis, an early, definitive diagnosis of IE may not be possible because it takes time for cultures to be identified as positive for bacterial growth and for echocardiographic changes to occur. However, in patients admitted to outside

Table 18.2 Modified Duke criteria for diagnosing infective endocarditis

Definite infective endocarditis
Pathologic criteria
1. Microorganism detected by culture or histologic examination of a vegetation, an embolized vegetation, or an intracardiac abscess
2. Pathologic lesions (a vegetation or intracardiac abscess) confirmed by histologic examination showing active endocarditis
Clinical criteria[a]
1. Two major criteria
2. One major criterion and three minor criteria
3. Five minor criteria
Possible infective endocarditis
1. One major criterion and one minor criterion
2. Three minor criteria
Rejected
1. Firm alternate diagnosis explaining manifestations of infective endocarditis
2. Resolution of infective endocarditis syndrome with antibiotic therapy for ≤4 days
3. No pathologic evidence of infective endocarditis at surgery or autopsy, with antibiotic therapy for ≤4 days
4. Does not meet criteria for possible infective endocarditis, as above

[a]See Table 18.3 for definitions of major and minor criteria. These criteria have been universally accepted and are in current use [22]. Reprinted [with minor modifications] from Li et al. [24] (copyright © 2000, Oxford University Press) with permission from the publisher

facilities and then transferred to tertiary care centers for more specialized care, blood cultures may now be positive, echocardiographic findings may be distinct, or empiric treatment for IE may have begun before transfer. Therefore, it is appropriate for emergency clinicians to be familiar with the 2000 modified Duke diagnostic criteria for IE [24] (Tables 18.2 and 18.3) [23].

Recognizing Life-Threatening Presentations of IE

In addition to the common symptoms of IE reviewed above, patients with life-threatening IE can have new heart failure symptoms and may have a sepsis-like presentation. Although nearly all patients with IE have fever, only 25–50% of children with IE have heart failure, and only 0–25% have chest pain [21]. A focal neurologic deficit may be important if it is associated with an ongoing or recurrent embolic event. As vegetations grow, they may break off and embolize to the lungs in right-sided IE or to the central nervous system, spleen, or extremities in left-sided IE. These events may predominate in some patients; therefore, patients with fever and central nervous system symptoms (including severe headache, sterile meningitis, or focal neurologic signs), pneumonia, or pulmonary embolism should have immediate evaluation for IE [25, 26].

Table 18.3 Major and minor criteria in the Modified Duke Criteria for diagnosing infective endocarditis

Major criteria
1. Blood culture positive for IE
(a) Typical microorganisms consistent with IE from two separate blood cultures
(i) Viridans streptococci (including nutritionally variant strains A*biotrophia* species)
(ii) *Streptococcus bovis*
(iii) AACEK group
(iv) *Staphylococcus aureus*
(v) Community-acquired enterococci, in the absence of a primary focus
(b) Microorganisms consistent with IE from persistently positive blood cultures, defined as follows:
At least 2 positive cultures of blood drawn either >12 h apart
or
All of 3 or a majority of ≥4 separate cultures of blood
(c) Single positive blood culture for *Coxiella burnetii* or
IgG antibody titer >1:800
2. Evidence of endocardial involvement by positive echocardiogram for IE (transesophageal echocardiography recommended in patients with prosthetic valves, transthoracic echocardiography as first test in other patients) defined as follows:
(i) Oscillating intracardiac mass on valve or supporting structures, in the path of regurgitant jets, or on implanted material (in the absence of an alternative anatomic explanation)
(ii) Abscess
(iii) New or partial dehiscence of prosthetic valve
New valvular regurgitation (worsening or changing of preexisting murmur not sufficient)
Minor criteria
1. *Predisposition*: Predisposing heart condition or injection drug use
2. *Fever*: temperature > 38° C
3. *Vascular phenomena*: Major arterial emboli, septic pulmonary infarcts, mycotic aneurysm, intracranial hemorrhage, conjunctival hemorrhages, Janeway lesions
4. *Immunologic phenomena*: Glomerulonephritis, Osler nodes, Roth spots, rheumatoid factor
5. *Microbiological evidence*: Positive blood culture but does meet a major criterion as noted above[a] or serological evidence of active infection with organism consistent with infective endocarditis

AACEK indicates *Aggregatibacter* (formerly*) parainfluenzae*, *Aggregatibacter* (formerly *Actinobacillus*) *actinomycetemcomitans*, *Cardiobacterium hominis*, *Eikenella corrodens*, and *Kingella kingae*; *IgG* immunoglobulin G, *TEE* transesophageal echocardiography, and *TTE* transthoracic echocardiograph. These criteria have been universally accepted and are in current use [22]. Reprinted [with minor modifications] from Li et al. [24] (copyright © 2000, Oxford University Press) with permission from the publisher

Managing of Infective Endocarditis in the Emergency Department

Initial Assessment and Evaluation

When IE is suspected, the most urgent evaluation in the emergency department is hemodynamic status. If heart failure is suspected, echocardiographic imaging and several closely spaced blood cultures should be obtained without delay, in addition to routine tests, such as a complete blood count with differential to assess for anemia and thrombocytopenia and a metabolic panel including renal function assessment. Hemodynamic support such as administering vasopressors and transfer to a critical care unit may be necessary including immediate empiric antimicrobial therapy (see below). Patients with confirmed heart failure may require urgent cardiac surgery [9, 21, 22].

Treating Infective Endocarditis

The American Heart Association has issued and updated comprehensive guidelines for treating IE [9, 22, 23]. Presumptive antibiotic treatment is based on the patient's age, clinical presentation, preexisting cardiac status, recent surgery, and local antimicrobial sensitivity. Antimicrobial therapy should begin only after appropriate blood cultures have been obtained. Until the cultures can be evaluated, empiric therapy is generally required [22]. Renal function should be assessed if vancomycin or gentamicin is administered. Reviewing and defining the choice of parenteral therapy with an infectious disease specialist is recommended [9, 22]. Finally, empiric therapy should be revised to a focused, narrowed therapy for any specific pathogen identified by blood culture or by other laboratory methods.

For patients with an acute clinical presentation (days) with suspected or proven native valve infection, empiric coverage for *S. aureus*, streptococci, and aerobic gram-negative bacilli may include intravenous (IV) vancomycin and cefepime. For patients with a subacute (weeks) presentation of native valve infection, empirical coverage of *S. aureus*, viridans group streptococci, AACEK, and enterococci with IV vancomycin and ampicillin-sulbactam (Unasyn®) is reasonable [22].

For patients with suspected or proven prosthetic valve infection, treating *Staphylococcus*, enterococci, and aerobic gram-negative bacilli is reasonable if the onset of symptoms is within 1 year of surgical placement of the valve. This regimen may include IV vancomycin, rifampin, gentamicin, and cefepime. However, if the onset of symptoms is >1 year after valve placement, IV vancomycin and ceftriaxone may be appropriate to cover staphylococci, viridans group streptococci, and enterococci [22].

Surgical Evaluation

In the emergency department, immediate consultation with cardiology and cardiovascular surgery may be warranted in several groups of patients:

- Patients with left-sided native valve endocarditis, prosthetic valve endocarditis (PVE), and, rarely, right-sided native valve IE, who may benefit from early valve surgery
- Patients with suspected or confirmed IE with symptoms or signs of heart failure [9, 21, 22]
- Patients with new heart block and annular or aortic abscess or destructive penetrating lesions
- Patients with PVE and heart failure secondary to valve dehiscence, intracardiac fistula, or severe prosthetic valve dysfunction and those with relapsing PVE
- Patients with recurrent emboli and persistent or enlarging vegetations despite appropriate antimicrobial therapy and those with severe valvular regurgitation and mobile vegetations at least 10 mm in diameter
- Patients with right-sided IE with tricuspid valve vegetations at least 20 mm in diameter and recurrent pulmonary embolism despite antimicrobial therapy
- Patients with IE caused by fungal pathogens or highly resistant bacterial pathogens recovered from blood cultures or previously documented at the outside referring center [9, 22, 27–29].

Complications of Infective Endocarditis

Complications of IE include valve damage, spread of infection (perivalvular), or heart failure. Heart failure may result from the incompetence of the valve after infection of the chordae tendineae with rupture or by obstructive lesions (vegetations) or other damage to key cardiac structures. Perivalvular infection extension may result in cardiac abscess, fistula, or pseudoaneurysm [21]. Additionally, in PVE, infection may cause the prosthesis to become unstable [9]. Emboli from right-sided endocarditis may cause necrotizing pneumonia and prolonged fever, whereas emboli from left-sided endocarditis can lead to systemic emboli to central nervous system, visceral organs, limbs, and coronary arteries. Septic emboli may result in hemorrhage, infarct, or abscess in intra-abdominal organs [9, 21, 22, 26]. When these septic emboli travel to the central nervous system, they may result in stroke symptoms or mycotic aneurysm [9, 21, 22, 26]. Renal failure can occur from immune complex deposition or as an adverse side effect of therapy [21].

Outcomes and Preventing Infective Endocarditis

More than 90% of children with native valve endocarditis due to viridans group streptococci can be cured. Cure rates for enterococci IE vary from 75 to 90% when treated with synergistic antibiotics; cure rates are lower for *S. aureus*, in the range of 60–75%. Gram-negative bacilli IE cure rates are even lower at less than 50%; fungal IE cure rates are under 20% [21].

The 2007 American Heart Association guidelines recommend antibacterial prophylaxis before high-risk dental procedures in the highest-risk groups. These groups include patients with a history of cardiac valve repair with prosthetic valve or material, previous IE, and certain congenital heart diseases (unrepaired cyanotic CHD, repaired CHD with prosthetic material or a device during the first 6 months post-procedure, repaired CHD with residual defects at the site adjacent to the site of the prosthetic patch or device) and recipients of heart transplants who have cardiac valvulopathy [9, 22, 30].

Infective Endocarditis Clinical Pearls

- Incidence of infective endocarditis in children has increased over the past few decades due to improved survival of children with congenital heart disease, use of prosthetic devices for correcting heart defects, and more frequent and prolonged use of central venous catheters.
- Incidence of infective endocarditis is highest in children with congenital heart disease. Surgery for congenital heart disease is a major risk factor.
- Turbulent flow in the heart from an area of high pressure to an area of low pressure damages the endothelium in the down-pressure area which becomes a nidus for infection and subsequent vegetation.
- *Staphylococcus aureus* has replaced viridans group *Streptococcus* (VGS) as the most common cause of infective endocarditis in children with underlying heart disease after the first year of life. Gram-negative oropharyngeal flora, the so-called AACEK (previously HACEK) organisms, are a less common cause of infective endocarditis in children. Rarely, fastidious pathogens, previously referred to as nutritionally variant streptococci (NVS), now comprised of *Abiotrophia* species, can cause infective endocarditis.
- Infective endocarditis can present as subacute illness progressing over a few weeks or as acute illness with sepsis-like presentation. Subacute presentation may include with nonspecific symptoms such as low-grade fever, malaise anorexia/weight loss, headache, and arthralgia. Physical signs are mainly the manifestations of valvular damage, embolic phenomenon, and immune complex-mediated involvement of different body systems.
- The hallmark diagnosis of infective endocarditis is serial positive blood cultures obtained, over a period of time, from different venipuncture sites. Blood count may show anemia and thrombocytopenia. The erythrocyte sedimentation rate is typically elevated. Urinalysis may show hematuria, and serum complement concentration may be low.

- Echocardiography is paramount to evaluating infective endocarditis in children. Two-dimensional imaging can detect vegetations as small as 2 mm. Transthoracic echocardiography is usually adequate for initial rapid imaging (sensitivity is 80% in children). Transesophageal echocardiography can be useful in evaluating patients with congenital heart disease or with complex cardiac anatomy.
- The Modified Duke Criteria are useful in making or rejecting the diagnosis of infective endocarditis. Major criteria are based on blood cultures and echocardiography results. Minor criteria are based on predisposing heart condition, fever, and signs of vascular and immunologic phenomena.
- Patients with life-threatening infective endocarditis can have heart failure symptoms and may have sepsis-like presentation. The most urgent evaluation in the emergency department is hemodynamic status. If heart failure is suspected, echocardiography and several closely spaced blood cultures should be obtained without delay. Hemodynamic support and transfer to a critical care unit may be necessary.
- Presumptive antibiotic treatment is based on the patient's age, clinical presentation, preexisting cardiac status, recent surgery, and local antimicrobial sensitivity. Reviewing and defining the choice of parenteral therapy with an infectious disease specialist is warranted. The American Heart Association has issued and updated comprehensive guidelines for treating infective endocarditis.
- In the emergency department, immediate consultation with cardiology and cardiovascular surgery may be warranted in several groups of patients including those with left-sided native valve endocarditis, prosthetic valve endocarditis, heart failure, recurrent emboli and those with tricuspid valve vegetation at least 20 mm in diameter.

References

1. Awadallah SM, Kavey RE, Byrum CJ, Smith FC, Kveselis DA, Blackman MS. The changing pattern of infective endocarditis in childhood. Am J Cardiol. 1991;68:90–4.
2. Ferrieri P, Gewitz MH, Gerber MA, et al. Unique features of infective endocarditis in childhood. Pediatrics. 2002;109:931–43.
3. Day MD, Gauvreau K, Shulman S, Newburger JW. Characteristics of children hospitalized with infective endocarditis. Circulation. 2009;119:865–70.
4. Rosenthal LB, Feja KN, Levasseur SM, Alba LR, Gersony W, Saiman L. The changing epidemiology of pediatric endocarditis at a children's hospital over seven decades. Pediatr Cardiol. 2010;31:813–20.
5. Johnson JA, Boyce TG, Cetta F, Steckelberg JM, Johnson JN. Infective endocarditis in the pediatric patient: a 60-year single-institution review. Mayo Clin Proc. 2012;87:629–35.
6. Pant S, Patel NJ, Deshmukh A, et al. Trends in infective endocarditis incidence, microbiology, and valve replacement in the United States from 2000 to 2011. J Am Coll Cardiol. 2015;65:2070–6.
7. Gupta S, Sakhuja A, McGrath E, Asmar B. Trends, microbiology, and outcomes of infective endocarditis in children during 2000–2010 in the United States. Congenit Heart Dis. 2017;12:196–201.
8. Coward K, Tucker N, Darville T. Infective endocarditis in Arkansan children from 1990 through 2002. Pediatr Infect Dis J. 2003;22:1048–52.
9. Baltimore RS, Gewitz M, Baddour LM, et al. Infective endocarditis in childhood: 2015 update: a scientific statement from the American Heart Association. Circulation. 2015;132:1487–515.

10. Stull TL, Lipuma JJ. Endocarditis in children. 2nd ed. New York: Raven Press; 1992.
11. Saiman L, Prince A, Gersony WM. Pediatric infective endocarditis in the modern era. J Pediatr. 1993;122:847–53.
12. Rushani D, Kaufman JS, Ionescu-Ittu R, et al. Infective endocarditis in children with congenital heart disease: cumulative incidence and predictors. Circulation. 2013;128:1412–9.
13. Morris CD, Reller MD, Menashe VD. Thirty-year incidence of infective endocarditis after surgery for congenital heart defect. JAMA. 1998;279:599–603.
14. Daher AH, Berkowitz FE. Infective endocarditis in neonates. Clin Pediatr (Phila). 1995;34:198–206.
15. Oelberg DG. Neonatal endocarditis–neither rare nor fatal. Clin Pediatr (Phila). 1998;37:747–8.
16. Opie GF, Fraser SH, Drew JH, Drew S. Bacterial endocarditis in neonatal intensive care. J Paediatr Child Health. 1999;35:545–8.
17. Moreillon P, Que YA. Infective endocarditis. Lancet. 2004;363:139–49.
18. Alshammary A, Hervas-Malo M, Robinson JL. Pediatric infective endocarditis: has Staphylococcus aureus overtaken viridans group streptococci as the predominant etiological agent? Can J Infect Dis Med Microbiol. 2008;19:63–8.
19. Feder HM Jr, Roberts JC, Salazar J, Leopold HB, Toro-Salazar O. HACEK endocarditis in infants and children: two cases and a literature review. Pediatr Infect Dis J. 2003;22:557–62.
20. Stockheim JA, Chadwick EG, Kessler S, et al. Are the Duke criteria superior to the Beth Israel criteria for the diagnosis of infective endocarditis in children? Clin Infect Dis. 1998;27:1451–6.
21. Levasseur SS, Saiman L. Endocarditis and other intravascular infections. In: Long SS, Pickering LK, Prober CG, editors. Principles and practice of pediatric infectious diseases. 4th ed. Philadelphia: Elsevier Saunders; 2012. p. 256–65.
22. Baddour LM, Wilson WR, Bayer AS, et al. Infective endocarditis in adults: diagnosis, antimicrobial therapy, and management of complications: a scientific statement for healthcare professionals from the american heart association. Circulation. 2015;132:1435–86.
23. Baddour LM, Wilson WR, Bayer AS, et al. Infective endocarditis: diagnosis, antimicrobial therapy, and management of complications: a statement for healthcare professionals from the Committee on Rheumatic Fever, Endocarditis, and Kawasaki Disease, Council on Cardiovascular Disease in the Young, and the Councils on Clinical Cardiology, Stroke, and Cardiovascular Surgery and Anesthesia, American Heart Association: endorsed by the Infectious Diseases Society of America. Circulation. 2005;111:e394–434.
24. Li JS, Sexton DJ, Mick N, et al. Proposed modifications to the Duke criteria for the diagnosis of infective endocarditis. Clin Infect Dis. 2000;30:633–8.
25. Tan M, Armstrong D, Birken C, et al. Bacterial endocarditis in a child presenting with acute arterial ischemic stroke: should thrombolytic therapy be absolutely contraindicated? Dev Med Child Neurol. 2009;51:151–4.
26. Thuny F, Di Salvo G, Belliard O, et al. Risk of embolism and death in infective endocarditis: prognostic value of echocardiography: a prospective multicenter study. Circulation. 2005;112:69–75.
27. Aksoy O, Sexton DJ, Wang A, et al. Early surgery in patients with infective endocarditis: a propensity score analysis. Clin Infect Dis. 2007;44:364–72.
28. Cabell CH, Abrutyn E, Fowler VG Jr, et al. Use of surgery in patients with native valve infective endocarditis: results from the International Collaboration on Endocarditis Merged Database. Am Heart J. 2005;150:1092–8.
29. Wang A, Pappas P, Anstrom KJ, et al. The use and effect of surgical therapy for prosthetic valve infective endocarditis: a propensity analysis of a multicenter, international cohort. Am Heart J. 2005;150:1086–91.
30. Wilson W, Taubert KA, Gewitz M, et al. Prevention of infective endocarditis: guidelines from the American Heart Association: a guideline from the American Heart Association Rheumatic Fever, Endocarditis and Kawasaki Disease Committee, Council on Cardiovascular Disease in the Young, and the Council on Clinical Cardiology, Council on Cardiovascular Surgery and Anesthesia, and the Quality of Care and Outcomes Research Interdisciplinary Working Group. J Am Dent Assoc. 2007;138:739–45; 47–60.

19 Inflammatory Heart Diseases in Children

Adam L. Ware, Dongngan T. Truong, and Lloyd Y. Tani

Inflammatory illnesses, such as rheumatic fever, Kawasaki disease, and viral myocarditis, can cause substantial acute cardiovascular damage and lead to longstanding complications in children. The acute presentations of these conditions are variable and can range from mild, nonspecific symptoms to life-threatening cardiovascular collapse. The emergency department is often the first point of medical care for these patients, and early recognition and treatment of the underlying inflammation are essential to preventing cardiac damage.

Rheumatic Fever

Clinical Vignette

An 8-year-old-girl was admitted to the emergency department because of uncontrollable arm movements. Her parents reported that she had a 4-week history of worsening coordination and fidgeting. She has been tripping over objects and bumping into walls and is unable to sit still. Her teachers recently commented on a decline in her penmanship and said that she is more disruptive and moody in class. She has no remarkable medical history and no recent illnesses, except for a sore throat and fever several months ago that resolved spontaneously. Physical examination revealed a new 3/6 high-pitched systolic murmur at the apex that radiates to the left axillae.

A. L. Ware, M.D. (✉) • D. T. Truong, M.D. • L. Y. Tani, M.D.
Department of Pediatrics, Division of Pediatric Cardiology, University of Utah School of Medicine, Primary Children's Hospital, Salt Lake City, UT, USA
e-mail: adam.ware@hsc.utah.edu; dongngan.truong@hsc.utah.edu; Lloyd.Tani@hsc.utah.edu

© Springer International Publishing AG, part of Springer Nature 2018

A. P. Sarnaik et al. (eds.), *Cardiac Emergencies in Children*,
https://doi.org/10.1007/978-3-319-73754-6_19

The Pathophysiology of Rheumatic Fever

Acute rheumatic fever (ARF) is an acute inflammatory illness that follows group A streptococcal (GAS) pharyngitis caused by an abnormal immune response in a susceptible host. The immune response may cause inflammation of the heart, joints, brain, or connective tissue. Certain strains of GAS are more likely to cause ARF. These rheumatogenic strains express specific virulence factors, including the M protein, on the cell surface [1]. The pathogenesis of ARF is not completely understood, but current models suggest that after exposure to certain streptococcal antigens, a process known as "molecular mimicry" can begin an abnormal cellular and humoral immune response. Antibodies directed at GAS cross-react with host antigens, including cardiac antigens, initiating an inflammatory cascade. Endothelial cell damage leads to infiltration of additional inflammatory cells, and exposed cardiac proteins further activate the immune system in a process known as "epitope spreading." Serial exposure to the GAS antigen may lead to recurrence of ARF and increase the likelihood of persistent and evolving cardiac changes manifesting as chronic rheumatic heart disease (RHD). The dominant abnormality in RHD is mitral valve dysfunction with variable combinations of insufficiency and stenosis. The aortic valve is less commonly affected. Although the incidence of ARF has declined sharply in developed countries, ARF leading to RHD remains the leading cause of heart failure in children and adolescents in the developing world [2].

The Acute Presentation of Rheumatic Fever

Acute rheumatic fever typically presents in children 5–15 years of age, although it occasionally affects younger children and older adolescents or young adults. The five major diagnostic criteria are carditis, arthritis, chorea, subcutaneous nodules, and erythema marginatum: the "Jones criteria." Carditis and arthritis are the most common and are seen in 50–70% and 35–66% of cases, respectively. Chorea (10–30%) is less common, and subcutaneous nodules (0–10%) and erythema marginatum (<6%) are rare [3]. Most symptoms appear 10 days to 5 weeks after GAS pharyngitis, with chorea presenting up to 6 months after the initial illness. The GAS pharyngitis that precedes ARF may be mild or even subclinical. Patients most commonly seek medical care for joint pain and inflammation. Patients with cardiac involvement may present due to heart failure symptoms related to marked valve regurgitation or a new murmur detected on physical examination.

The Jones criteria have been used since 1944 and have been revised several times, most recently in 2015 (Table 19.1) [3]. The diagnosis of ARF is based on the presence of two major criteria or one major criterion and two minor criteria, in addition to evidence of a preceding GAS infection. Given the wide global variability in the incidence of ARF, the latest revision of the Jones criteria suggests that children should be categorized as low risk or moderate to high risk for ARF and that different diagnostic criteria should be used according to these categories (Table 19.1). Risk stratification is based on the population incidence of ARF and RHD. Low-risk

Table 19.1 Revised Jones criteria for diagnosing acute rheumatic fever in patients with evidence of a preceding group A streptococcal infection

Low-risk populations[a]	Moderate-to-high-risk populations
Major criteria	
Carditis[b] • Clinical or subclinical	Carditis • Clinical or subclinical
Arthritis • Polyarthritis only	Arthritis • Monoarthritis or polyarthritis • Polyarthralgia[c]
Chorea	Chorea
Erythema marginatum	Erythema marginatum
Subcutaneous nodules	Subcutaneous nodules
Minor criteria	
Polyarthralgia	Monoarthralgia
Fever (≥38.5 °C)	Fever (≥38 °C)
ESR ≥60 mm/h and/or a CRP concentration ≥ 3.0 mg/dL[d]	ESR ≥30 mm/h and/or a CRP concentration ≥ 3.0 mg/dL[d]
Prolonged PR interval, after accounting for age variability (unless carditis is a major criterion)	Prolonged PR interval, after accounting for age variability (unless carditis is a major criterion)

A diagnosis of initial acute rheumatic fever requires two major manifestations or one major plus two minor manifestations. A diagnosis of recurrent acute rheumatic fever requires two major manifestations, one major and two minor manifestations, or three minor manifestations

CRP C-reactive protein, *ESR* erythrocyte sedimentation rate

[a]Low-risk populations are those with an ARF incidence ≤2 per 100,000 school-aged children or an all-age rheumatic heart disease prevalence of ≤1 per 1000 population per year

[b]Subclinical carditis indicated by echocardiographic evidence of valvulitis

[c]Polyarthralgia should only be considered as a major manifestation in moderate-to-high-risk populations after excluding other causes. Additionally, joint manifestations can be considered in either the major or minor categories but not both in the same patient

[d]CRP concentration must be greater than the laboratory's upper limit of normal. Also, because ESR may evolve during the course of ARF, peak ESR values should be used

patients reside in populations with an annual incidence of fewer than 2 cases of ARF per 100,000 school-aged children or an all-age prevalence of RHD of not more than 1 per 1000 population. Children clearly not from a low-risk population should be considered at moderate to high risk. The definition of major and minor criteria varies based on the child's risk stratification (Table 19.1) [3]. Populations from most developed countries, including the USA, are considered to be low risk.

Carditis is the most common major feature of ARF. Carditis typically presents as a valvulitis with new-onset mitral insufficiency, with or without aortic valve insufficiency (Fig. 19.1). Mitral insufficiency is almost universal in ARF patients with carditis, presenting in up to 95% of carditis cases [2]. Aortic insufficiency is less common and usually presents in combination with mitral insufficiency. Mild valve insufficiency may not be recognized without an echocardiogram and is usually asymptomatic. Moderate and severe mitral insufficiency can lead to pulmonary congestion and edema, so affected patients may present with cough, dyspnea on exertion, shortness of breath, and orthopnea. Pericarditis and myocarditis may be

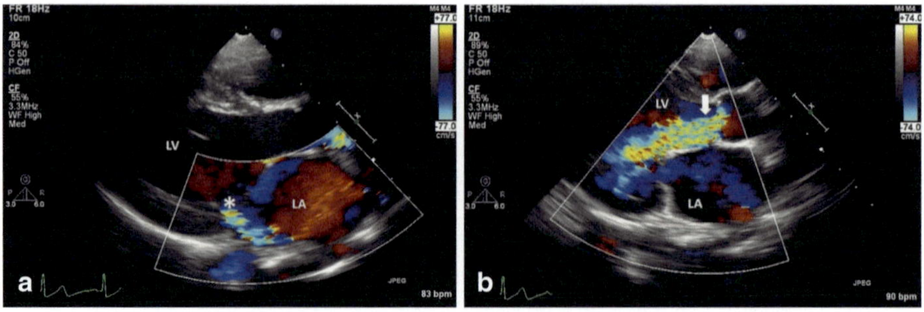

Fig. 19.1 (**a**) Mitral insufficiency (asterisk) and (**b**) aortic insufficiency (arrow) in an 8-year-old boy with acute rheumatic fever at presentation. *LA* left atrium, *LV* left ventricle

present, but in the absence of valve insufficiency, they should not be considered a major manifestation of the Jones criteria. Pericarditis of ARF is rarely associated with large effusions or tamponade. Biopsies may reveal evidence of myocarditis, but unlike other forms of myocarditis, myocyte necrosis does not occur, and troponin concentrations are not elevated [2]. All patients with carditis should be referred to a cardiologist.

Subclinical carditis has been described in rheumatic fever, and strict echocardiographic criteria have been established to diagnose features of carditis that may be inaudible. For this reason, all patients with confirmed or suspected ARF should undergo echocardiography. Clinical or subclinical carditis is a major criterion for the diagnosis of ARF in both risk groups.

Arthritis is a common feature of ARF and one that needs to be assessed carefully. The differential diagnosis for arthritis is broad and creates the potential for misdiagnosis. Additionally, salicylates and other nonsteroidal anti-inflammatory drugs relieve the pain, and ready access to these medications may alter the natural course of the arthritis. The classic presentation is a migratory polyarthritis of the large joints. The polyarthritis manifests as swollen and erythematous joints with pain that is often out of proportion to the physical findings. In addition to polyarthritis, aseptic monoarthritis has been described in high-risk populations. Polyarthralgia is a minor criterion in low-risk populations and a major criterion in high-risk populations. Post-streptococcal reactive arthritis should not be mistaken for the arthritis or polyarthralgia of ARF. As opposed to the arthritis of ARF, post-streptococcal reactive arthritis tends to involve small joints, is more persistent, and is less responsive to anti-inflammatory medications.

As exemplified in the clinical vignette above, chorea is the involuntary and purposeless movements of the trunk and extremities, as well as muscle weakness and emotional lability. It is a late finding in ARF, occurring 2–6 months after the initial GAS pharyngitis. Physical exam findings consistent with chorea include "milkmaid's grip," or irregular contractions of the fingers when squeezing an object; "pronator sign," or the pronation of hands when extended above the head; and "spooning," or the hyperextension of the fingers when the hands are extended forward while the eyes are closed. Parents may notice increased emotional lability or

Table 19.2 Tests for diagnosing suspected rheumatic fever

Laboratory tests • Evidence of inflammation: elevated C-reactive protein concentration, erythrocyte sedimentation rate, or white blood cell count • Evidence of group A streptococcal infection: elevated anti-streptolysin O or anti-DNase B titers, rapid streptococcal antigen test, throat culture • Consider additional infectious work-up: blood culture or viral PCR testing to rule out other diagnoses
Chest radiography (if evidence of carditis)
Electrocardiography
Echocardiography

new difficulties with fine muscular coordination, such as degraded penmanship or the ability to button clothing. Chorea of ARF must be differentiated from other inherited and acquired neurologic disorders as described in the section below. Consulting with a neurologist is strongly encouraged.

The dermatologic findings in ARF include erythema marginatum and subcutaneous nodules. Erythema marginatum consists of a bright-pink, macular, nonpruritic, and often evanescent rash with serpiginous borders and a pale center. The rash is usually on the trunk and proximal extremities and rarely affects the face. The subcutaneous nodules are small, firm, painless nodules on the bony portions of the extensor surfaces of the joints and on the spinous processes of the back. They are not transient and may last for weeks. The cutaneous manifestations of ARF are usually associated with carditis and are rarely the only major criteria for diagnosis [3].

As with the major criteria, the minor criteria vary based on risk category (Table 19.1). As mentioned earlier, polyarthralgia is a minor criterion in low-risk patients. Fever is a consistent feature of ARF, and in high-risk populations, a lower fever is a minor criterion. Laboratory evidence of systemic inflammation is common and also varies based on the pretest probability of ARF. In the absence of an elevated C-reactive protein (CRP) concentration or erythrocyte sedimentation rate (ESR), the diagnosis of ARF is unlikely, except in cases presenting with chorea or indolent carditis. Finally, conduction abnormalities can be seen in ARF, with the most common being first-degree atrioventricular block, although a more advanced atrioventricular block can be seen as well.

Laboratory evidence of a preceding streptococcal infection from a positive throat culture, rapid strep test, or an elevated or rising anti-streptolysin O or anti-DNAse B titer is required for the diagnosis of ARF (Tables 19.1 and 19.2). However, evidence of a prior GAS infection may be absent in patients presenting with chorea or chronic valve insufficiency (chronic RHD), given the delayed presentation of these conditions.

The Differential Diagnosis of Rheumatic Fever

The differential diagnosis of ARF largely depends on the patient's primary symptoms. The carditis of ARF should be distinguished from other causes of new valvar regurgitation, such as infective endocarditis or progressive valve insufficiency related to an underlying congenital abnormality. Innocent murmurs are common in school-aged children and should be differentiated from the regurgitant murmurs associated with ARF. Arthritis should be distinguished from a post-streptococcal reactive arthropathy, connective tissue diseases, and infectious causes, including viral arthropathies and septic arthritis. Isolated chorea should lead to a thorough investigation of inherited causes, such as Huntington disease, Wilson disease, Lesch-Nyhan syndrome, ataxia-telangiectasia, and Friedreich's ataxia. Autoimmune disorders, such as lupus, endocrine and metabolic disorders, psychological disorders, and toxin or drug exposure should also be ruled out.

Managing Rheumatic Fever in the Emergency Department

The essential first step in managing inflammatory diseases with potential cardiac involvement such as ARF is to recognize the clinical features and diagnose the condition correctly. Initial treatment of ARF is aimed at eliminating the immune response, decreasing inflammation, and addressing valve insufficiency.

All patients with a diagnosis of ARF should be treated with antibiotics for GAS (Table 19.3). Patients with joint symptoms should be started on aspirin or other nonsteroidal anti-inflammatory medications. Treatment of chorea depends on the severity of symptoms; a neurology consultation should be strongly considered. Any patient in whom ARF is suspected should undergo echocardiography, and a cardiologist should be consulted if carditis is present. Patients with ARF and mild-to-moderate carditis should be treated with high-dose aspirin (80–100 mg/kg/day divided every 6 h in children or 4–8 g/day in adolescents and adults). In patients with moderate-to-severe carditis, many experts recommend a course of steroids (some recommend prednisone 2 mg/kg/day for 2 weeks followed by taper), although there is no evidence of clear benefit. Patients with subclinical and very mild carditis may be followed closely as outpatients, whereas those with moderate-to-severe carditis should be monitored as inpatients. Patients with signs of hemodynamic compromise related to marked valvular dysfunction should be admitted to an intensive care unit.

Ruptured mitral valve chordae can lead to severe valvular insufficiency and flail mitral leaflets. Patients presenting with severe valve insufficiency and hemodynamic compromise with severe heart failure should be evaluated for urgent surgical intervention. In this setting, medical management should not delay surgical repair. Until surgery, systemic vasodilators, such as nitroprusside or milrinone, may be considered to reduce afterload. These medications may promote antegrade flow and thereby decrease mitral insufficiency; however, the use of vasodilators in this setting is often limited by systemic hypotension.

Ongoing Management of Rheumatic Fever

All patients with ARF should be evaluated for cardiac involvement, and those with carditis should be referred to a cardiologist. For patients treated with salicylate or

Table 19.3 Primary and secondary prophylaxis for rheumatic fever

Primary prophylaxis of GAS pharyngitis	Secondary prophylaxis[a]
Amoxicillin • 50 mg/kg orally once daily × 10 days (max dose 1 g/dose	**Benzathine penicillin G** • Patients ≤27 kg: 600,000 U IM every 3–4 weeks • Patients >27 kg: 1.2 million U IM every 3–4 weeks
Or	
Phenoxymethylpenicillin (penicillin V) • Patients ≤27 kg: 250 mg orally BID or TID × 10 days • Patients >27 kg: 500 mg orally BID or TID × 10 days	**Phenoxymethylpenicillin (penicillin V)** • 250 mg orally BID
Or	
Benzathine penicillin G • Patients ≤27 kg: 600,000 U IM × 1 dose • Patients >27 kg: 1.2 million U IM × 1 dose	**Sulfadiazine** • Patients ≤27 kg: 0.5 g orally daily • Patients >27 kg: 1 g orally daily
Or	
Cephalexin • 25–50 mg/kg/day orally divided BID × 10 days (max dose 1000 mg/day)	
Beta-lactam-allergic patients	
Azithromycin • 12 mg/kg/dose orally × 1 day (max dose 500 mg/dose) and then 6 mg/kg/dose orally × 4 days (max dose 250 mg/dose) **Clarithromycin** • 7.5 mg/kg/dose (maximum 250 mg/dose) orally BID × 10 days **Clindamycin** • 7 mg/kg/dose (maximum 300 mg/dose) orally TID × 10 days	**Azithromycin** • 5 mg/kg (max dose 250 mg) orally daily

[a]Duration of secondary prophylaxis:

- Carditis with residual rheumatic heart disease: 10 years from last episode or until 40 years old (whichever is longest)
- Carditis with no residual rheumatic heart disease: 10 years or until 21 years old (whichever is longest)
- No carditis: 5 years or until 21 years old (whichever is longest)

steroids, the optimal duration of therapy is unknown. Some experts recommend discontinuing treatment when concentrations of acute-phase reactants return to normal or after 4–6 weeks. Patients treated with prolonged high-dose salicylates should have salicylate concentrations between 20 and 30 mg/dL [2]. If steroids were prescribed initially, salicylates should be prescribed before discontinuing steroids to prevent rebound inflammation. Heart failure may need to be managed in patients with moderate-to-severe valve insufficiency; in which case, oral diuretics and afterload reduction may be necessary. Given the risk of progressive mitral insufficiency, some physicians recommend restricting patient activity during the acute phase of the illness.

All patients with ARF require long-term secondary prophylaxis against repeat GAS infections (Table 19.3). The duration of secondary prophylaxis is based on the degree of RHD. The importance of secondary prophylaxis should be emphasized at each encounter because the risk of RHD increases with each recurrence of ARF [2].

Complications of Acute Rheumatic Fever

The primary goal of early treatment and secondary prophylaxis in ARF is to prevent chronic RHD, which remains the leading cause of heart failure in children and adolescents worldwide. Like carditis of ARF, the primary manifestations of RHD in children include mitral and aortic insufficiency. In addition, mitral and aortic stenosis can develop over time and may present decades after the initial episode. These complications are more likely after severe initial carditis or frequent recurrences of ARF.

Rheumatic Fever Clinical Pearls

- Acute rheumatic fever most commonly affects children between 5 and 15 years old
- Cardiac involvement (carditis) may be clinical or subclinical and is related to regurgitation of the mitral or aortic valves
- Echocardiograms should be obtained in all patients with confirmed or suspected ARF
- Cardiac involvement may persist or evolve into chronic rheumatic heart disease
- Joint symptoms have a broad differential diagnosis and may lead to misdiagnosis
- Patients presenting with chorea or indolent carditis may have no evidence of GAS infection

Kawasaki Disease

Clinical Vignette

A 5-year-old boy presented to the emergency department after 9 days of persistent fever. On day 4 of his illness, his pediatrician noted fever and pain in the lower back and abdomen, diagnosed acute otitis media, and prescribed amoxicillin. On day 6 of his illness, the patient returned to his pediatrician with persistent fever, back pain, and a new peeling rash on his lower back. His antibiotic was changed to cefuroxime. By day 9 of his illness, still febrile, he was referred to the emergency department. A physical examination noted an irritable child with bilateral non-suppurative conjunctivitis, erythematous and cracked lips, and a macular rash on his lower back. His white blood cell count was 17,000, hematocrit was 38, and platelet count was 755,000. Urinalysis revealed 16 WBC per high-power field with no bacteria. Results of a comprehensive metabolic panel were normal. An echocardiogram showed a giant aneurysm of the left anterior descending coronary artery with thrombus formation.

The Pathophysiology of Kawasaki Disease

Kawasaki disease (KD) is a self-limited systemic vasculitis that occurs most often in infants and young children and affects the medium-sized muscular arteries. The vascular changes most often affect the coronary arteries, potentially resulting in aneurysm formation with the subsequent risk of thrombus formation or arterial narrowing [4]. Kawasaki disease was first described in 1967, yet the underlying cause remains unknown, although several hypotheses have proposed infectious, environmental, and autoimmune triggers of acute KD.

The acute inflammatory phase of KD involves both the adaptive and innate arms of the immune system. An initial influx of neutrophils and $CD8^+$ T cells leads to a necrotizing arteritis. Aneurysms typically form in the acute phase and may be related to hemodynamic stresses because aneurysms are more commonly found in the proximal coronary arteries and at the branch points. Altered blood flow, particularly stasis, can cause thrombus formation and myocardial ischemia or infarction. Subacute vasculitis begins weeks after the initial episode but may last for months or years. Finally, luminal myofibroblastic proliferation narrows the vessel lumen and can also result in coronary stenosis and ischemic heart disease [4].

The Acute Presentation of Kawasaki Disease

Kawasaki disease is a clinical diagnosis and typically presents in children less than 5 years old, although it can present in older children. The principal symptoms are the diagnostic criteria. The diagnosis of complete or "classic" KD can be made if there is fever lasting at least 5 consecutive days with at least four of five additional symptoms: bilateral, non-suppurative, conjunctival injections; oral mucosal changes; polymorphous rash; extremity changes, often as palmar and/or solar erythema and edema; and cervical lymphadenopathy (Fig. 19.2). These symptoms are often not concurrent, and a careful history is essential to elicit the diagnostic signs. Some experts suggest that the diagnosis can be made by day 4 of fever if four principal symptoms are clearly present. If less than 4 of the criteria for complete KD are present, the diagnosis of incomplete KD can be considered if at least two of the principal symptoms are present with additional laboratory or echocardiographic criteria (Fig. 19.3). Coronary artery dilation confirms the diagnosis of incomplete KD.

Although most patients with KD do not have cardiac symptoms, a small subset present with acute KD shock syndrome. This syndrome is characterized by a more severe carditis, with decreased systolic and diastolic function. Kawasaki disease shock syndrome is not common, with one center describing shock symptoms in 7% of 187 KD patients over 4 years [5]. Some degree of left ventricular systolic dysfunction or mitral insufficiency may be present in up to 20% of acute KD patients. Patients with hemodynamic compromise related to KD are more likely to have laboratory findings supporting a greater degree of inflammation, higher rates of recrudescent fevers after treatment with intravenous immune globulin (IVIG), and a higher rate of coronary artery aneurysms [5, 6].

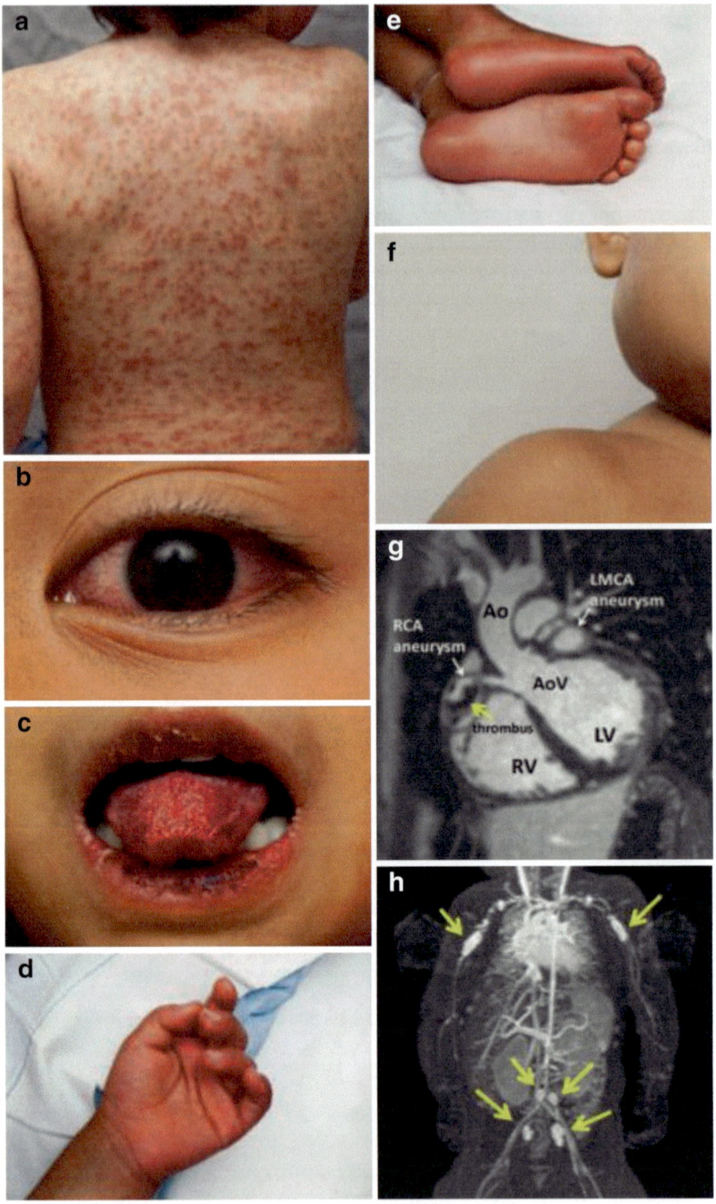

Fig. 19.2 Classic clinical features of Kawasaki disease. (**a**) Rash characterized by maculopapular, diffuse erythroderma, or multiforme-like erythema. (**b**) Bilateral conjunctivitis and bulbar conjunctival injection without exudate. (**c**) Oral changes include cheilitis (erythema and cracking of the lips), strawberry tongue, and erythema of the oral and pharyngeal mucosa. (**d**) Palmar and (**e**) plantar erythema, which is usually accompanied by swelling and resolves with subsequent periungual desquamation in the subacute phase. (**f**) Cervical adenopathy, which is usually a unilateral node no more than 1.5 cm in diameter. (**g**) Coronary artery anuerysm in the right coronary artery with a nonocclusive thrombus and the left main coronary artery demonstrated on magnetic resonance imaging. *Ao*, aorta; *AoV*, aortic valve; *LV*, left ventricle; *RV*, right ventricle. (**h**) Peripheral artery anuerysms in the axillary, subclavian, iliac, and femoral arteries. Images reused with permission from American Heart Association

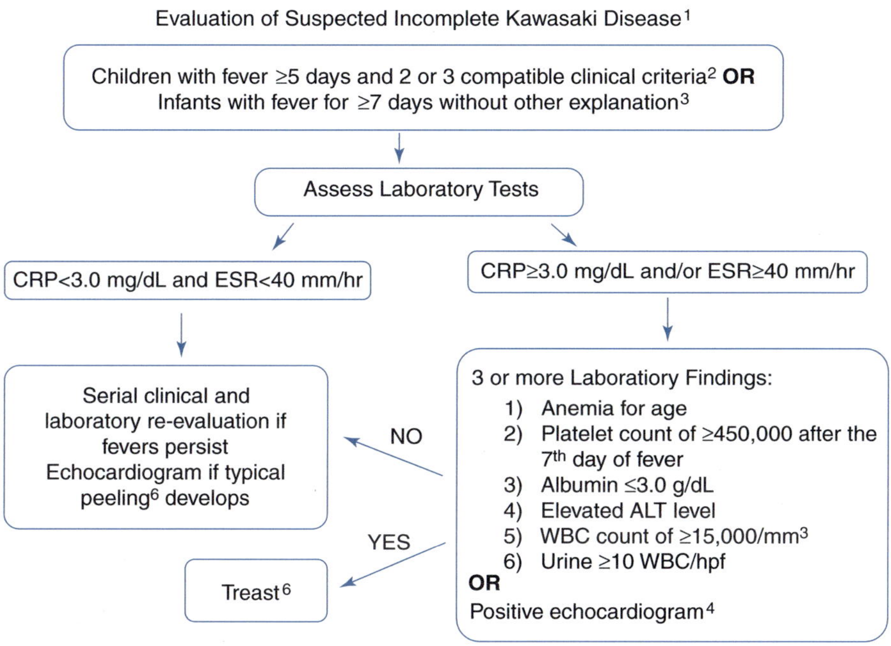

Fig. 19.3 Evaluation of suspected incomplete Kawasaki disease. (1) In the absence of a "gold standard" for diagnosis, this algorithm cannot be evidence based but rather represents the informed opinion of the expert committee. Consultation with an expert should be sought any time assistance is needed. (2) Clinical findings of Kawasaki disease are listed in Table 19.3. Characteristics suggesting that another diagnosis should be considered include exudative conjunctivitis, exudative pharyngitis, ulcerative intraoral lesions, bullous or vesicular rash, generalized adenopathy, or splenomegaly. (3) Infants ≤6 months of age are the most likely to develop prolonged fever without other clinical criteria for Kawasaki disease; these infants are at particularly high risk of developing coronary artery abnormalities. (4) Echocardiography is considered positive for purposes of this algorithm if any of three conditions are met: *Z* score of left anterior descending coronary artery or right coronary artery ≥2.5; coronary artery aneurysm is observed; or ≥3 other suggestive features exist, including decreased left ventricular function, mitral regurgitation, pericardial effusion, or *Z* scores in left anterior descending coronary artery or right coronary artery of 2–2.5. (5) If the echocardiogram is positive, treatment should be given within 10 days of fever onset or after the 10th day of fever in the presence of clinical and laboratory signs (C-reactive protein [CRP], erythrocyte sedimentation rate [ESR]) of ongoing inflammation. (6) Typical peeling begins under the nail beds of fingers and toes. *ALT* indicates alanine transaminase, *WBC* white blood cells. Image reused with permission from the American Heart Association

Patients with KD typically have remitting episodes of high fever. The fever is present for at least 5 consecutive days and, in the absence of treatment, lasts an average of 10 days but can persist for up to a month [4].

Conjunctival injection may be one of the earliest principal features and can occur shortly after the onset of fever. The injection is nonexudative and limbic-sparing. The limbus is a relatively avascular area around the iris and is thus spared from the inflammation. The conjunctivitis can resolve rapidly and may not be present at the time of clinical evaluation.

Mucosal changes consist of brightly erythematous lips, tongue, buccal mucosa, and pharynx. The lips are often dry and cracked, and the tongue has been described as "strawberry" because of the erythema and prominent papillae. Discrete ulcerative lesions and a pharyngeal exudate are not typical of KD.

The rash is nonspecific and is typically maculopapular. Several variations have been identified, but vesicular or bullous rashes are not among them [4]. The rash usually begins in the perineum and spreads to the chest and extremities. Desquamation can occur both on the extremities, typically periungual, and in the perineum.

Extremity changes manifest as erythema and induration of the palms and soles. The interphalangeal joints may also be swollen. Children will often avoid using their hands or weight-bearing because of the pain.

Cervical lymphadenopathy is typically unilateral. The affected lymph node should measure at least 1.5 cm and is typically not tender. Cervical lymphadenopathy is the least common of the principal features.

There is no pathognomonic test for KD, but blood and urine tests can aid in the diagnosis and are particularly helpful in the setting of incomplete KD, where they are part of the diagnostic algorithm (Fig. 19.3). During the acute presentation, laboratory evidence of systemic inflammation is nearly universal, with at least moderate elevations in CRP concentration and ESR. After treatment with IVIG, CRP concentrations are more representative of the patient's inflammation because IVIG can actually increase ESR. Anemia and hypoalbuminemia are common. White blood cell counts can be increased and demonstrate a neutrophil predominance. Thrombocytosis typically appears during the second week of the illness. Liver function tests, including serum concentrations of transaminases and gamma-glutamyltranspeptidase, can also be elevated.

Noncardiac features of KD have also been described. Children may have prodromal symptoms of abdominal pain and diarrhea that precede fever. Hydrops of the gallbladder is well described and can present in up to 15% of patients. Children with fever and irritability often undergo a lumbar puncture to rule out meningitis which reveals aseptic meningitis. Urethritis and phimosis can occur during the acute phase and are often the impetus to obtain a urinalysis, which may show a sterile pyuria. Kawasaki disease has also been diagnosed in patients with simultaneous macrophage-activation syndrome.

The Differential Diagnosis of Kawasaki Disease

Diagnosing KD can be difficult, given the overlap of symptoms with infectious and rheumatologic conditions. Distinguishing among infectious diagnoses can be particularly challenging because these conditions may also present with fever, inflamed mucosa, nonspecific rashes, and changes in extremities. Common infections that may mimic these findings include staphylococcal and streptococcal skin infections as well as many viruses. Testing for viral infections, such as adenovirus, Epstein-Barr virus, and enterovirus, may be helpful. However, persistent fever, clinical features of a viral illness, and positive viral testing should not be dismissed as being inconsistent with KD if the clinical criteria for KD are met. Many patients with KD have a concomitant infectious or viral illness, and a positive viral study does not rule out KD [7]. Drug reactions, toxic shock syndrome, Stevens-Johnson syndrome, and staphylococcal scalded skin syndrome may present with similar cutaneous findings and desquamation. Rheumatologic conditions, such as juvenile rheumatoid arthritis, may present with elevated inflammatory markers and joint changes.

Children at both ends of the typical age spectrum for KD including those less than 6 months and greater than 5 years should be evaluated cautiously because they more commonly present with incomplete KD. Fever in an infant may prompt an infectious work-up, including analysis of cerebrospinal fluid and urine. A sterile pleocytosis or pyuria may be a sign of KD. Adolescents with fever and acalculous cholecystitis should also be evaluated for KD.

Managing Kawasaki Disease in the Emergency Department

As described above, KD patients can present with hemodynamic compromise and shock. In this setting, vasoactive infusions may be necessary along with *careful* volume resuscitation. These symptoms often prompt sepsis evaluations, and KD should be on the differential for patients with prolonged fever and aseptic meningitis or sterile pyuria. Any patient with hemodynamic compromise should be admitted to an intensive care unit for monitoring, treatment, and cardiology consultation. Patients in KD shock typically present with more severe inflammation and are more likely to be resistant to treatment with IVIG. They are also at higher risk for coronary artery aneurysms [5].

The challenge for the emergency physician confronting KD is not usually managing a critically ill child but rather recognizing the clinical features that may suggest KD, particularly in children outside of the typical age range for KD or who present with incomplete KD. A high index of suspicion is essential for timely diagnosis, hospital admission, and beginning therapy. The diagnosis of KD should be considered in any infant with a prolonged fever. A diagnosis of a viral syndrome does not rule out KD.

Ongoing Management of Kawasaki Disease

Intravenous immune globulin plus aspirin is the mainstay of therapy in treating KD and has greatly decreased the incidence of coronary artery aneurysms [8, 9]. Once diagnosed, the patient should be admitted and treatment begun. An echocardiogram is not necessary before starting therapies. Treatment should be started as soon as the diagnosis is made and ideally no later than 10 days after onset of the fever. If the diagnosis is not made until 10 days after the onset of fever, treatment should be reserved for patients with ongoing fever or evidence of systemic inflammation and those with evidence of coronary artery aneurysms. A 2 g/kg dose of IVIG should be infused over 10–12 h. Some centers recommend pretreatment with acetaminophen and diphenhydramine before beginning the infusion, given the risk of a hypersensitivity reaction including anaphylaxis. A slow infusion also prevents excessive volume load in a potentially poorly functioning left ventricle. A hemolytic reaction can occur after IVIG infusion and cause worsening anemia. After completing the initial infusion of IVIG, the patient should be monitored for recrudescence of fever for 36 h. If fever recurs, most experts recommend repeating a dose of IVIG and considering other therapies [4].

In addition to IVIG, aspirin should be given to all patients diagnosed with KD to decrease inflammation. A dosage of 80–100 mg/kg/day in four divided doses is commonly recommended, although lower doses of 30–50 mg/kg/day are used in other countries, with no evidence supporting one dose or the other. When the fever has been absent for 48–72 h, the patient is transitioned to low-dose aspirin (3–5 mg/kg/day) for its antiplatelet activity, although some experts suggest use of high-dose aspirin until the 14th day of illness. Low-dose antiplatelet aspirin is given at least until the patient is evaluated clinically and echocardiographically 6–8 weeks after the initial diagnosis. Systemic anticoagulation is reserved for patients with giant or complex coronary artery aneurysms because they have the highest risk of coronary artery thrombosis [4].

Complications of Kawasaki Disease

The most feared complication of KD is coronary artery aneurysms (Fig. 19.4). These coronary abnormalities typically present during the acute/subacute phase and may regress with treatment. Aneurysms are most likely to occur in children less than 6 months old or more than 8 years old and in boys. Aneurysms are classified based on the coronary artery Z score for body surface area and by their absolute dimensions. Aneurysms are classified as small (Z score ≥2.5 to <5), medium (Z score ≥5 to <10 and absolute diameter <8 mm), and large or giant (Z score ≥10 or absolute diameter ≥8 mm). Morbidity occurs primarily in patients with giant aneurysms and

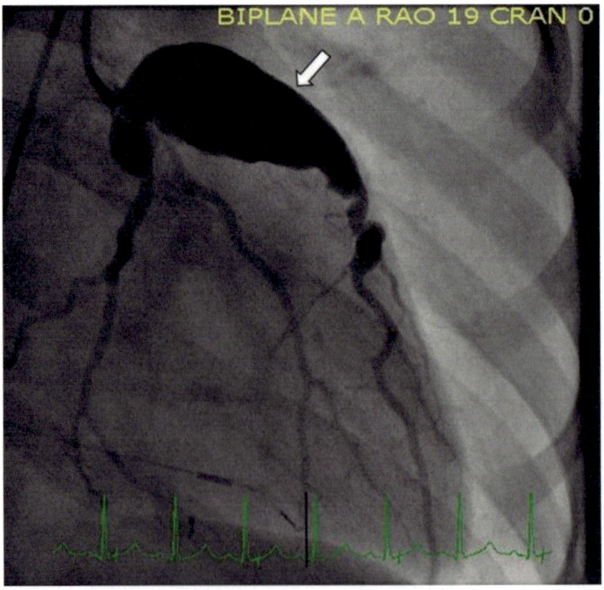

Fig. 19.4 A giant coronary artery aneurysm in the left main coronary artery with thrombus formation (arrow) in a 6-year-old boy with Kawasaki disease

Table 19.4 Suggested tests for diagnosing suspected Kawasaki disease

Lab evaluation
• C-reactive protein, erythrocyte sedimentation rate • Complete blood count (anemia and thrombocytopenia) • Comprehensive metabolic panel (hypoalbuminemia and elevated liver function tests) • Urinalysis with microscopy (sterile pyuria)
Echocardiogram (sedated if needed)
Electrocardiogram

is related to the development of coronary stenoses and myocardial ischemic events. One study placed the cardiac event-free rate at 30 years at only 36% in those with giant aneurysms [10].

Patients with KD and current or regressed coronary artery aneurysms are at higher risk for early coronary artery disease and should have lifelong follow-up. These patients should be screened and treated for additional coronary artery disease risk factors. Individuals presenting with a history of KD and chest pain should be evaluated for acute coronary syndrome (Table 19.4).

Kawasaki Disease Clinical Pearls

- Kawasaki disease should be on the differential for any infant or child with prolonged fever
- Infants less than 6 months old typically present with incomplete Kawasaki disease
- A subset of patients with Kawasaki disease may present with a shock-like clinical picture due to myocarditis and ventricular dysfunction
- Exudative conjunctivitis and pharyngitis make the diagnosis of Kawasaki disease less likely
- Confirmed diagnosis of a respiratory virus does not rule out Kawasaki disease because the conditions can coexist
- Patients presenting with chest pain and a history of Kawasaki disease should be evaluated for acute coronary syndrome

Myocarditis

Clinical Vignette

A 10-year-old boy presents to the emergency department with a 5-day history of fever, cough, rhinorrhea, and abdominal pain. On day 4 of his illness, shortness of breath and exercise intolerance worsened. On day 5, he became lethargic and his mental status changed. On presentation, he was tachycardiac, tachypneic, and hypotensive with poor perfusion. An electrocardiogram revealed low-voltage QRS complexes with diffuse ST segment elevations. Troponin concentrations were elevated at 2.1 ng/mL. An echocardiogram revealed decreased left ventricular function with an ejection fraction of 18%.

Table 19.5 Causes of myocarditis

Infectious • **Viral:** Parvovirus B19, human herpesvirus 6, Epstein-Barr virus, adenovirus, enterovirus, HIV, influenza A and B, varicella, respiratory syncytial virus • **Bacterial:** *Streptococcus* species, *Staphylococcus* species, *Mycobacterium* species, *Borrelia* species, *Mycoplasma pneumoniae*, *Treponema pallidum* • **Fungal:** *Candida* species, *Aspergillus* species, *Cryptococcus* species, *Histoplasma* species, *Coccidioides* species, *Nocardia* • **Parasitic:** *Trypanosoma cruzi*, visceral larva migrans, schistosomiasis
Noninfectious • **Medications:** anthracyclines, doxorubicin, phenytoin, aminophylline, phenytoin • **Toxins:** cocaine, ethanol, carbon monoxide, copper, iron, lead, arsenic • **Hypersensitivity reactions:** penicillin, tetracycline, sulfonamides, cephalosporins, diuretics, tricyclic antidepressants, nonsteroidal anti-inflammatory drugs, benzodiazepines, clozapine, methyldopa
Autoimmune: systemic lupus erythematosus, Churg-Strauss syndrome, inflammatory bowel disease, Wegner granulomatosis, sarcoidosis, dermatomyositis, thyrotoxicosis

The Pathophysiology of Myocarditis

Myocarditis is an inflammatory disease of the myocardium [11]. The inflammatory agent is most commonly viral, although other infectious agents, autoimmune conditions, and toxins can be responsible (Table 19.5). During the acute phase, local injury to myocytes activates the innate immune system. Toll-like receptors trigger the release of inflammatory cytokines. The subacute phase is marked by the arrival of additional inflammatory cells from both the innate and adaptive immune systems. These cells contribute to the inflammatory milieu and can directly damage myocytes. Like other inflammatory heart conditions, molecular mimicry may contribute to ongoing inflammation when exposed cardiac proteins, particularly myosin, lead to ongoing inflammation due to the autoimmune response.

The chronic phase of myocarditis may have several outcomes. Clearing the antigen with minimal damage to the myocytes will lead to complete recovery. Antigenic clearing with severe myocyte damage will lead to fibrotic changes and subsequent dilated cardiomyopathy. Pathologic cardiac remodeling is also likely if myocyte inflammation persists because of ongoing exposure to the antigen or autoimmune-mediated myocyte damage [12].

The Acute Presentation of Myocarditis

The clinical presentation of myocarditis is variable and can range from unrecognized asymptomatic cases to those with heart failure, life-threatening arrhythmias, or hemodynamic collapse. The age distribution is bimodal, with most children presenting in infancy or mid-teens. Four predominant clinical presentations are usually discussed in the literature: acute myocarditis, fulminant myocarditis, acute chest pain with features of acute coronary syndrome, and sudden death.

Acute myocarditis classically presents with progressive heart failure symptoms weeks to months after a viral infection. Exercise intolerance, dyspnea, and fatigue are all common features. Depending on the degree of heart failure, the physical examination may reveal normal to varying degrees of tachycardia, tachypnea, pallor, and poor perfusion. A gallop rhythm and a new mitral insufficiency murmur may be present. Echocardiograms commonly show LV dilation and dysfunction in acute myocarditis.

Fulminant myocarditis has a more severe presentation, in which patients present with rapidly progressive heart failure symptoms days to weeks after a respiratory or gastrointestinal viral illness. Ventricular dysfunction can be serious, and patients may present in cardiogenic shock with multi-organ failure. Ventricular arrhythmias are common and typically present as ventricular tachycardia. In contrast to the echocardiographic findings of acute myocarditis, fulminant myocarditis presents with a normal ventricular chamber size, severely decreased systolic function, and septal thickening secondary to myocardial edema. Children may be more likely than adults to present with fulminant myocarditis [13].

Patients in the acute phase of myocarditis can present with substantial chest pain and clinical findings suggesting an acute coronary syndrome. Chest pain is the predominant symptom, with ECG findings showing diffuse ST segment elevations or depressions (Fig. 19.5). Cardiac biomarker concentrations may be elevated, with troponin being more commonly elevated than creatine kinase [14]. Cardiac biomarker concentrations are not uniformly elevated in fulminant myocarditis. Echocardiography typically reveals normal or mildly decreased ventricular function. Cardiac catheterization is often performed in these patients but does not demonstrate coronary artery disease. However, coronary vasospasm has been

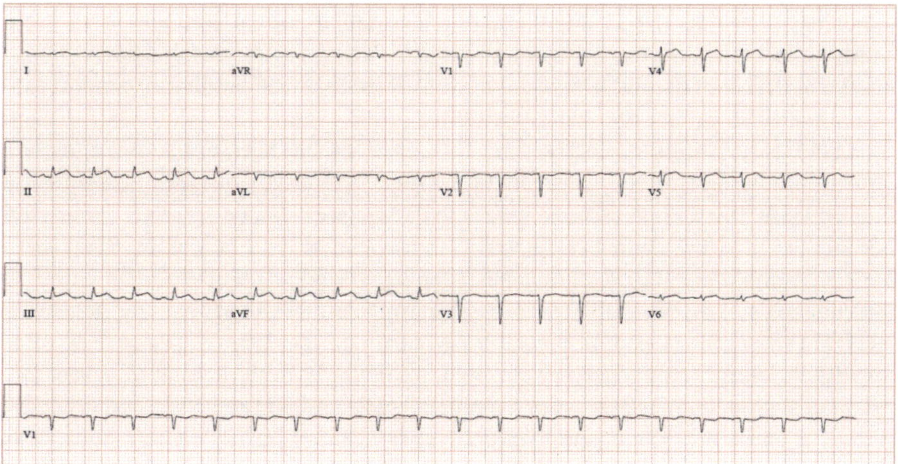

Fig. 19.5 Low-voltage QRS complexes, ST segment changes, and Q waves characteristic of myocarditis in a 12-year-old girl with myocarditis

Table 19.6 Suggested tests for diagnosing suspected myocarditis in the emergency department

Laboratory tests
• C-reactive protein concentration, erythrocyte sedimentation rate, complete blood count, comprehensive metabolic panel, troponin concentration, B-type natriuretic peptide concentration
Infectious screen
• Blood culture, viral PCR testing
Chest radiography
Echocardiography
Electrocardiography

PCR polymerase chain reaction

found in patients with suspected myocarditis during intracoronary acetylcholine testing [12].

Sudden cardiac death from fatal arrhythmias can be the initial presentation of myocarditis. In adolescents and children, myocarditis is thought to be the primary cause of sudden death in 5–8% of cases. The incidence may be higher in infants because myocarditis has been implicated as a cause of sudden infant death syndrome. In one single-center autopsy study, 43% of 62 patients had a positive PCR viral assay [15].

Diagnosis can be challenging in patients with myocarditis because no single test is uniformly positive. In the emergency department, appropriate tests include ECG, blood tests, and echocardiography (Table 19.6).

An abnormal electrocardiogram in children with myocarditis may be the most common clinical finding. However, no single pathologic ECG finding has been consistently associated with myocarditis. The most common abnormalities are in the ST segment and T waves and can include ST elevation and T wave inversion. Q waves are variably present, as are low-voltage QRS waves. Varying degrees of heart block have been described, and premature ventricular contractions and more severe ventricular tachyarrhythmias can be present. Patients with sustained arrhythmias have a high risk of cardiac arrest and may need mechanical circulatory support [16]. A normal ECG cannot rule out myocarditis.

Laboratory results typically show evidence of cardiac injury, inflammation, infection, and electrolyte disturbances. Cardiac biomarker concentrations, including troponin T and I and creatine kinase (MB fraction), can be elevated. Some studies suggest that the degree of elevation is associated with outcomes. Troponin T concentration above 0.052 ng/mL has been suggested as an appropriate cutoff for the diagnosis of myocarditis [15]. However, myocarditis can occur in the absence of elevated troponin concentrations. B-type natriuretic peptide (BNP) or N-terminal pro-BNP concentrations may be elevated, particularly in the setting of severe ventricular dysfunction. Inflammatory markers, such as CRP and ESR, are often elevated, as are WBC counts and liver enzyme concentrations, but all are nonspecific for myocarditis. Electrolytes should be evaluated and corrected to minimize the risk of ventricular arrhythmias. The patient should be evaluated for infectious disease, and PCR-based viral testing is often performed. The meaning of a positive viral study in noncardiac tissue is unclear. Prospective studies of adults comparing serologic viral diagnoses to PCR analyses of endomyocardial biopsy samples have reported a correlate virus in only 4% of patients. Alternatively, in another study of 21 children with clinical myocarditis, viral PCR testing of serum samples for cardiotropic viruses was positive in 43%, whereas these viruses were present in only 3% of 75 children undergoing viral testing for a fever [15].

Cardiac imaging is important in diagnosing myocarditis. A chest radiograph will be abnormal in up to 90% of patients. The most common finding is cardiomegaly, but pleural effusions and pulmonary edema are also common. An echocardiogram typically reveals ventricular dilation and dysfunction. Global dysfunction is more common, but regional wall motion abnormalities may be present. As described above, echocardiography can help distinguish acute from fulminant myocarditis. Additional echocardiographic findings may include mitral insufficiency and pericardial effusions. Outside the emergency department, cardiac MRI evaluating myocyte inflammation and edema is used for diagnosing myocarditis and determining prognosis.

The Differential Diagnosis of Myocarditis

Given the nonspecific features of myocarditis, medical professionals should consider this diagnosis in any patient presenting with features of heart failure. Myocarditis was responsible for new-onset LV dysfunction in up to 20% of children in the UK [15]. Additional factors should also be considered for patients with new-onset ventricular dysfunction (Table 19.5). Genetic mutations in cardiac proteins, such as titin, lamin, or myosin, can cause dilated cardiomyopathy. Mitochondrial myopathies or X-linked conditions, such as Barth syndrome, can lead to similar cardiac phenotypes.

Additional diagnoses to consider include autoimmune disorders, such as polymyositis, Churg-Strauss syndrome, Wegener's granulomatosis, systemic lupus erythematosus, and sarcoidosis. Inborn errors of metabolism, including glycogen storage diseases, are rare but can lead to cardiac dysfunction. Nutritional deficiencies in vitamins or minerals, such as thiamine and zinc, are rare and more related to alcoholism in adults. Antineoplastic drugs, particularly anthracyclines, commonly lead to LV dysfunction. Acute coronary syndromes are rare in children, but patients with chest pain, ECG abnormalities, and elevated troponin concentrations should be evaluated for coronary artery abnormalities and, in rare cases, for spontaneous coronary artery dissection.

Managing Myocarditis in the Emergency Department

Initial treatment of myocarditis is aimed at supporting cardiac output. Pediatric heart failure guidelines suggest milrinone or dobutamine as first-line agents for children with decompensated heart failure, with epinephrine reserved for patients with refractory hypotension and poor end-organ perfusion [17]. Dosages of epinephrine should be escalated cautiously because of its propensity to increase myocardial oxygen consumption. Respiratory support with noninvasive positive-pressure or mechanical ventilation is often necessary for patients with hemodynamic compromise during the acute phase. Mechanical circulatory support, including extracorporeal membrane oxygenation or ventricular assist devices, should be considered, particularly in patients with fulminant myocarditis, because 70–90% of these patients recover cardiac function and are transplant-free at long-term follow-up [15]. Antiarrhythmic medications may be necessary in the acute phase. Digoxin is not recommended in this phase because it has increased myocardial injury in animal studies [15]. Patients in this phase with less-severe symptoms at presentation but concerns for myocarditis should be admitted to the hospital given the possibility of ventricular arrhythmias. All patients with myocarditis should be seen by a cardiologist, especially in the event of ventricular dysfunction, arrhythmias, or hemodynamic compromise.

Ongoing Management of Myocarditis

Myocarditis is typically diagnosed definitively after the patient is stabilized in the emergency department. Historically, the gold standard for suspected myocarditis was an endomyocardial biopsy that met certain histologic criteria. However, biopsy-derived diagnoses can be challenging because of the nonuniform inflammation of the myocardium, as well as the risk associated with biopsy in very young patients and during the acute phase of illness. Cardiac MRI is increasingly used in cases of suspected myocarditis. New MRI diagnostic criteria, known as the Lake Louise criteria, can be used to diagnose myocarditis. These criteria are based on MRI evidence of myocardial inflammation on T2 signaling, global early gadolinium enhancement, or focal late gadolinium enhancement [18].

Ongoing evaluation of cardiac function is essential to determine appropriate therapies. Fluid status should be monitored carefully, and IV loop diuretics are first-line treatment for patients with fluid overload. Patients with persistent heart failure are commonly transitioned to treatments that often include angiotensin converting enzyme inhibitors and beta-blockers. In murine models, both of these drugs were associated with decreased inflammation, myocardial fibrosis, and autoantibody production [15]. Aldosterone antagonists may also be considered for patients with persistent heart failure symptoms based on improved survival in studies of adults. Escalation or weaning of clinical support is based on the clinical response to treatment.

Patients presenting with acute or fulminant myocarditis are commonly treated with IVIG and, less frequently, with steroids despite limited efficacy data. Among children enrolled in the National Heart, Lung, and Blood Institute-funded Pediatric Cardiomyopathy Registry, the use of IVIG did not improve LV function or survival [15]. The use of immunomodulator therapy and specific regimens vary by institution.

Complications of Myocarditis

The most important complications of myocarditis include persistent cardiac dysfunction, chronic heart failure, and persistent and/or progressive heart failure requiring consideration of heart transplantation. Cardiac transplant rates in patients with myocarditis range from 4 to 18%. Most children with myocarditis will recover normal cardiac function with about half regaining a normal ejection fraction after 3 years [15].

Myocarditis Clinical Pearls

- The clinical presentation of myocarditis is variable and may include acute-onset chest pain, progressive heart failure, or sudden death
- Troponin concentrations are more commonly elevated than are creatine kinase concentrations, but cardiac biomarkers may be negative
- Electrocardiographic changes in myocarditis include ST segment changes, low-voltage QRS complexes, heart block, or abnormal Q waves
- Patients in whom myocarditis is suspected should be admitted during the acute phase and monitored for cardiac arrhythmias
- Cardiology consultation should be sought for patients with myocarditis

References

1. Marijon E, Mirabel M, Celermajer DS, Jouven X. Rheumatic heart disease. Lancet. 2012;379(9819):953–64.
2. Tani LY. Rheumatic fever and rheumatic heart disease. In: Allen HD, Shaddy RE, Penny DJ, Cetta F, Feltes TF, editors. Moss and Adams' heart disease in infants, adolescents, and children, including the fetus and young adult. 9th ed. Philadelphia: Wolters Kluwer; 2016. p. 1373–404.
3. Gewitz MH, Baltimore RS, Tani LY, et al. Revision of the Jones criteria for the diagnosis of acute rheumatic fever in the era of Doppler echocardiography a scientific statement from the American Heart Association. Circulation. 2015;131:1806–18.
4. Newburger JW, Takahashi M, Gerber MA, et al. Diagnosis, treatment, and long-term management of Kawasaki disease: a statement for health professionals from the Committee on Rheumatic Fever, Endocarditis and Kawasaki Disease, Council on Cardiovascular Disease in the Young, American Heart Association. Circulation. 2004;110:2747–71.
5. Kanegaye JT, Wilder MS, Molkara D, et al. Recognition of a Kawasaki disease shock syndrome. Pediatrics. 2009;123:e783–9.
6. Printz BF, Sleeper LA, Newburger JW, et al. Noncoronary cardiac abnormalities are associated with coronary artery dilation and with laboratory inflammatory markers in acute Kawasaki disease. J Am Coll Cardiol. 2010;57:86–92.
7. Turnier JL, Anderson MS, Heizer HR, Jone P-N, Glode MP, Dominguez SR. Concurrent respiratory viruses and Kawasaki disease. Pediatrics. 2015;136:e609–14.
8. Newburger J, Takahashi M, Burns JC, et al. The treatment of Kawasaki syndrome with intravenous gamma globulin. N Engl J Med. 1986;315:341–7.
9. Cohen E, Sundel R. Kawasaki disease at 50 years. JAMA Pediatr. 2016;170(11):1093–9.
10. Newburger JW, Takahashi M, Burns JC. Kawasaki disease. J Am Coll Cardiol. 2016;67:1738–49.
11. Canter CE, Simpson KP. Diagnosis and treatment of myocarditis in children in the current era. Circulation. 2014;129:115–28.

12. Sagar S, Liu PP, Cooper LT. Myocarditis. Lancet. 2012;379:738–47.
13. Cooper LT. Myocarditis. N Engl J Med. 2009;360:1526–38.
14. Caforio ALP, Pankuweit S, Arbustini E, et al. Current state of knowledge on aetiology, diagnosis, management, and therapy of myocarditis: a position statement of the European Society of Cardiology Working Group on Myocardial and Pericardial Diseases. Eur Heart J. 2013;34:2636–48.
15. Simpson KE, Anwar S, Canter CE. Myocarditis. In: Allen HD, Shaddy RE, Penny DJ, Feltes TF, Cetta F, editors. Moss and Adams' heart disease in infants, adolescents, and children, including the fetus and young adult. 9th ed. Philadelphia: Wolters Kluwer; 2016. p. 1313–30.
16. Priori SG, Blomström-Lundqvist C, Mazzanti A, et al. 2015 ESC guidelines for the management of patients with ventricular arrhythmias and the prevention of sudden cardiac death—addenda. Eur Heart J. 2015;36:2793–867.
17. Kirk R, Dipchand AI, Rosenthal DN, et al. The International Society for Heart and Lung Transplantation guidelines for the management of pediatric heart failure: executive summary. J Hear Lung Transplant. 2014;33:888–909.
18. Friedrich MG, Sechtem U, Schulz-Menger J, et al. Cardiovascular magnetic resonance in myocarditis: a JACC white paper. J Am Coll Cardiol. 2009;53:1475–87.

Cardiac Emergencies in Countries with Limited Resources

20

Manish Chokhandre, Rekha Solomon, and Swati Garekar

Introduction

The incidence of congenital heart disease worldwide is known to be relatively unaffected by economic disparity. The challenges faced by physicians of the third world are due to paucity of resources and trained personnel in the field of pediatric cardiology.

It is estimated that nearly 100,000 babies with critical congenital heart disease are born annually in India. There are approximately 30 dedicated cardiac centers to cater to this population. This coupled with the numerous intangible effects of a less literate population poses a barrier to the care provided.

This chapter is an overview of common or important heart diseases seen by the third-world physicians. A few are primarily cardiac, while the rest are where the cardiac manifestation is a part of systemic involvement. The underlying theme is that vaccination, better nutrition, general hygiene, and timely care can either prevent these diseases or ensure a better outcome (Fig. 20.1).

M. Chokhandre, M.D. • S. Garekar, B.C. (Pediatr. Cardiol.) (✉)
Fortis Hospital, Mumbai, India

R. Solomon, M.D.
BJ Wadia Hospital for Children, Mumbai, India

© Springer International Publishing AG, part of Springer Nature 2018
A. P. Sarnaik et al. (eds.), *Cardiac Emergencies in Children*,
https://doi.org/10.1007/978-3-319-73754-6_20

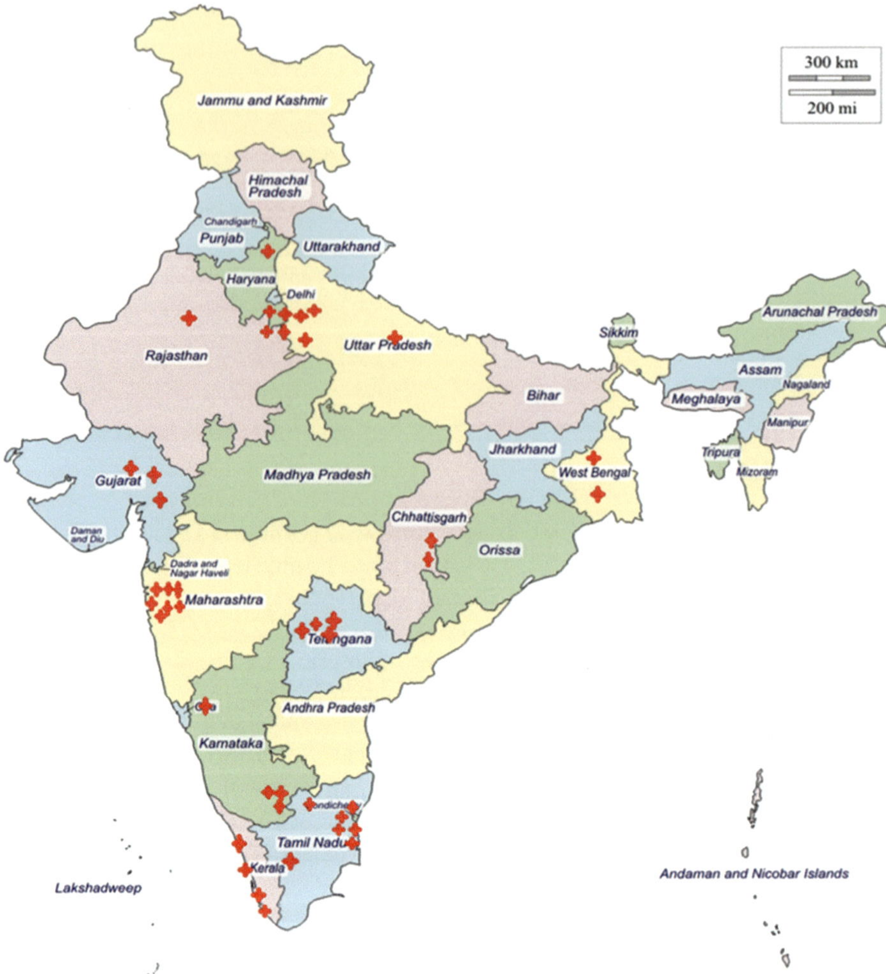

Fig. 20.1 Map of India showing location (red asterisk) of dedicated pediatric cardiac surgery centers in India (2016)

Case: Late Presentation of Large Shunts

Clinical Vignette

A 3-year-old child presents to the emergency department with a 4-day history of fever, cough, and breathing difficulty. He has history of recurrent respiratory infections and poor weight gain. He weighs 6 kg (birth weight 2.4 kg) and stays in a remote village. On examination, he is cachectic without any dysmorphic features. His systemic examination is significant for respiratory distress, bounding pulses, bilateral crepitations, laterally displaced apical impulse, grade 3/6 systolic murmur in the left infraclavicular area, and hepatomegaly. Chest X-ray shows cardiomegaly and right upper zone consolidation.

He is intubated and ventilated. His echocardiogram shows a large patent ductus arteriosus (PDA) with severe pulmonary hypertension. He undergoes successful device closure of patent ductus arteriosus after pneumonia is resolved.

Pathophysiology

A large PDA begins shunting a significant amount of blood into the pulmonary circuit once the pulmonary vascular resistance falls to adult levels by age 6 weeks. This correlates clinically with onset of repeated respiratory tract infections, breast-feeding difficulty (suck-rest-suck cycle), and failure to gain weight. The large shunt results in volume overload of the left atrium and ventricle. This places an additional metabolic demand on the child. Each respiratory infection worsens the heart failure and slows weight gain further. This forms a vicious cycle which may be life threatening.

The unrestricted shunt of a large PDA at the arterial level implies severe, flow-related pulmonary hypertension. An uncorrected PDA leads to pulmonary vascular obstructive changes sooner than in a ventricular septal defect.

Local factors in the third world preclude diagnosis and management in a timely manner.

Clinical Manifestations

Baseline tachycardia, bounding pulses, heaving apex, cardiomegaly, and hepatomegaly. A machinery murmur in the left infraclavicular area is typically not heard in a large PDA; the systolic component only is heard.

Laboratory Investigations

Chest X-ray: cardiomegaly and pulmonary plethora (Fig. 20.2)

Echocardiogram: large PDA. Peak systolic gradient of less than 20 mmHg and even lesser diastolic gradient across the PDA. Enlarged left atrium and ventricle and severe pulmonary hypertension

ECG: Increased mid-precordial QRS voltages and tall R waves in V5-6. Broad P wave (p mitrale) in V1

Additional tests as applicable for a child with severe malnourishment

Clinical pitfalls: the absence of a loud murmur may mask the underlying large PDA. Each respiratory tract infection may get treated in isolation. The failure to thrive may be falsely attributed to prevalent malnourishment in the community

Diagnostic clues: history of repeated lower respiratory tract infections, failure to thrive, and signs of heart failure (mild tachypnea, baseline tachycardia, murmur, congestive hepatomegaly)

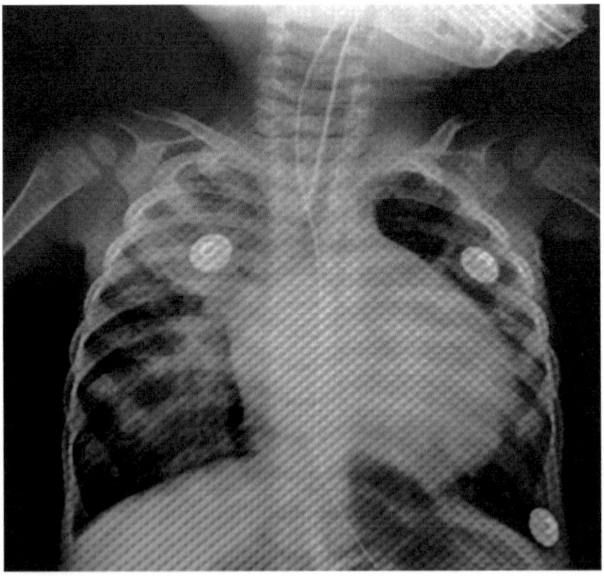

Fig. 20.2 Chest radiograph showing cardiomegaly and right midzone and upper zone consolidation

Emergency Management Principles

Respiratory support as required. IV fluid restriction. Administer medications for congestive heart failure. Early referral for transcatheter or surgical closure of PDA

Clinical Pearl

A triad of repeated lower respiratory tract infections, failure to thrive, and heart failure suggest a large intracardiac shunt.

Case: Dilated Cardiomyopathy in the Third World

Clinical Vignette

A 9-month-old child presents with irritability, decreased oral intake, mild nasal discharge, and cough for the past 3 days. Physical examination is significant with a heart rate of 180/min, bilateral fine crepitations, and mild hepatomegaly. There is no murmur. Peripheral pulses are well felt, and peripheral pulse oximetry reading is normal. In the emergency room, he has a short generalized tonic/clonic convulsion. The arterial blood gas shows metabolic acidosis and low ionized calcium. The chest X-ray shows cardiomegaly and normal pulmonary vascular markings. An echocardiogram shows a dilated left ventricle with poor contractility. Blood investigations reveal depressed calcium and vitamin D levels, the supplementation of which results in normalization of left ventricular function. He is diagnosed with vitamin D deficiency causing dilated cardiomyopathy (DCM).

Etiology and Pathophysiology

Sufficient calcium stores are essential for contractility of muscles including cardiac myocytes. Reduced maternal vitamin D levels result in deficient calcium stores in the infant. The effect is compounded by poor exposure to sunlight in exclusively breast-fed dark-skinned babies. The poor extracellular calcium stores interfere with myocardial contractility. The initial compensation is via an increase in the resting heart rate and stretching of the muscles, and the condition remains subclinical. A common upper respiratory illness unmasks the underlying cardiomyopathy as myocardial function worsens.

Clinical Manifestations

Irritability, poor feeding, and tachycardia out of proportion to febrile illness. Look for signs of calcium and vitamin D deficiency (frontal bossing, wide open anterior fontanel, wrist widening, Harrison sulcus, double malleoli, etc.).

Laboratory Investigations

Blood tests: serum total and ionized calcium, serum 25-hydroxyvitamin D levels, serum parathyroid hormone levels, serum magnesium, serum phosphorus, serum alkaline phosphatase, and serum albumin levels

The entire work-up for dilated cardiomyopathy is appropriate. As there is widespread deficiency of calcium and vitamin D in the population, it is vital to investigate for other causes of DCM.

ECG: prolonged QTc. The normal value for infants <6 months is 490 ms. For age more than 6 months, the cutoff for girls is 470 ms, and for boys it is 450 ms.

Echocardiogram: a dilated (>+2 z score) left ventricle with globally reduced contractility. It is essential to document coronary anatomy (Fig. 20.3).

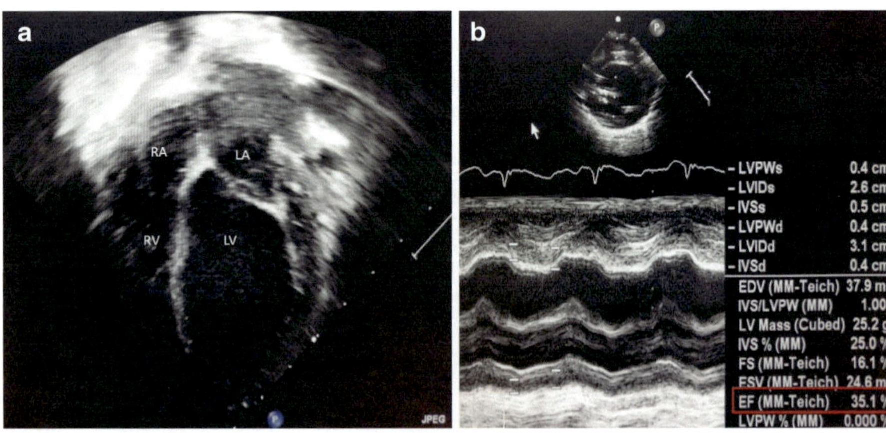

Fig. 20.3 (**a**) Echocardiogram (apical four-chamber view) of a 9-month old infant showing dilated (and dysfunctional) left ventricle due to vitamin D deficiency. (**b**) M-mode of the same patient showing reduced left ventricular systolic function (left ventricular ejection fraction—35%)

Emergency Stabilization

Institute inotropic support of the heart including calcium in the form of intravenous infusion with monitoring of serum calcium concentrations. Institute vitamin D supplementation.

Drug Table 20.1

Name	Dose range	Side effects	Remarks
Calcium	IV: (dose expressed in mg of calcium gluconate) IV: 100–200 mg/kg/dose over 5–10 min; follow with an infusion with a maximum dose of 500 mg/kg/day Oral: (dose expressed as elemental calcium) 45–65 mg/kg/day in four divided doses	Hypotension; IV extravasation may cause tissue necrosis	1 g calcium gluconate = 90 mg elemental calcium = 4.5 mEq calcium IV to be given with heart rate monitoring
25-Hydroxyvitamin D_3	*Daily regime for therapy* <1 month: 1000 IU/day for 2–3 months 1–12 months: 1000–5000 IU/day orally for 2–3 months >12 months: 5000 IU/day orally for 2–3 months	Weakness, nausea, dry mouth, constipation, muscle pain, bone pain	Maintenance therapy dose is 400–1000 IU/day Supplement the mother in breastfeeding infants
25-Hydroxyvitamin D_3	*Weekly regime for therapy* 50,000 IU once a week orally for 6 weeks		

Clinical pitfalls: a dilated and poorly contractile left ventricle may be secondary to myocarditis or other causes. Multiple serum calcium and ionized calcium levels may have to be obtained. A random single test may be normal.

Diagnostic clues: history of poor vitamin D and calcium intake during pregnancy and lactation period. History of maternal malnutrition, head-to-toe cloth cover for the mother at all times due to religious reasons, and faulty feeding practices. Signs of rickets on physical examination.

Clinical Pearls

Suspect calcium/vitamin D deficiency as a cause of DCM in the appropriate clinical scenario. Persistent tachycardia in the absence of a usual cause and cardiomegaly on chest radiograph are pointers to possible cardiac dysfunction.

It is vital to rule out all treatable causes of DCM before labeling the child as having idiopathic DCM.

Case: Stroke and the Heart in Childhood

Clinical Vignette

A 2-year-old boy with unrepaired tetralogy of Fallot presents with a 1-day history of weakness of the right side of his body. There is no history of fever. He is cyanosed and plethoric and has clubbing. His peripheral pulse oximetry reading is 65%. He has an ejection systolic murmur in the pulmonary area with single second heart sound. He has right-sided weakness (2/5) with brisk reflexes and up-going plantar reflex. MRI brain reveals an infarct in the left middle cerebral artery territory. His echocardiogram shows tetralogy of Fallot with pulmonary atresia with non-confluent branch pulmonary arteries. There are no vegetations.

Etiology of Stroke

Unrepaired cyanotic heart defects or Eisenmenger syndrome: cardiac embolism, venous thrombosis, and brain abscess

Cardiac procedures: Extracorporeal membrane oxygenation (ECMO), ventricular assist device, and cardiac catheterization

Infective endocarditis

Dilated cardiomyopathies with poor ejection fraction

Chronic arrhythmias

Paradoxical embolism through a patent foramen ovale

Pathophysiology of Stroke in Unrepaired CHD

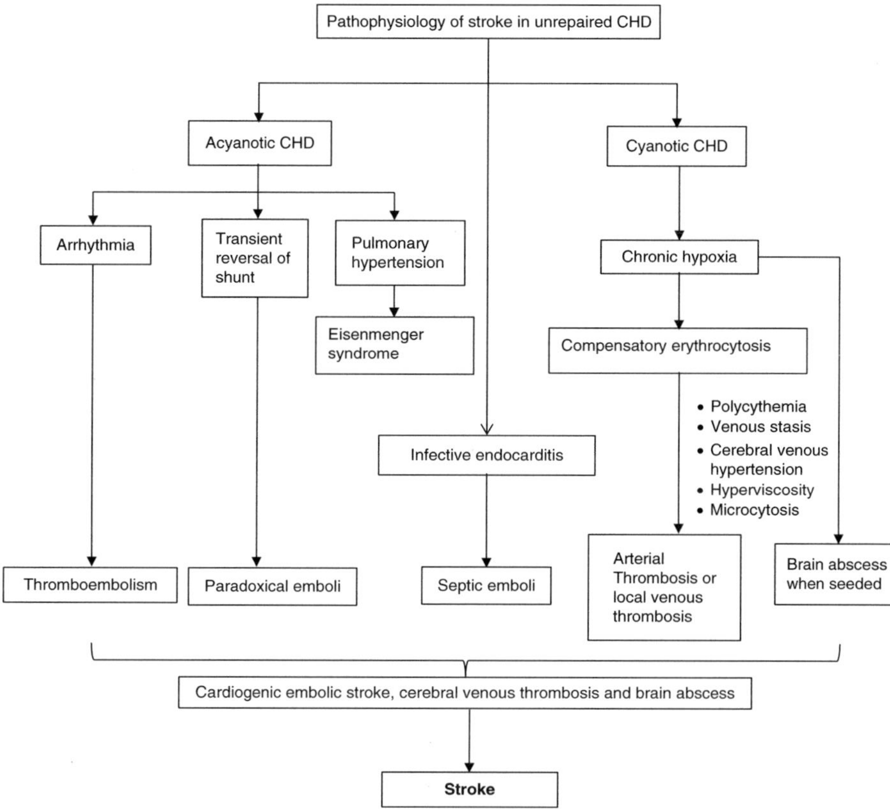

Laboratory Investigations

Blood tests: CBC (polycythemia, microcytosis). Blood culture: If neuroimaging and echocardiogram are not immediately available, it is safer to obtain blood culture and start antibiotics as per local guidelines. Baseline PTT and thrombophilia testing as necessary

Echocardiogram: to delineate the heart disease and look for vegetation or thrombus

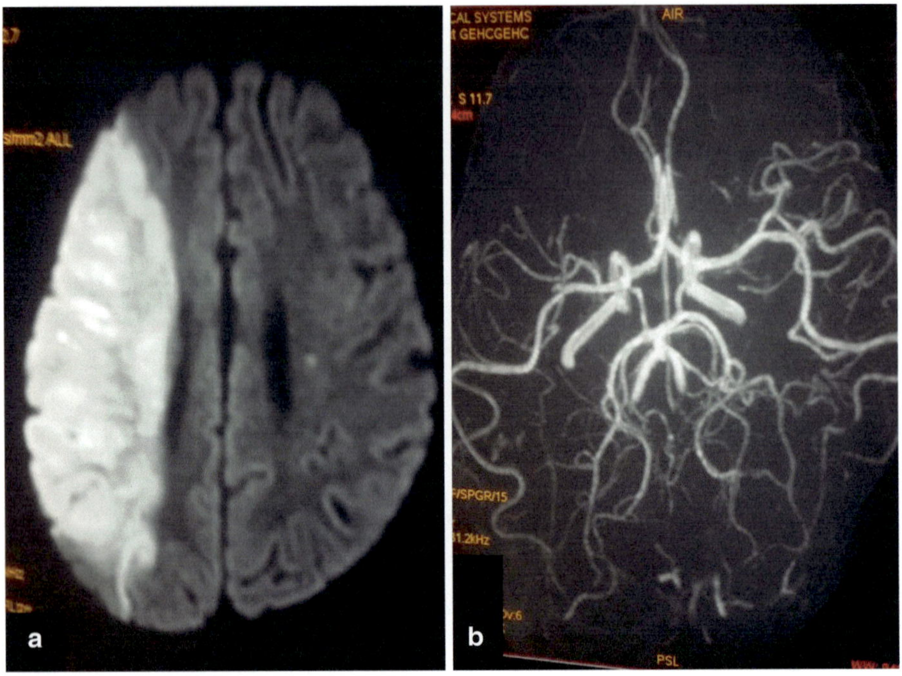

Fig. 20.4 (**a**) Magnetic resonance imaging of a 2-year-old boy with tetralogy of Fallot suggestive of ischemic infarct in right middle cerebral artery territory (right frontotemporal and parietal lobes). (**b**) Magnetic resonance angiogram of the same patient showing paucity of flow in cortical branches of right middle cerebral artery

CT Brain with contrast or magnetic resonance imaging (MRI) with MRA (magnetic resonance angiography) and MRV (magnetic resonance venography) (Fig. 20.4)

Clinical Manifestations

Headache and vomiting, focal neurologic deficit, and seizures are common presenting symptoms. Infratentorial brain abscesses may be asymptomatic until tonsillar herniation occurs.

Emergency Management

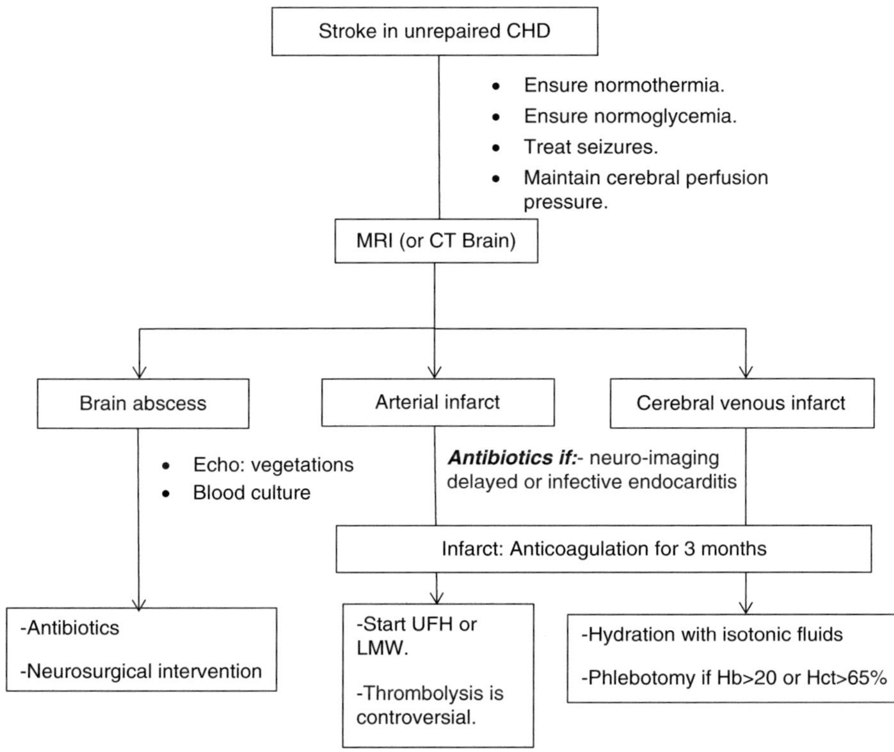

As hyperviscosity poses continued risk of venous thrombosis intravenous hydration should be initiated swiftly and phlebotomy should be considered.

Iron deficiency has been shown to increase predilection toward stroke. Many children with cyanotic heart disease are deficient in iron in addition to having polycythemia. These patients should receive oral iron supplementation.

Children with stroke or brain abscess should be evaluated for congenital heart disease and referred for appropriate surgical correction if necessary.

Drug Table 20.2

Drug	Dose	Side effects	Remarks
Unfractionated heparin	Loading dose: 75 U/kg IV over 10 min Maintenance dose: 25 U/kg IV for <1 year 20 U/kg for >1 year Usually 1–2 weeks till LMWH is therapeutic	Bleeding	Target PTT: 60–85 s (4 h after loading dose, 4 h after every dose change)
Low molecular weight heparin	<2 months: 3 mg/kg/day in two divided doses subcutaneously >2 months: 2 mg/kg/day in two divided doses subcutaneously	Bleeding	Target level of anti-Xa (4 h after dose): 0.5–1 U/mL

Diagnostic Pitfalls

Any child with stroke warrants a careful cardiac evaluation to rule out cardiac etiology.

Clinical Pearls

Antibiotics should be started in a patient with CHD and stroke if neuroimaging is delayed and presence of a brain abscess is not ruled out.

Phlebotomy should be reserved for symptomatic children with hematocrit >65% and has to be accompanied by careful hydration.

Case: Fulminant Native Valve Infective Endocarditis in a Previously Healthy Child

Clinical Vignette

A previously healthy 10-year-old boy presents with a 10-day history of high grade fever and a rash. Physical examination is significant for ecchymotic spots all over the body and a swollen and painful left knee joint. There is mild splenomegaly. ECG shows a second-degree heart block type 1. A diagnosis of infective endocarditis (IE) is entertained, and appropriate antibiotics are started after obtaining blood culture. An echocardiogram shows a perivalvar vegetation of the aortic valve. Over the course of the next 48 h, the patient's condition deteriorates; complete heart block and moderate aortic regurgitation develop. The patient is taken to the operating room for high-risk aortic valve surgery.

Etiology

Eight to ten percent of cases of IE occur in children with no underlying structural heart defect. The aortic and mitral valves are most commonly affected, and *Staphylococcus aureus* bacteremia is the most common cause. In the third world, chances of partially treated local bacterial infections becoming systemic are higher due to limited laboratory testing, indiscriminate antibiotic use, patient noncompliance, medication costs, and doctor shopping.

Pathophysiology

Initial pathogen colonization requires damaged endothelium. Nonbacterial thrombotic endocarditis occurs at that site which then serves as a nidus for colonization of bacteria with adhesins. Macroscopic vegetations are the end result. These interfere with valve function, causing regurgitation and eventually cardiac failure. A periannular vegetation may damage the annulus and, in case of aortic valve, may destroy conduction tissue. Large vegetations (>10 mm) are likely to embolize anywhere in the body. Systemic effects are also caused by sepsis and immune complex-mediated vasculitis.

Clinical Manifestations

Bradycardia, wide pulse pressure, and diastolic murmur of aortic regurgitation along with lack of response to antibiotics are signs of fulminant involvement of the aortic valve (Fig. 20.5). Skin manifestations of IE include red-purple, slightly

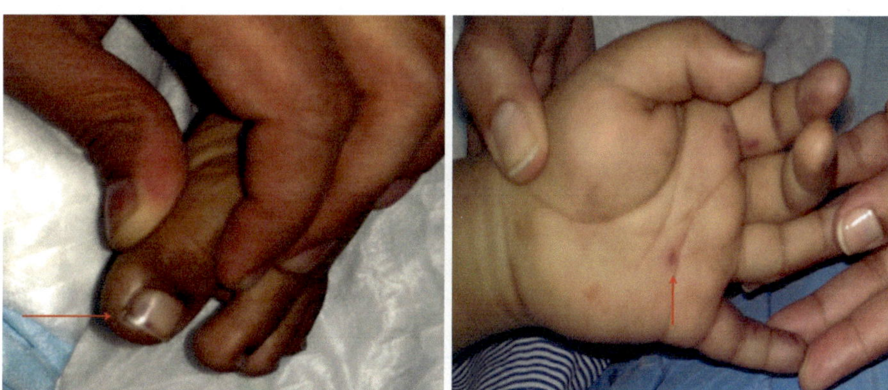

Fig. 20.5 Skin lesions of IE. Subungual splinter hemorrhages (left) and hemorrhagic coarse petechial lesions on palms—Janeway lesions (right)

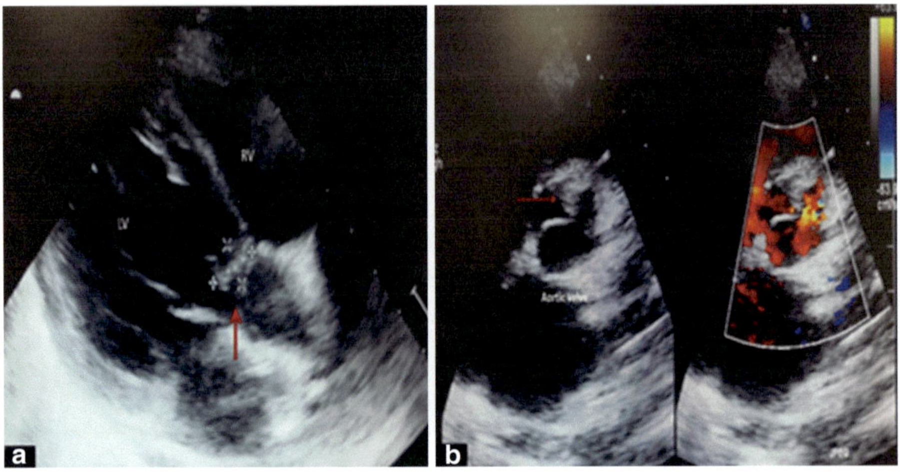

Fig. 20.6 (**a**) Echocardiogram (parasternal long-axis view) showing vegetation (arrow) in left ventricular outflow tract arising from base of the aortic valve. (**b**) Echocardiogram (parasternal short-axis view at level of aortic valve) showing vegetation and abscess (arrow) near aortic valve annulus

raised, painful papules (Osler's nodes), splinter hemorrhages in the nail beds, and painless hemorrhagic petechial lesions mostly on palms and soles referred to as Janeway lesions (Fig. 20.5).

Laboratory Investigations

Echocardiogram shows the affected valve. Particular attention must be paid to the aortic annulus, in the presence of aortic vegetation. Valvar regurgitation can be assessed and quantified adequately as well (Fig. 20.6).

Additional imaging may be required to identify the source of initial bacteremia.

Clinical pitfalls: the initial presentation of fever and rash may get mistaken for collagen vascular disease or streptococcal septic shock syndrome. This is more likely to happen in the absence of history of a congenital heart disease or a murmur.

Diagnostic clues: second-degree or higher heart block in the setting of high fever and other evidence of infective endocarditis

Emergency Management Principles

Supportive care by use of inotropes, ventilator, appropriate antibiotics, early review for surgical intervention; temporary transvenous pacemaker as needed

Clinical Pearls

Diagnosis of native valve IE requires a high index of suspicion.

Prolonged fever and rash in the setting of rhythm disturbances or a murmur are pointers to native valve IE.

Early surgical intervention is lifesaving.

Case: Tuberculosis and the Heart

Clinical Vignette

A 12-year-old girl presents with a 7-day history of dyspnea and progressive swelling of feet. She has a history of tuberculosis in the recent past. She has raised jugular venous pressure, diminished heart sounds, tender hepatomegaly, full flanks, and pitting edema up to the midshins. The echocardiogram confirms thickened pericardium with hyperechogenicity and functional indices consistent with constrictive pericarditis.

Etiology

Tuberculous pericarditis (TP) is characterized by pericardial inflammation due to *Mycobacterium tuberculosis* (MTB) and may progress to constrictive pericarditis. It is an important cause of constrictive pericarditis in the third world.

Pathophysiology and Clinical features

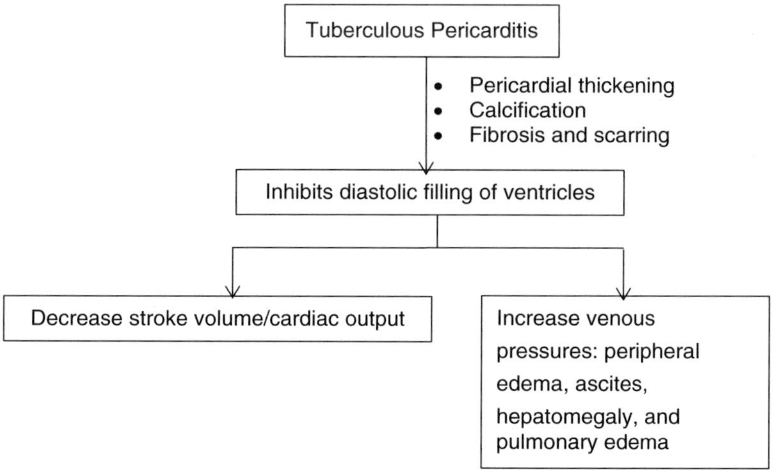

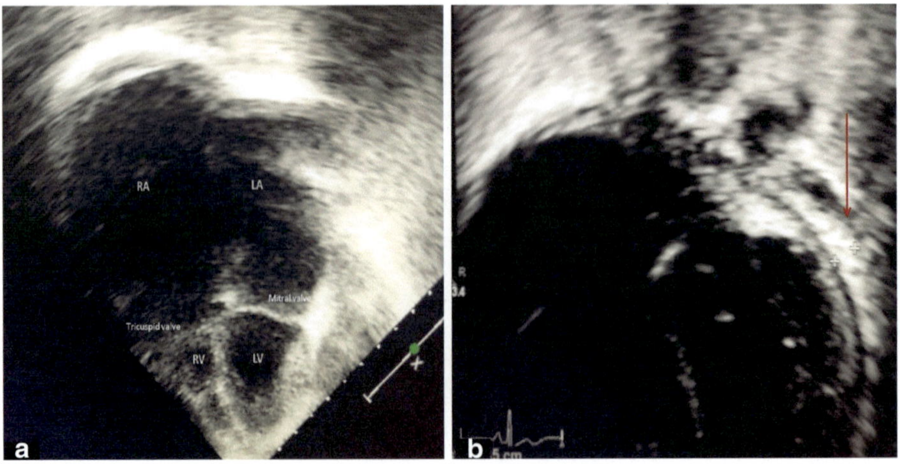

Fig. 20.7 (**a**) Echocardiogram (apical four-chamber view) showing dilated right and left atria. (**b**) Echocardiogram showing thickened and calcified (arrow) pericardium

Laboratory Investigations

- Blood tests: CBC, ESR, Mantoux test, and HIV testing.
- Pericardial fluid for microscopy, AFB smear, and MTB PCR (RIF assay) and MTB culture and sensitivity. Pericardial biopsy specimen for histopathology (caseous granuloma).
- CT thorax.
- ECG: nonspecific and highly variable (low voltage, biatrial enlargement) atrial arrhythmias are frequent.
- CXR: pulmonary venous congestion, pleural effusion, atrial enlargement, and pericardial calcification.
- Echocardiogram: normal ventricular chamber size, biatrial enlargement, dilated IVC without respiratory variation, and dense and immobile pericardium. Decrease in ventricular filling during inspiration (Fig. 20.7).

If diagnosis is uncertain: cardiac CT, cardiac MRI, and cardiac catheterization

Diagnostic clues: right heart failure signs in a patient from area with endemic MTB, with a history of TB or TB contact

Management

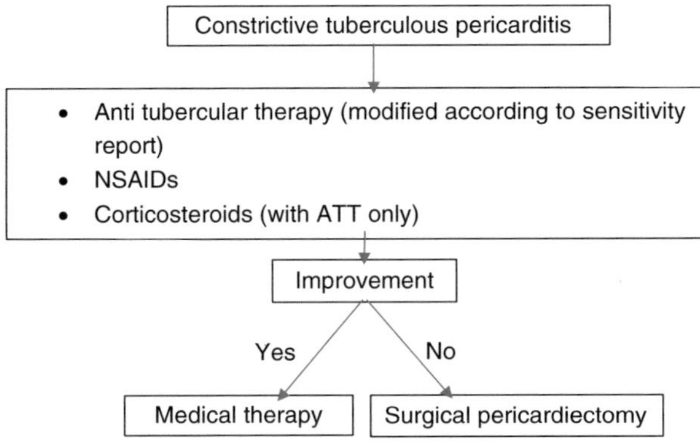

Surgical pericardiectomy: the calcified and fibrous portion of the diseased pericardium or the entire infected pericardium is removed through thoracotomy or sternotomy.

Emergency Management Principles

Judicious use of diuretics

Drug Table 20.3

Drug	Dose	Side effects	Remarks
Indomethacin	1–2 mg/kg/day in two to four divided doses (max 4 mg/kg/day) for 3–4 weeks maximum	Nausea, vomiting diarrhea, renal impairment	Monitor platelet count and renal function tests
Prednisone	1–2 mg/kg/day in three divided doses	Glucose intolerance, increased blood pressure, Cushingoid state, hirsutism	
Dexamethasone	0.2 mg/kg/day IV/IM in three to four divided doses	Convulsions, glucose intolerance, irritability	

Diuretics: see Table 20.7.

Antituberculous treatment: various antituberculous drug combinations and treatment duration of different lengths (6, 9, 12 months) have been used successfully. The choice for combination of drugs and duration of therapy should depend on culture and sensitivity pattern and as per local guidelines/ WHO recommendations.

Steroids: the use of corticosteroids in pulmonary TB without antituberculous management will exacerbate the underlying TB infection.

Clinical pitfalls: the weight gain and full appearance of the child due to constrictive pericarditis can be mistaken for a drug reaction.

> **Clinical Pearls**
> Tuberculous pericarditis is likely in a patient with history of TB, who presents with symptoms and signs of right heart failure.
>
> A detailed echocardiogram is essential to diagnose constrictive pericarditis.
>
> Steroids have to be accompanied by antituberculous treatment, in the management of tuberculous pericarditis.

Case: Myocarditis in the Setting of Common Infectious Diseases

> **Clinical Vignette**
> A previously healthy 10-year-old girl presents with a 5-day history of high fever and myalgia and shortness of breath. She appears toxic, dyspneic, and febrile. She has a pulse rate of 134/min, BP of 74/50 mm Hg, cold extremities, and a saturation of 94%. There is pallor, bilateral chest crackles, gallop rhythm, and moderate hepatomegaly. Fluid resuscitation is initiated, but there is persistence of hypotension. Echocardiogram reveals a mildly dilated left ventricle with moderate dysfunction. Blood investigations reveal positive dengue serology.

Etiology

Dengue is a mosquito-borne tropical disease caused by the dengue virus. Dengue is a major cause of seasonal morbidity and mortality in Southeast Asia.

The Pathophysiology of Myocardial Cell Injury in Dengue

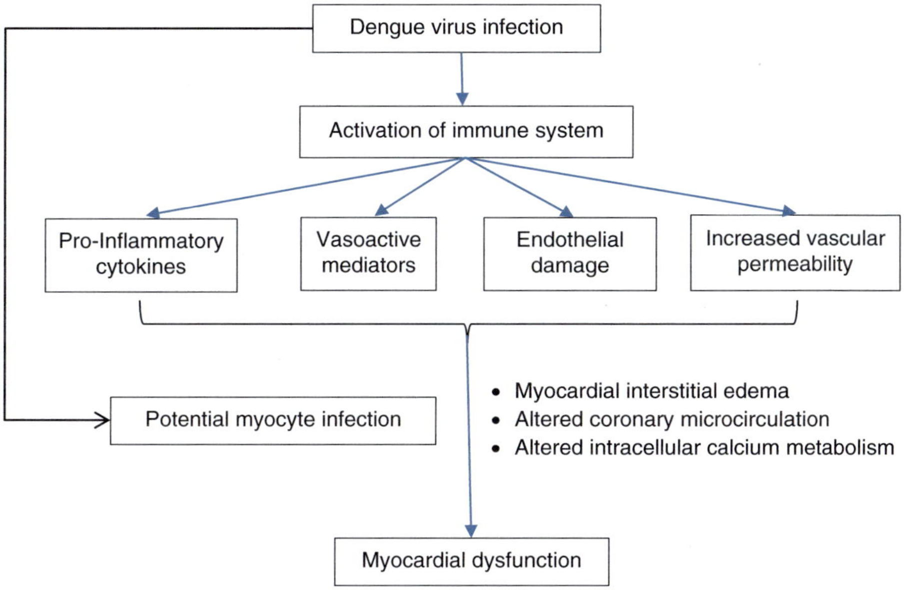

Clinical Manifestations

The initial manifestations are fever, myalgia, nonspecific headache and backache, and rash. The later manifestations of respiratory distress, arrhythmias, and cardiogenic shock are primarily seen in patients reinfected with the virus of a different strain.

Laboratory Investigations

Complete blood count. Serial monitoring of hematocrit and platelets. Dengue IgM and IgG antibodies, and viral RNA testing by PCR/RT-PCR and NS1 antigen. Cardiac enzymes include CPK (MB), troponin T, and BNP levels.

ECG: sinus bradycardia, conduction abnormalities, AV block, acute atrial fibrillation, ventricular arrhythmia, and acute myocardial infarction

Echocardiography: diminished LV function and dilatation

Emergency Management Principles

Dengue myocarditis: cardiac dysfunction as a cause of pulmonary edema rather than fluid overload is suggested by persistent hypotension despite fluid replacement and serial improvement in hematocrit. This mandates routine anti-failure medications and inotropes. Supportive mechanical ventilation and antiarrhythmic agents may be required. Severe symptomatic bradycardia will need a temporary intravenous pacemaker. Fulminant dengue myocarditis unresponsive to inotropes may warrant a trial of steroid therapy and intravenous immunoglobulins (IVIG). However this is controversial.

Drug Table 20.4

Name	Dose range	Side effect	Remarks
Dopamine	IV infusion @ 5–10 mcg/kg/min	Tachyarrhythmias, vasoconstriction, gangrene of extremities, palpitation	Increases cardiac output and blood pressure
Dobutamine	IV infusion @ 5–10 mcg/kg/min	Chest pain, headache, palpitation, ventricular dysrhythmias	Increases cardiac output, to manage short-term cardiac decompensation
Adrenaline	IV infusion @ 0.05–0.6 mcg/kg/min	Pallor, tachycardia, anxiety, headache	Increases myocardial oxygen consumption
Noradrenaline	IV infusion @ 0.05–0.6 mcg/kg/min	Headache, palpitation, irritability, pallor	Increases cardiac output, causes vasoconstriction at a higher dose
Milrinone	Loading dose: 50 mcg/kg IV over 10 min IV infusion @ 0.2–0.7 mcg/kg/min	Hypotension, headache, ventricular dysrhythmia	Can be used in normotensive state. Increases cardiac output and stroke volume, decreases SVR
Intravenous immunoglobulin	1 gm/kg/day IV for 2 days Start initial infusion at rate 0.5 mg/kg/min for 30 min, if tolerated gradually increase	Chills, chest tightness, breathlessness, fever, rash, anaphylaxis, muscle ache	Max infusion rate is 3 mg/kg/min
Corticosteroids IV methyl prednisolone	10 mg/kg/day IV in two divided doses for 3 days	Fluid retention, alteration in glucose tolerance, hypertension, abdominal distention	Start with oral prednisolone after 3 days of IV
Prednisolone	2 mg/kg/day oral in two divided doses for 3 days	Fluid retention, alteration in glucose tolerance, hypertension, abdominal distention behavioral changes, increased appetite, Cushingoid state, hirsutism	Start weaning prednisone by decreasing it 0.2 mg/kg biweekly till it is completely weaned off (6 weeks)

Clinical pitfall: myocarditis in dengue may occur in isolation or in the setting of severe capillary leak, bleeding, and multi-organ dysfunction. Fluid intolerance in a bleeding child may be a warning sign of myocardial dysfunction.

Clinical Pearls

Disproportionate sinus tachycardia, conduction blocks, and SVT/VT are pointers to myocardial involvement.

Occurrence of pulmonary edema and persistent hypotension with fluid resuscitation in the presence of a rising hematocrit may be a sign of cardiac involvement.

Early use of inotropes and judicious fluid resuscitation are lifesaving.

High index of suspicion of myocarditis should be maintained and confirmed by echocardiogram early in the course.

Case: Cardiac Stigmata of Human Immunodeficiency Virus (HIV) Infection/Acquired Immunodeficiency Syndrome (AIDS)

Clinical Vignette

A 10-year-old boy presents with fever, cough, and chest pain on and off for 4 months. His mother reports that he has had bilateral leg swelling for the last month. His weight is 19 kg and he appears emaciated. There is generalized edema. His pulses are weak and thready, heart rate is 130/min, and blood pressure is 80/60 mm Hg. His peripheries are cold. There is jugular venous distension, muffled heart sounds, and tender hepatosplenomegaly. Chest X-ray shows cardiomegaly. Echocardiogram reveals large pericardial effusion with evidence of tamponade. Bedside pericardial fluid drainage is accomplished. Work-up for the emaciated state reveals HIV/AIDS.

Etiology

The survival of children living with HIV/AIDS has increased with the availability of highly active antiretroviral therapy (HAART). Pericardial involvement has decreased post-HAART. Depressed CD4 counts, malignancies, and opportunistic infections are common settings where pericardial effusion is found.

Pathophysiology of Pericardial Tamponade

The fluid accumulated in the pericardial space exerts pressure on the cardiac chambers resulting in suboptimal filling (expansion) of the atria and ventricles. One effect of this is decreased venous return leading to elevated systemic venous pressure. The other effect is diminished ventricular stroke volume.

Clinical Manifestations of Pericardial Tamponade

Signs of low cardiac output are seen. Classic triad (Beck's triad) of hypotension, muffled heart sounds, and jugular venous distention should raise immediate suspicion of pericardial tamponade. Pulsus paradoxus may be elicited: with the patient breathing normally, measure BP manually. Note difference in systolic BP at two points (while deflating cuff slowly), one when Korotkoff sounds are heard intermittently and two when they are heard continuously. If the difference in systolic BP is >10 m Hg, it is diagnostic of pulsus paradoxus.

Lab Investigations

CBC, ESR, work-up for tuberculosis, and virology

Chest XR: cardiomegaly (Fig. 20.8)

Echocardiography: large pericardial effusion with collapse of right atrial free wall, RV diastolic collapse, dilated IVC, exaggerated respiratory variation in mitral, tricuspid inflow velocities (Fig. 20.9)

ECG: Low voltage, PR segment depression

Fluid analysis for Gram stain, culture, and cytology; pericardial biopsy

Clinical pitfall: cardiac tamponade has to be an important differential diagnosis in any situation with catecholamine resistant shock.

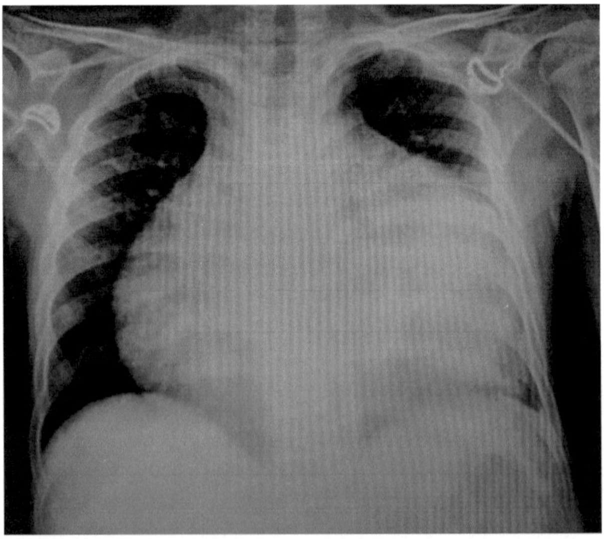

Fig. 20.8 Chest radiogram of a child showing huge cardiomegaly due to massive pericardial effusion

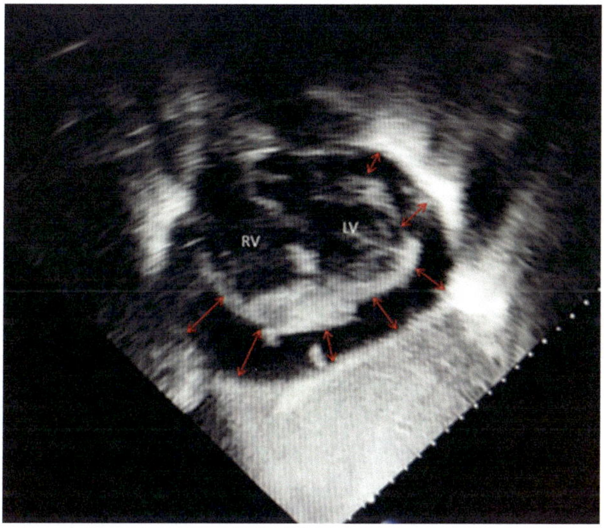

Fig. 20.9 Echocardiogram (subcostal view) showing large global pericardial effusion (arrow)

Emergency Management Principles

- Pericardiocentesis
- Hydration if hypovolemic, inotropes, and antibiotics (these are temporizing measures and should not be allowed to substitute for or to delay pericardiocentesis)
- Mechanical ventilation
- Antiretroviral therapy (HAART)

Pericardiocentesis: to be performed under echocardiographic guidance, with the patient in a head high, 30-degree elevation.

- Identify the anatomic landmarks, and select the site for needle insertion (subxiphoid or apical). Sterilize the area and inject a local anesthetic.
- Introduce a wide-bore needle attached with a syringe into the marked space. Aspirate during needle advancement, and stop advancing once fluid return is seen (watch for ectopic beats on ECG monitoring).
- Advance a J-tipped guidewire into the needle into the pericardial space. Replace the needle with dilators. After adequate dilatation, replace the dilator with a pigtail catheter over the guidewire into the pericardium. Attach a collecting bag to the pigtail catheter and secure the catheter.

Clinical Pearls

In the setting of HIV, it is imperative to rule out coexisting tuberculosis.

Beck's triad is diagnostic of cardiac tamponade.

Differentiation from constrictive pericarditis is important and can be made on echocardiogram.

Emergency pericardiocentesis is lifesaving.

Case: Cardiac Manifestations of the Unimmunized Child

Case 1

Clinical Vignette

A 10-day-old term newborn presents to the emergency department with a 3-day history of fever, irritability, and feeding difficulty. The newborn was delivered at home by a traditional birth attendant. Cow dung was applied to the raw umbilical stump (a common practice in remote villages of India). On examination, the baby is irritable with inconsolable cry. There is purulent umbilical stump discharge. Opisthotonus, trismus, and hyperreflexia are noted. A diagnosis of tetanus is made. He is managed with ventilatory support, antibiotics, and muscle relaxants. Two weeks later, the neonate developed severe hypertension and tachycardia with alternating relative hypotension and bradycardia.

Etiology and Pathophysiology

Tetanus is caused by *Clostridium tetani*, an anaerobic, Gram-positive rod, and is an exotoxin-mediated disease. Tetanospasmin blocks the release of neurotransmitter from the presynaptic inhibitory neurons resulting in reflex irritability and autonomic hyperactivity. One third of patients presenting with muscle spasms progress to autonomic instability 1–3 weeks later.

Laboratory Investigations

Tetanus is a clinical diagnosis. Some rarely performed investigations are wound culture and electromyogram. A serum anti-tetanus toxin level of $\geq$0.1 IU/mL is protective and makes the diagnosis of tetanus unlikely.

Diagnostic clues: the importance of eliciting perinatal and maternal immunization history (neonatal tetanus) or history of injury and immunization status of patient (tetanus in the child) cannot be overemphasized. In the presence of positive history, a clinical examination for trismus, muscle spasms, and rigidity is confirmatory for tetanus.

Emergency Management Principles

General measures: the patient should be kept in a quiet and shaded room. Nutritional care and prevention of bed sores are essential.

Wound care: all wounds should be cleaned thoroughly and debrided if necessary.

Tetanus immunoglobulin (TIG): administer human TIG 500 units by IM/IV as soon as possible. In addition to TIG, age-appropriate tetanus toxoid-containing vaccine should be administered.

Management Algorithm for Autonomic Instability

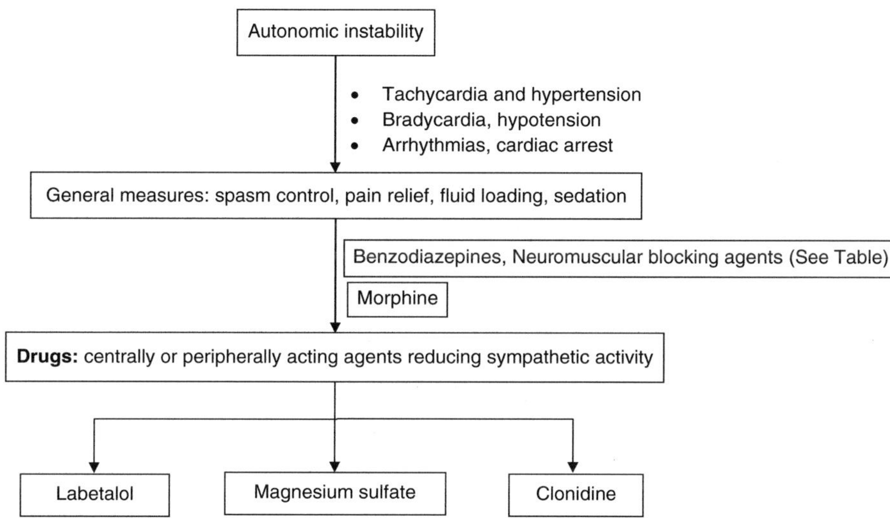

Drug Table 20.5

Name	Dose range	Side effect	Remarks
Tetanus immunoglobulin (TIG)	500 IU single dose IM/IV	Allergic reactions, anaphylaxis	Active immunization should begin as soon as condition stabilizes
Metronidazole	15–30 mg/kg/day oral/IV in two to three divided doses for 10–14 days	Headache, nausea, vomiting, heartburn	Preferred drug
Midazolam	0.1–0.8 mg/kg/h continuous IV infusion	Drowsiness, restlessness, injection site reactions	Rapid onset of action Alternatives: diazepam, lorazepam
Baclofen	<16 years: 500 mcg IT (intrathecal) >16 years: 800 mcg IT	Respiratory depression, hypotension, delirium, secondary CNS infection	
Vecuronium	0.015–0.1 mg/kg/h continuous IV infusion	Prolonged use causes muscle weakness and atrophy	Relatively few cardiovascular side effects
Magnesium sulfate	Loading dose of 50 mg/kg IV followed by a maintenance infusion of 30–50 mg/kg/h titrated against clinical effect	Flushing, hypotension, muscle weakness, diarrhea, hypocalcaemia	Serum magnesium levels should be monitored 6 h
Morphine	0.1–0.5 mg/kg/h continuous IV infusion	Hypotension, sedation, GI disturbances	Reduces sympathetic alpha-adrenergic tone

(continued)

Drug Table 20.5 (continued)

Name	Dose range	Side effect	Remarks
Clonidine	2 mcg/kg/day IV or oral in three divided doses	Hypotension, rash, dry mouth, vomiting	
Labetalol	0.2–2 mg/kg/h continuous IV infusion	Profound hypotension, pulmonary edema, hepatic impairment	

Clinical Pearls

Diagnosis of tetanus is made clinically.

History of home delivery, unsterile umbilical cord care, and difficulty feeding followed by rigidity are important indicators in neonatal tetanus.

Intravenous magnesium sulfate and fluid resuscitation are essential.

The delay in diagnosis may have significant impact on long-term outcome.

Case 2

Clinical Vignette

A previously healthy 7-year-old boy presents in cardiovascular collapse. There is a 7-day history of fever along with progressive swelling of the neck making it difficult for him to swallow. The child is unimmunized. Examination reveals bradycardia (pulse 38) and poor perfusion. There is bilateral tender cervical lymphadenopathy and neck edema (bull neck). There is a membrane over the right tonsil and posterior pharyngeal wall. ECG shows complete heart block. A diagnosis of nasopharyngeal diphtheria complicated by myocarditis and heart block is made.

Etiology

Diphtheria is a vaccine-preventable disease caused by toxin of *Corynebacterium diphtheriae*, a Gram-positive bacillus. Only toxigenic strains cause severe disease affecting multiple systems (kidneys, nervous system, and heart). The cardiac complications can range from myocardial dysfunction to rapidly progressive fatal complete heart block. Diphtheritic myocarditis occurs in 10–20% of patients. Cardiovascular involvement is the most common cause of death in diphtheria.

Pathophysiology

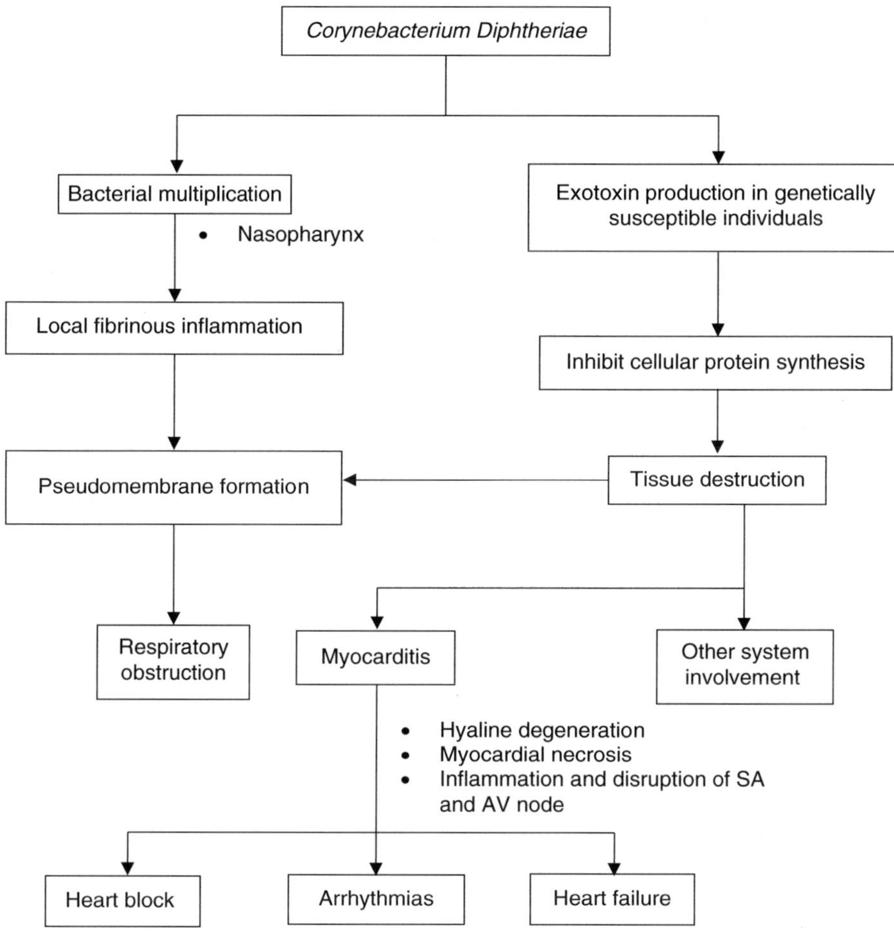

Clinical Manifestations

Local infection develops into nasal discharge/sore throat, membrane of nasal septum/tonsils/soft palate along with malaise, anorexia, and low-grade fever. There is characteristic "bull-neck" appearance because of local edema and lymphadenopathy in tonsillopharyngeal diphtheria. Severe airway obstruction complicates severe laryngeal diphtheria. Diphtheritic myocarditis can occur early in the course of the illness or weeks later, presenting as abnormal cardiac rhythms and features of congestive cardiac failure or shock leading to death.

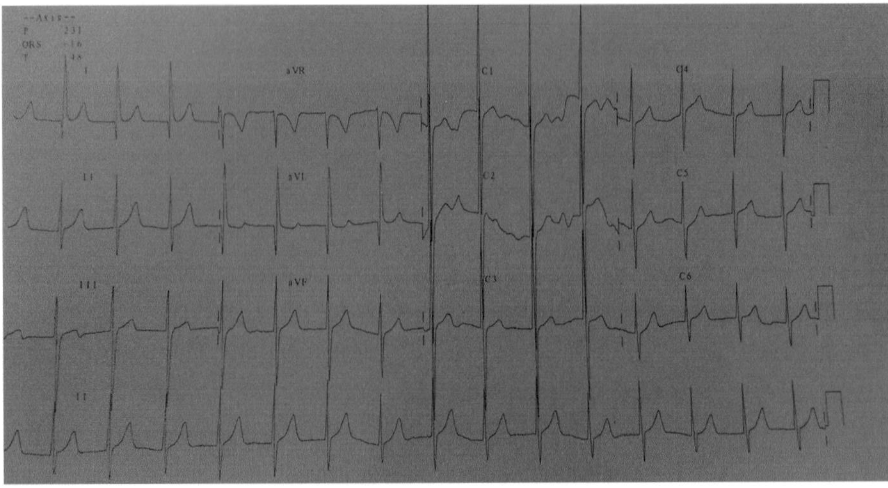

Fig. 20.10 Electrocardiogram of a patient suffering from diphtheritic myocarditis (second week of illness) showing complete heart block

Laboratory Investigations

Diagnosis of diphtheria is usually made on the basis of clinical presentation.

Pharyngeal swab/culture. Isolated diphtheria bacilli must be tested for toxin production. Respiratory secretions: polymerase chain reaction test for diphtheria toxin genes, isolation of *C. diphtheria* from cultures of specimens from close contacts.

Electrocardiogram: may show ventricular tachycardias and conduction blocks/ complete heart block (Fig. 20.10)

Echocardiography: ventricular dilatation and dysfunction

Emergency Management Principles

General measures: isolation, diphtheria antitoxin, and antibiotics

Drug Table 20.6

Drug	Dose	Side effects	Remarks
Diphtheria antitoxin	Nasopharyngeal disease—40,000 to 60,0000 units IV infusion Systemic disease—80,000 to 100,000 units	Anaphylactic reactions, serum sickness, febrile reaction	Equine serum product; prior sensitivity testing essential
Erythromycin	40 mg/kg/day (max 2 g/ day) Oral or IV for 14 days *40 mg/kg/day (max 2 g/day to close contacts orally for 7–10 days*	GI disturbances, QT prolongation	Disease is usually not contagious 48 h after antibiotics are instituted

Management of Diphtheritic Myocarditis and Complete Heart Block

Diphtheritic Myocarditis

Conventional heart failure therapy: use of diuretics, ACE inhibitors, and digoxin

Drug Table 20.7

Drug	Dose and duration	Side effects	Remarks
Furosemide	0.5–2 mg/kg/dose IV two to three times a day 1–4 mg/kg/day orally divided in three to four doses	Electrolyte imbalance, metabolic alkalosis, ototoxicity	
Spironolactone	1–3 mg/kg/day orally divided in 2–3 doses	Vomiting, diarrhea, dizziness, gynecomastia	Enhances potassium retention
Chlorothiazide	20–40 mg/kg/day orally in two divided doses	Vomiting, diarrhea, muscle pain	Delayed onset of action and less potent compared to furosemide
Digoxin	*Rapid digitalization*: 25–40 μg/kg (1/2 dose initially, followed by 1/4 q 12 h × 2): *Infant or child* *Note: These doses are PO; IV dose is 75% of PO dose* *Maintenance dose* 5–10 μg/kg/day orally in two divided doses	Nausea, vomiting, diarrhea, headache, rhythm disturbances, toxicity Trough serum level: 1–2 ng/mL in >6 months old	In active myocarditis, avoid digitalis or use of a lower dose due to fear of precipitating fatal arrhythmias. **Contraindicated in heart block** Hypokalemia and hypercalcemia exacerbate digitalis toxicity
Enalapril/ captopril	*Enalapril*: 0.08–0.5 mg/kg/ day orally in two divided doses *Captopril*: children >1 year, 2.5–6 mg/kg/day in two to four divided doses	Cough, hypotension, angioedema	Additional benefit of cardiac remodeling
Carvedilol	Initial dose 0.1 mg/kg/day (maximum: 6.25 mg) orally in two divided doses. Increase to maximum of 0.5–1 mg/kg/day over 8–12 weeks	Chest pain, hypotension, bradycardia, edema, nausea, micturition disorders	Nonselective receptor blocking as well as free radical scavenging effects

Antiarrhythmic agents in patients with significant atrial and ventricular arrhythmias should be used as appropriate.

Complete heart block: temporary pacemaker implantation, to be followed by permanent implantation as required.

Temporary transvenous pacemaker implantation procedure (Fig. 20.11)

1. Site: jugular vein, femoral vein
2. Pass the pacing catheter under fluoroscopic guidance, to the apex of the right ventricle. In an emergency, the highest output should be tried first; it should then be gradually reduced until the capture is lost
3. Check for capture and sensing threshold and stability of capture on pacemaker box
4. Secure position of pacing catheter

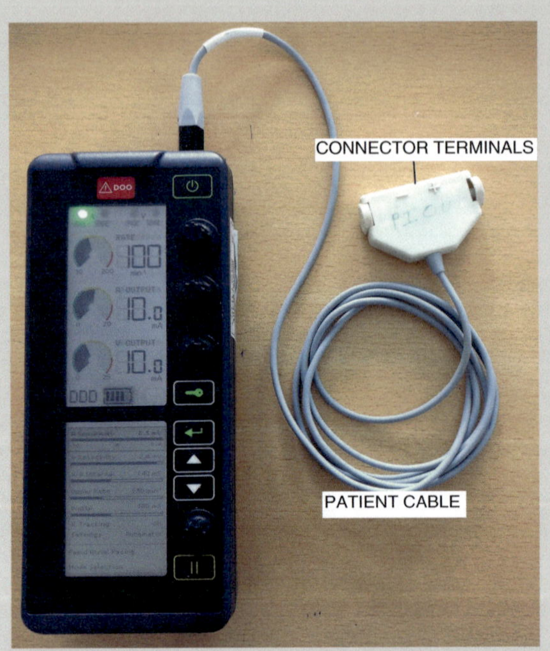

Fig. 20.11 Image showing pacemaker box with patient cable with connector

Clinical Pearls

Conduction system disturbance is a marker of severe myocardial damage. Early recognition and control of symptomatic bradycardia or ventricular tachycardias may be lifesaving. Complete heart block necessitates a temporary pacemaker placement.

Clinical pitfalls: High index of suspicion is required in culture-negative diphtheria infection- associated complete heart block, as delay in diagnosis may prove fatal

Diagnostic clues: neck swelling, tonsillopharyngeal membrane, and bulbar palsy

Bibliography

1. Consensus on timing of intervention for common congenital heart disease. Working Group on Management of Congenital Heart Diseases in India. Indian Pediatr. 2008;45(2):117–26.
2. Karabayir N, Kelesoglu E, Bornau H, Oztarhan K, Aktas D, et al. Dilated cardiomyopathy due to vitamin D deficiency. Int J Clin Cardiol. 2016;3:84.
3. Sinclair AJ, Fox CK, Ichord RN, Almond CS, Bernard TJ, Beslow LA, et al. Stroke in children with cardiac disease: report from the International Pediatric Stroke Study Group Symposium. Pediatr Neurol. 2015;52(1):5–15.
4. Baltimore RS, Gewitz M, Baddour LM, Beerman LB, Jackson MA, Lockhart PB, Pahl E, Schutze GE, Shulman ST, Willoughby R Jr, on behalf of the American Heart Association Rheumatic Fever, Endocarditis, and Kawasaki Disease Committee of the Council on Cardiovascular Disease in the Young and the Council on Cardiovascular and Stroke Nursing. Infective endocarditis in childhood: 2015 update: a scientific statement from the American Heart Association. Circulation. 2015;132:1487–515.
5. Leontyev S, Borger MA, Modi P, Lehmann S, Seeburger J, Doenst T, Mohr FW. Surgical management of aortic root abscess: a 13-year experience in 172 patients with 100% follow-up. J Thorac Cardiovasc Surg. 2012;143(2):332–7.
6. Porta-Sánchez A, Sagristà-Sauleda J, Ferreira-González I, Torrents-Fernández A, Roca-Luque I, García-Dorado D. Constrictive pericarditis: etiologic spectrum, patterns of clinical presentation, prognostic factors, and long-term follow-up. Rev Esp Cardiol (Engl Ed). 2015;68(12):1092–100.
7. Miranda CH, Borges Mde C, Matsuno AK, Vilar FC, Gali LG, Volpe GJ, Schmidt A, Pazin-Filho A, Silva FM, Castro-Jorge LA, Oliveira MF, Saggioro F, Martines RB, Fonseca BA. Evaluation of cardiac involvement during dengue viral infection. Clin Infect Dis. 2013;57(6):812–9.
8. Alqaqa A, Suleiman A, Birnhak S, Tariq S, Sison R, Hamdan A, DeBari VA, Shamoon F. Cardiac sequelae of human immunodeficiency virus disease. Am J Med Sci. 2014;348(1):82–6.
9. MJ V, Ramakrishnan S, Kothari SS, Parashar A, Juneja R, Saxena A. Complete heart block due to diphtheritic myocarditis in the present era. Ann Pediatr Cardiol. 2013;6(1):34–8.
10. Rodrigo C, Fernando D, Rajapakse S. Pharmacological management of tetanus: an evidence-based review. Crit Care. 2014;18(2):217.

21 Evaluation and Management of Pediatric Chest Pain, Syncope, and Murmur in the Emergency Department

Shahnawaz M. Amdani and Robert D. Ross

Chest Pain

Case

A 12-year-old African American male presents to the emergency department (ED) with complaints of chest pain for the last 2 days. He is an active basketball player and said that the chest pain started while he was watching TV at night. He denies any other symptoms and says "the pain is bothering me."

Chest pain has gained notoriety as an early symptom for myocardial infarction in adults. Although the etiology of chest pain in pediatrics is very different, this concern still remains among patients, parents, and often emergency and primary care physicians. Moreover, the rare but highly publicized cases of sudden cardiac death in athletes add to their fears and provoke expensive and often unnecessary cardiology consultations and testing.

Contrary to the belief at large in the community, the etiology of chest pain in pediatric patients is mostly non-cardiac (>95%). While chest pain due to cardiac etiology is rare (1–4%), it is important for physicians evaluating children with chest pain to be able to distinguish cardiac from non-cardiac etiologies and when to refer and/or investigate further [1–3].

S. M. Amdani, M.B.B.S., M.D.
Division of Pediatric Cardiology, Children's Hospital of Michigan, Carman and Ann Adams Department of Pediatrics, Wayne State University School of Medicine, Detroit, MI, USA

R. D. Ross, M.D. (✉)
Pediatrics, Division of Cardiology, Children's Hospital of Michigan and Wayne State University School of Medicine, Detroit, MI, USA
e-mail: RRoss@dmc.org

© Springer International Publishing AG, part of Springer Nature 2018

A. P. Sarnaik et al. (eds.), *Cardiac Emergencies in Children*,
https://doi.org/10.1007/978-3-319-73754-6_21

Non-cardiac Chest Pain

Non-cardiac chest pain could be due to various causes:

1. ***Musculoskeletal***: Most adolescents presenting to the emergency department will have a musculoskeletal cause for their chest pain (50–70%). It is more commonly seen in teen athletes or teens involved in activities such as weight lifting. It is usually a result of costochondritis, precordial catch syndrome, slipping rib syndrome, or skeletal trauma. Classically, the patients will complain of localized muscle tenderness, occurring at rest, pinpointing the exact area of pain, and describing it as "sharp" or "stabbing" in nature. It often gets worse with body movements including respiratory effort. There is usually no association of worsening with activity and no other coexistent symptoms (sweating, "feeling of impending doom," feelings of passing out). Many adolescents and children have idiopathic (no associated cause) chest pain.
2. ***Gastrointestinal***: In children, GERD (gastroesophageal reflux disease) often produces symptoms that may be confused with chest pain. The burning sensation is often in the chest as a result of reflux of acidic stomach content into the esophagus, which may be interpreted as "chest pain" by children. A careful history elucidating a history of intake of fried or spicy foods and caffeine and an association of symptoms after meals might give the clinician a clue about this diagnosis. With the growing obesity pandemic in the pediatric population, emergency and primary care physicians should be familiar with the diagnosis and management of GERD [4].
3. ***Respiratory***: An often underrecognized but widely present etiology in children presenting with chest pain to the ED is asthma. Prevalence of exercise-induced asthma in children presenting with chest pain can be as high as ~70% [5]. Such patients will classically give history of "chest tightness," coughing, shortness of breath, and occasionally wheezing during or immediately following exercise. These patients may have a history of childhood asthma and often have other features of atopy like eczema and food allergies and often a positive family history of asthma or atopic and allergic diseases. These patients may be diagnosed by an exercise stress test with pre- and postexercise pulmonary function testing, which will demonstrate the obstructive airway pattern after exercise, which reverses with the administration of a bronchodilator.

   Children with pneumonia may have pleuritic chest pain from inflammation that may present as diffuse, sharp/stabbing chest pain, exacerbated by deep breathing. Other less common causes including pneumothorax, empyema, and lung abscess should be kept in mind while evaluating a "sick-looking child" with chest pain, and these can be demonstrated on a CXR. Also, sickle cell disease patients with acute chest syndrome may present with excruciating chest pain but often have a positive past medical history of having this disease.
4. ***Psychogenic and other causes***: Children with non-cardiac chest pain often have underlying anxiety [6]. This may be a setup for a vicious cycle of pain leading to anxiety, which further worsens the pain. A careful history about general well-being

of the child and an insight into the social situation of the family along with a family history of recent stress or mental disorders may guide the clinician to making this diagnosis. The physician should also take a good history for the use of recreational drugs as cocaine abuse may cause true coronary spasm and myocardial infarction.

Diagnosis and Management

History

In most cases of chest pain presenting to the ED or the clinic, a careful history directed at the details of chest pain is a quintessential first step at narrowing the diagnosis. This should include the location, intensity, quality, radiation, and aggravating/alleviating factors. In addition, a complete past medical history (prior congenital heart disease, prior cardiac surgeries or transcatheter interventions, history of Kawasaki disease, history of asthma/sickle cell disease), family history (history of dilated/hypertrophic cardiomyopathy, sudden cardiac death, arrhythmias, or accidental deaths), and social history (history of recreational drug use, history of smoking) are required.

Focused Physical Examination

1. ***General examination***: Evaluate for signs of atopy (eczematous patches, allergic shiners, nasal breathing); appearance (sick looking – pericarditis/myocarditis, empyema/lung abscess); distress (sweating, difficulty breathing), leaning forward while sitting (pericarditis); or the presence of fever (infectious etiology).
2. ***Respiratory examination***: Evaluate for wheezing (asthma) and decreased breath sounds (pneumonia, pleural effusion).
3. ***Cardiac examination***: Evaluate for localized palpable tenderness of the chest wall (costochondritis/skeletal trauma), a gallop rhythm (dilated cardiomyopathy), pericardial friction rub (pericarditis/myopericarditis), systolic murmur best heard at the mid- to upper sternal border accentuated by clenching fist/squatting (hypertrophic cardiomyopathy), irregular heartbeat (arrhythmia), or poor pulses (myocarditis, dilated cardiomyopathy). Typical costochondritis pain is localized to the size of a quarter or less and reproducible on palpation.

Testing

Most children with chest pain in the emergency room will usually get an ECG, and most will be able to be reassured when this is normal. Abnormal findings to pursue with a cardiology consultation would be marked bradycardia or tachycardia, abnormal QRS axis, significant hypertrophy, or ischemic ST segment changes that are not early repolarization. Many will require a CXR for respiratory symptoms associated with the pain, and a normal heart size and silhouette are reassuring. Any abnormal lung findings such as pneumonia, pneumothorax, or effusions should be addressed. Significant cardiomegaly warrants further cardiology evaluation. Many emergency room physicians have been trained in portable echo techniques, and scanning those with cardiomegaly may reveal a pericardial effusion, which should prompt an immediate evaluation by cardiology. In the absence of signs or symptoms of a true cardiac chest pain, troponin levels are not useful. Unlike adults where an elevated troponin often suggests an acute coronary syndrome, in pediatric patients, the most common cause is either myocarditis or pericarditis [7].

Management

In most cases of typical non-cardiac chest pain, reassurance and NSAIDs are sufficient. For recurrent or persistent pain, ibuprofen three times a day for 3 days is effective. However, since there is significant patient, parental, and caregiver anxiety, this reassurance should be approached with compassion. If the history and physical examination points to a non-cardiac cause, the patient and the family should be reassured that the child has a "benign" cause of chest pain. If a specific cause is identified, further management should be directed accordingly. For patients with GERD, a histamine-2 blocker or a proton pump inhibitor may be used. Patients with exercise-induced asthma will benefit from an inhaled albuterol, 15–20 min prior to gym class or scheduled activity. Patients with pneumonia, pneumothorax, empyema, or lung abscess may need to be admitted to the hospital for therapy such as intravenous antibiotics, a chest tube, or even surgical drainage for complete resolution. Patients with sickle cell disease presenting as acute chest syndrome need intense pain management along with antibiotics and transfusions. Patients with psychogenic chest pain may benefit from counseling.

Patients with true cardiac pain must be seen immediately by pediatric cardiology. Examples include myocardial ischemia in patients with a history of Kawasaki disease with coronary involvement, previous coronary artery surgery such as the arterial switch for transposition of the great vessels or ALCAPA repair, or ischemia from acute myocarditis. Other cardiac conditions that can present with acute chest pain are HOCM, post-pericardiotomy syndrome and Marfan syndrome with aortic aneurysm and/or dissection. If ischemic pain is truly suspected, then appropriate measures prior to the arrival of cardiology would be obtaining a stat 12-lead ECG, sending cardiac enzymes, and then subsequently providing morphine, oxygen, nitroglycerin, and aspirin. If there is any hemodynamic instability, then PALS/ACLS guidelines should be followed.

Patient Follow-Up

The 12-year-old male likely has musculoskeletal chest pain, or costochondritis. Patient and parent education, rest, and analgesic will be the correct management.

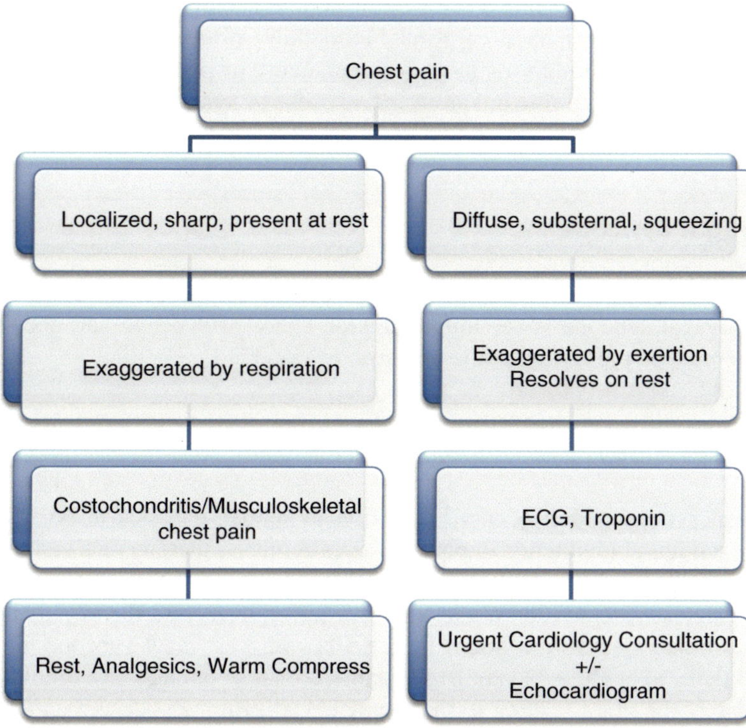

Algorithm for Evaluation of Pediatric Chest Pain

Syncope

Case 1

An 11-year-old female presents to the ED after "passing out" at church. On arrival to the emergency department (ED), she is awake and in no distress. She states that she was standing in church when she started feeling dizzy, felt nauseous, and saw a "curtain fall in front of her eyes" after which she fell to the ground and doesn't remember anything else after that. Her mother who was standing by her side reports that she did not observe any shaking movements and she did not bite her tongue or become incontinent but did appear quite pale when she woke up after a few seconds.

Case 2

An 18-year-old female presents to the ED after "feeling dizzy" and "passing out." She states that she was washing dishes and doesn't remember what happened but then woke up lying on the ground. She has a bruised forehead. She is alert and in no distress in the ED. On further questioning, she states that she has history of tetralogy of Fallot and had two "heart surgeries" as a baby. She last saw a cardiologist 3 years ago.

Syncope is defined as and a transient loss of consciousness with loss of muscular tone due to decreased cerebral blood flow following which recovery is spontaneous [8]. Although the most common cause of pediatric syncope is vasovagal, it is important to rule out any cardiac cause of syncope, as the implications are very different.

Vasovagal Syncope

This is also known as neurocardiogenic syncope, reflex syncope, and common fainting. Vasovagal syncope is the most common cause of syncope and accounts for 40–50% of cases presenting to the pediatric ED [9–12].

Pathophysiology

Vasovagal syncope often occurs in relation to sudden changes in postural tone. During standing, blood tends to pool in the extremities, thereby decreasing venous return to the heart. Normally, the baroreceptors respond to this leading to arterial and venous vasoconstriction along with increasing heart rate thereby maintaining adequate blood flow to the brain. In patients with vasovagal syncope, often this reflex is delayed or altered leading to sustained venous pooling and continued hypoperfusion of the brain leading to the pre-syncopal symptoms described above and then sometimes to frank syncope. Once supine, the process reverses, and the heart no longer is required to pump blood against gravity to reach the brain. Other theories are that these patients have exaggerated vagotonia or reduced blood volumes predisposing them to syncope [13].

Clinical Features

A detailed history and physical examination are often the most important aspect for narrowing the differential and arriving at a diagnosis.

History

Adolescents seem particularly susceptible to vasovagal syncope as they are undergoing rapid growth and hormonal changes which may contribute to this phenomenon. Females are affected more often than males, and there is frequently a history of fainting in a parent. Patients frequently report premonitory symptoms of being light-headed, ringing in the ears, GI symptoms (nausea, vomiting), and often visual symptoms (floaters, blurry vision). This is often followed by brief loss of consciousness, and patients may report a headache after they wake up. Observers frequently note pallor with patients feeling "cold and clammy."

On further questioning, it is common that patients have not had adequate food or water intake through the day. They may have had a recent URI or were in a hot, humid environment. There are other stimuli such as yawning, tightly combing the hair, a hot shower, the sight of blood, sneezing, coughing, or urination that can trigger a syncopal episode.

If a syncopal episode occurs without any warning or prodromal symptoms, or during or immediately after an exertional activity, search for cardiac causes should be undertaken. Also, if there is significant bodily injury from the syncope, then further investigation is warranted. It is also essential to ask about family history as patients with cardiomyopathies or conditions like Marfan's syndrome often have a positive family history. A past history of Kawasaki disease or congenital heart disease is also important to elicit.

Physical Examination

Patients with vasovagal syncope typically have a normal cardiac examination by the time they arrive in the ED. Any abnormal findings should prompt evaluation for an underlying diagnosis:

1. ***Systolic ejection murmur***: hypertrophic cardiomyopathy, aortic stenosis
2. ***Tachycardia/gallop***: cardiomyopathy, myocarditis
3. ***Irregular rhythm***: arrhythmia
4. ***Pericardial rub/tachycardia/increased jugular venous distension***: pericarditis, myocarditis

Laboratory Tests

Laboratory tests have limited value in assessing a patient with vasovagal syncope. However, if other causes of syncope are suspected, then a CBC (ruling out anemia, infection), BUN/Cr (evaluating hydration status), CRP (myocarditis, pericarditis), and NT-pro BNP (cardiomyopathy, congestive heart failure) may aid in the diagnosis.

Electrocardiogram

ECG may be valuable in identifying cardiac causes of syncope.

1. ***Hypertrophic cardiomyopathy***: left ventricular hypertrophy, inverted T waves in inferolateral leads
2. ***Myocarditis***: sinus tachycardia, T wave inversions, low QRS voltage in the limb leads
3. ***Pericarditis***: sinus tachycardia, generalized ST elevation in all leads

4. ***Anomalous coronary artery origin***: deep and wide Q waves in leads I and aVL, T wave inversions in inferolateral leads, ST elevations in precordial leads
5. ***Arrhythmias***: long QT syndrome, SVT (narrow complex QRS tachycardia), atrial flutter (saw tooth appearance of atrial waves seen in inferior leads), VT (wide complex tachycardia, AV dissociation)
6. ***Pulmonary embolism***: RVH with strain pattern

Echocardiogram

In most cases of syncope in children, echocardiograms are not helpful or required. In the absence of a positive history, congenital heart disease, or Kawasaki disease and with a normal physical examination and electrocardiogram, the yield of an echocardiogram is extremely low [14]. If any findings on physical exam, ECG, or echocardiogram point to a cardiac cause, then an echocardiogram is indicated.

Management

In most cases of syncope in children, the cause is vasovagal. Patient and family reassurance and education are the only things required [11]. Instruction on increasing fluid intake (2–2.5 L of water a day) until the urine is clear, increasing salt intake, and avoiding caffeine are the cornerstone of management. Patients should be taught certain counterpressure maneuvers like arm folding and leg crossing. Also, patients should be encouraged to increase activity (to increase muscular tone and avoid venous pooling). Patients should also be told that such episodes tend to recur and one should either sit down and place their head low or lie down if they feel dizzy. If symptoms get worse despite their maneuvers or are associated with exertion and no warning or associated with seizures, then specialist consultations (cardiology, neurology) are warranted.

Patient Follow-Up

Case 1

The 11-year-old female had vasovagal syncope. She was advised to increase salt in the form of pretzels and water in her diet and has since remained symptom-free.

Case 2

The 18-year-old female with prior history of TOF repair was found on further evaluation (ECG, Holter monitoring) to have intermittent ventricular tachycardia. She underwent an electrophysiology study at which she was found to have inducible VT for which she underwent ICD implantation.

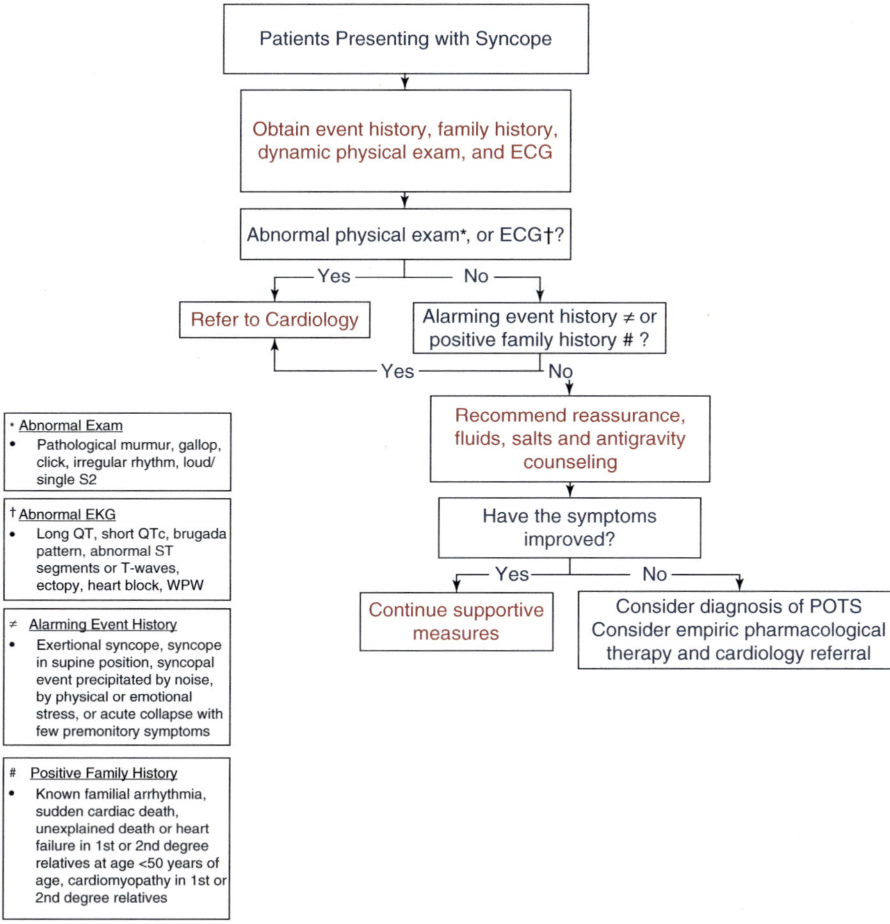

Algorithm for Evaluation of Pediatric Syncope
*POTS: Postural tachycardia syndrome is classically characterized by an abnormal increase in heart rate (30–40 bpm) in the absence of hypotension (>20 mm Hg drop in systolic blood pressure) with changing posture from supine to standing [15]
Reprinted from The Journal of Pediatrics, Vol-163, Issue-3, Kevin G. Friedman, Mark E. Alexander, Chest Pain and Syncope in Children: A Practical Approach to the Diagnosis of Cardiac Disease, Pages No 896–901.e3., Copyright (2013), with permission from Elsevier

Murmur

Case 1

A 6-week-old infant presents to the emergency room with difficulty feeding for 1 week. The mother says he is getting tired easily with feeds and has been sleeping more the last day. He has only wet his diaper once since early morning. On examination, the infant is listless and has subcostal and intercostal retractions. On auscultation, he has a 3/6 harsh holosystolic murmur best heard at the left lower sternal border. Mother reports a normal pregnancy and no prior medical illnesses.

Case 2

A 4-year-old female presents to the emergency room with fever and throat pain. The father states she has been tired and complaining that her "throat hurts" for the past 2 days. She has not been eating well since yesterday. She appears listless and on examination has a white exudate on the tonsils. On auscultation, a 1–2/6 vibratory systolic murmur is heard at the left lower sternal border. This murmur increases in intensity in the supine position. Father mentions that she has no chronic health problems and was previously healthy.

Introduction

Heart murmurs are perhaps the most common reason for referral to a pediatric cardiologist [16, 17]. Even though it's been over 200 years since René Laennec invented the first stethoscope, auscultation is still an art. An astute clinician can often arrive at the correct diagnosis with a good history and a complete physical examination [18]. Unfortunately, in this current era, the skills of auscultation are being lost as there is a wide availability of different diagnostic modalities and less time spent in effective physician-patient interaction.

As a primary care provider, it is important to use all possible information available to determine whether a given murmur heard on auscultation is physiologic or pathologic. There are some things to pay particular attention to.

History

1. *Failure to thrive, difficulty breathing, and easy fatigability with feeds:* suspect pulmonary overcirculation [ventricular septal defect (VSD), patent ductus arteriosus (PDA), atrioventricular septal defect (AVSD), aortopulmonary window (AP window)] or myocardial dysfunction [anomalous left coronary artery arising from pulmonary artery (ALCAPA), myocarditis].
2. *Cyanosis of tongue and buccal mucosa:* tetralogy of Fallot (TOF).
3. *Prior congenital heart disease:* Think of residual lesions or sequelae post repair of congenital heart defect.
4. *History of chromosomal anomalies or syndromes associated with congenital heart disease:*
   (a) **Down's syndrome:** atrioventricular septal defect (AVSD), ventricular septal defect (VSD)
   (b) **Infant of diabetic mother:** transposition of the great arteries (TGA), hypertrophic obstructive cardiomyopathy (HOCM)
   (c) **Holt-Oram:** atrial septal defect (ASD)
   (d) **Marfan's syndrome:** mitral valve prolapse (MVP), aortic dilation

   (e) **Williams syndrome:** peripheral pulmonary stenos is (PPS), supravalvular aortic stenosis
   (f) **Turner syndrome**: coarctation of the aorta
5. *No past medical history of disease or illness:* Still's murmur, venous hum
6. *Age:*
   (a) **Infancy:** The most common cause of a benign murmur is peripheral pulmonic stenosis, which is physiologic. This is a soft systolic ejection murmur heard at the upper sternal border radiating laterally and to the back. However, one has to be careful at this age group to exclude congenital heart disease resulting in pulmonary undercirculation (TGA, TOF) typically presenting in the first days-weeks of life or pulmonary overcirculation (VSD, PDA, ASD,) typically presenting around 6–8 weeks of age as pulmonary vascular resistance drops.
   (b) **Children and adolescents (1–18 years):** Usually in an otherwise healthy child, the most common cause is an innocent murmur or a Still's murmur. Such a murmur is usually soft, vibratory in nature, grade 2/6 in intensity, systolic, best heard at the left lower sternal border, and accentuated by having the patient lay supine. Often a venous hum (normal) can also be heard. However, valvular stenosis, infective endocarditis (new murmur appreciated in a patient with high fever), and rheumatic carditis (mitral regurgitation murmur in a child with recent history of streptococcal throat infection) may present in childhood and adolescent age group.

Physical Examination

1. *General appearance*:
   (a) **Mild-moderate respiratory distress:** pulmonary overcirculation [VSD, PDA, truncus arteriosus (TA)]
   (b) **Pale, listless child:** usually from systemic hypoperfusion (coarctation, severe aortic stenosis)
   (c) **Cyanotic child:** TGA, TOF
   (d) **Normal appearance:** Still's murmur, venous hum
2. *Respiratory examination*: While in most cases the respiratory examination is normal in patients with a heart murmur, it is often abnormal in patients with pulmonary overcirculation and may aid in the decision-making process.
3. *Cardiac examination*: This is most useful to arrive at a differential diagnosis and distinguish between a physiologic and a pathologic murmur. These are the most common findings associated with the following conditions:
   (a) **ASD:** Small ASD (often no murmur), large ASD [fixed split S2 and systolic ejection murmur at the left upper sternal border (LUSB)-functional pulmonary stenosis secondary to increased volume across valve].

(b) **VSD**: Loud holosystolic murmur best appreciated at the left lower sternal border (LLSB), diastolic rumble appreciated at the left apical area (functional mitral stenosis from increased volume across mitral valve). There may be a loud second heart sound if the defect is large leading to pulmonary hypertension.
(c) **PDA**: Continuous murmur best appreciated in the left infraclavicular area.
(d) **Aortic stenosis**: Systolic ejection murmur best appreciated at the right upper sternal border (RUSB) radiating to the carotids, frequently preceded by a systolic ejection click.
(e) **Pulmonary stenosis**: Systolic ejection murmur best appreciated at LUSB radiating to the back.
(f) **TOF**: Holosystolic murmur at LLSB, harsh systolic ejection murmur at LUSB radiating to the back.
(g) **TGA**: Single S2 and severe cyanosis with an otherwise normal exam.
(h) **Still's murmur**: Vibratory, systolic murmur best heard at LLSB, decreasing in intensity with sitting up from the supine position.
(i) **Venous hum**: Continuous low-grade murmur heard beneath the right or left clavicular area, decreasing in intensity with the head turned to the side of the murmur or lying down.
(j) **Rheumatic carditis**: Holosystolic murmur best heard at the apex radiating to the axilla (mitral regurgitation). Prominent diastolic murmur heard at the left midsternal border (aortic insufficiency).
(k) **Infective endocarditis**: Murmur often depends on valves involved.
(l) **Coarctation**: Systolic murmur from heard best at the upper left chest radiating to the back. Patient may have weak femoral pulses. Often, there is higher blood pressure in the right arm and then the left arm or legs.

Patient Follow-Up

Case 1

The 6-week-old infant had a large muscular VSD. Murmurs from left to right shunts are often not heard at the time of birth and become more prominent by 4–6 weeks of age as the pulmonary vascular resistance drops increasing the shunt and thus making the murmur more audible. This patient will require a cardiology consultation and an echocardiogram.

Case 2

The 4-year-old female had a Still's murmur, which is more prominent in the setting of fever, anxiety, or dehydration. Such murmurs classically increase in intensity with supine positioning. It is the sound from blood flow through the normal heart and vessels. This patient doesn't require any further evaluation unless the murmur persists over time or the nature of the murmur changes. Moreover, she should not be restricted from any physical activities.

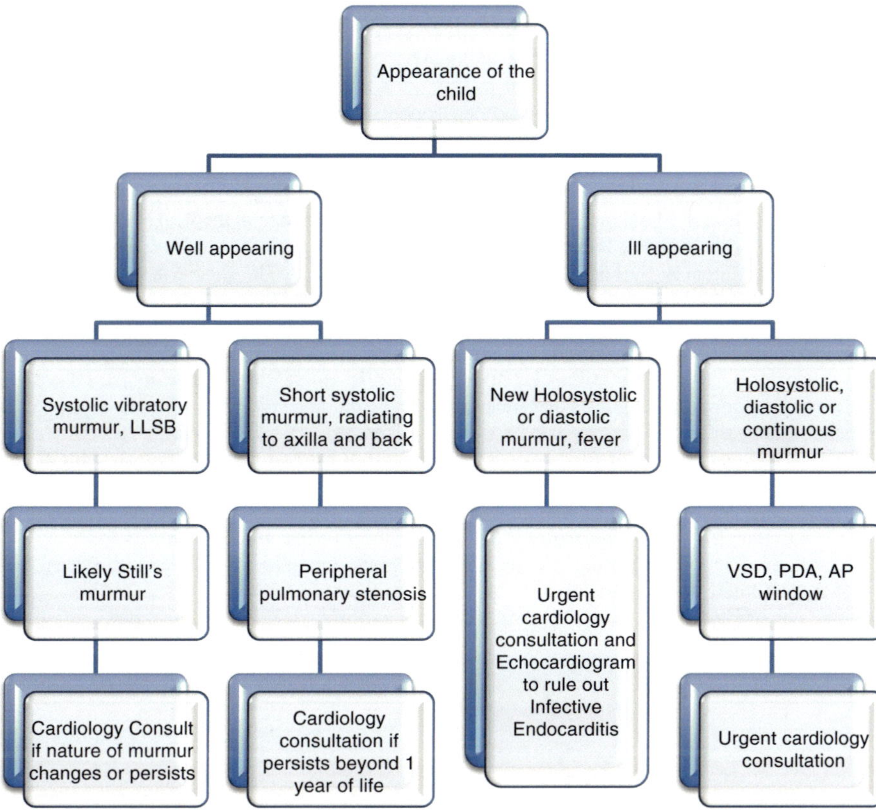

Approach to Evaluation of a Pediatric Patient with a Murmur

References

1. Saleeb SF, Li WY, Warren SZ, Lock JE. Effectiveness of screening for life-threatening chest pain in children. Pediatrics. 2011;128(5):e1062–8.
2. Friedman KG, Kane DA, Rathod RH, Renaud A, Farias M, Geggel R, Fulton DR, Lock JE, Saleeb SF. Management of pediatric chest pain using a standardized assessment and management plan. Pediatrics. 2011;128(2):239–45.
3. Selbst SM, Ruddy RM, Clark BJ, Henretig FM, Santulli T. Pediatric chest pain: a prospective study. Pediatrics. 1988;82(3):319–23.
4. Rudolph CD, Mazur LJ, Liptak GS, Baker RD, Boyle JT, Colletti RB, Gerson WT, Werlin SL. Guidelines for evaluation and treatment of gastroesophageal reflux in infants and children: recommendations of the North American Society for Pediatric Gastroenterology and Nutrition. J Pediatr Gastroenterol Nutr. 2001;32:S1–31.
5. Wiens L, Portnoy J, Sabath R, Ewing L, Gowdamarajan R, Scagliotti D. Chest pain in otherwise healthy children and adolescents is frequently caused by exercise-induced asthma. Pediatrics. 1992;90(3):350–3.
6. Lipsitz JD, Masia C, Apfel H, Marans Z, Gur M, Dent H, Fyer AJ. Noncardiac chest pain and psychopathology in children and adolescents. J Psychosom Res. 2005;59(3):185–8.

7. Brown JL, Hirsh DA, Mahle WT. Use of troponin as a screen for chest pain in the pediatric emergency department. Pediatr Cardiol. 2012;33(2):337–42.
8. Kapoor WN. Syncope. N Engl J Med. 2000;343(25):1856–62.
9. Massin MM, Bourguignont A, Coremans C, Comté L, Lepage P, Gérard P. Syncope in pediatric patients presenting to an emergency department. J Pediatr. 2004;145(2):223–8.
10. Pratt JL, Fleisher GR. Syncope in children and adolescents. Pediatr Emerg Care. 1989;5(2):80–2.
11. Driscoll DJ, Jacobsen SJ, Wollan PC. Syncope in children and adolescents. J Am Coll Cardiol. 1997;29(5):1039–45.
12. Serletis A, Rose S, Sheldon AG, Sheldon RS. Vasovagal syncope in medical students and their first-degree relatives. Eur Heart J. 2006;27(16):1965–70.
13. Mosqueda-Garcia R, Furlan R, Tank J, Fernandez-Violante R. The elusive pathophysiology of neurally mediated syncope. Circulation. 2000;102(23):2898–906.
14. Ritter S, Tani LY, Etheridge SP, Williams RV, Craig JE, Minich LL. What is the yield of screening echocardiography in pediatric syncope? Pediatrics. 2000;105(5):e58.
15. Olshansky B, Shen WK, Calkins H, Brignole M. 2015 Heart Rhythm Society expert consensus statement on the diagnosis and treatment of postural tachycardia syndrome, inappropriate sinus tachycardia, and vasovagal syncope. Heart Rhythm. 2015;12(6):e42.
16. Pelech AN. Evaluation of the pediatric patient with a cardiac murmur. Pediatr Clin N Am. 1999;46(2):167–88.
17. Newburger JW, Rosenthal A, Williams RG, Fellows K, Miettinen OS. Noninvasive tests in the initial evaluation of heart murmurs in children. N Engl J Med. 1983;308(2):61–4.
18. DeAngelis CD. Cardinal clinical signs in the differentiation of heart murmurs in children. Arch Pediatr Adolesc Med. 1996;150:169–74.

Index

© Springer International Publishing AG, part of Springer Nature 2018
A. P. Sarnaik et al. (eds.), *Cardiac Emergencies in Children*,
https://doi.org/10.1007/978-3-319-73754-6

I

Made in the USA
Monee, IL
15 September 2026

63227617R10247